Dialogs with Headache Patients

Dialogs with Headache Patients

Edited by

Mark W. Green and Robert Kaniecki

Cambridge Scholars Publishing

Dialogs with Headache Patients

Edited by Mark W. Green and Robert Kaniecki

This book first published 2022

Cambridge Scholars Publishing

Lady Stephenson Library, Newcastle upon Tyne, NE6 2PA, UK

British Library Cataloguing in Publication Data
A catalogue record for this book is available from the British Library

ISBN (10): 1-5275-8726-6
ISBN (13): 978-1-5275-8726-7

TABLE OF CONTENTS

PREFACE

CONVERSATIONS WITH HEADACHE PATIENTS

MARK W. GREEN, MD, FAAN
ROBERT G. KANIECKI, MD

As educators in the field of headache medicine we are commonly asked, "how do you explain that to a patient?" The "that" may involve issues surrounding diagnosis, testing, different treatment options, or even the basic explanations of the physiology behind the headache. Some patients may need to be reassured; others desire to learn more.

Patients often enter the headache specialist's office with a set of common questions. Health care providers are expected to be able to provide answers that are thorough and understandable. This book provides responses to patient concerns using a clear, conversational format. Providers and patients alike will benefit from this broad compilation of questions and answers. Some may be raised during the office encounter, while others may have been neglected and only considered afterwards. This text articulates many different aspects of patient's common concerns and can empower the patient to implement many solutions themselves.

The most common type of headache is a tension type headache; yet, by definition, these are not disabling and rarely prompt a visit to a health care provider. Migraine is by far the most common headache that prompts a visit, which is why so many of the conversations are dedicated to migraine-related issues. Since most migraineurs are women of child-bearing years, several sections are devoted to headaches and reproductive issues. Many other specific patient subgroups – children, transgenders, specific religious denominations – have different needs and different questions which are addressed in detail.

We invited experts with experience in clinical headache settings and asked them to provide their tips and insights. Bringing them together and editing their sections has been enjoyable and informative. There is much to learn within these pages, as none of us have "all the answers."

MIGRAINE IN A TRANSGENDER INDIVIDUAL

ANNA PACE, MD

ASSISTANT PROFESSOR
DEPARTMENT OF NEUROLOGY
CENTER FOR HEADACHE AND FACIAL PAIN
ICAHN SCHOOL OF MEDICINE AT MOUNT SINAI
NEW YORK CITY

I identify as transgender, and I just started on estrogen gender-affirming hormone therapy (GAHT). My migraine attacks have changed, and it seems like they are happening more frequently. Why is that?

There is a lot we know and don't know about how hormones affect the brain and the experience of migraine. We know that hormone fluctuations can trigger migraine in cisgender women especially during the menstrual cycle. Some women experience a migraine attack as estrogen levels drop during the cycle; it is that "delta", the change in the estrogen level, that can trigger pain. In other studies, at the basic hormone level, it appears that estrogen is pro-inflammatory, and high levels of estrogen can increase the likelihood of the chemical and electrical changes in the brain that cause migraine. Estrogen change or administration can also lead to aura, which some people with migraine have, but not all.

We don't have specific data in transgender individuals, but it has been suggested that hormones can affect the frequency of migraine attacks, sometimes for the better and sometimes for the worse. Since it seems estrogen can be pro-excitatory in the brain, transgender women on estrogen may notice an uptick in their migraine frequency when first starting on estrogen. The same possibility can happen in cisgender women on estrogen-containing birth control. One study showed that even non-migraine pain, such as musculoskeletal pain, may be increased in transgender women when they start estrogen.

I have migraines, but I have never had aura before. Since I am on estrogen, will I get an aura?

Since estrogen has been shown to increase the likelihood of aura, there is a possibility you may experience new aura when starting on estrogen or continuing on estrogen. Some examples of aura patients have described include seeing squiggly lines or zig-zags, rainbow shimmery arches of light, or black and white dots or spots in their vision. Usually, the aura comes right before a migraine headache, and can last for minutes to an hour, but for some people the aura happens without the headache. Not everyone on estrogen has aura though, so there is also a possibility you will not get aura. Each individual responds to hormone therapy differently, so it is important to monitor for new symptoms when starting on GAHT and follow up with your doctor if you do.

So, do all gender-affirming hormone therapies cause changes in migraine headaches?

Not necessarily. While some basic studies suggest estrogen is pro-inflammatory, other studies imply that testosterone can reduce pain processing. Some people who start on testosterone therapy may notice an improvement in migraine frequency or severity, while others, because hormone levels are changing, may notice an increase in attacks. Some people on GAHT experience no change in their migraine attacks at all. Each individual is different, and their response to GAHT can be different, so it is important to monitor headache frequency and attacks as one starts on hormone therapy.

Given we know that is the cycling or fluctuation in the level of hormones that can be triggers for migraine, it is possible that once transgender people are on stable hormone therapy, that that stability in hormone levels may lead to an improved headache frequency over the long term. What that means is, if you are in the beginning of your hormone therapy, your headaches may go up and down in terms of how often they are happening, but once your dosing regimen has been the same for a while and there have been no changes, your headache attacks may stabilize as well, and you will not notice as much of a roller-coaster ride with your frequency.

Do I need to stop hormone therapy because of my migraine attacks?

No! Transgender people with migraine do not have to choose between continuing hormone therapy and managing their migraines. Both can happen at the same time, and they should. Again, often when people are stable on gender-affirming hormone therapy and the doses do not change, migraine frequency can level off. Treatment for migraine should help support the continuation of hormone therapy, so long as the medications used to treat migraine do not interact with the hormones being given. Your endocrinologist and headache medicine specialist can work together to help monitor your hormones and your migraines.

What can I do to treat my migraines while I stay on estrogen?

There are many acute and preventive therapies that are available to treat migraine. Regardless of medication, one of the mainstays of migraine prevention is lifestyle modification. People with migraine, regardless of their gender identity, are encouraged to have a balanced diet and not miss meals, stay well hydrated, use less than 200mg of caffeine daily at the same amounts at the same time, try to keep active and exercise at least two to three times a week where possible. Getting adequate sleep, at sleeping the same hours each day, and stress reduction are also important. Minimizing triggers wherever possible will also help to keep migraine frequency at bay.

There are many oral and non-oral preventive treatment options to consider for migraine, as well as many acute therapies that come in a number of formulations. Nonpharmacologic options such as neuromodulation, nerve blocks, physical therapy, and behavioral therapies (such as biofeedback and cognitive behavioral therapy) are also excellent treatment options and should be considered. Choosing the right migraine therapy is best done together with your physician.

Will gender-affirming surgery affect my headaches also?

We do not have any data on gender-affirming surgeries, like "top" surgery, and migraine – but they do not seem to affect migraine frequency in a negative way. Some patients will experience a slight flurry of headaches immediately post-operatively, likely due to the stress of the surgery itself, not eating before the procedure, etc. But afterwards, many patients find their migraine frequency may improve. This may be due to a lot of factors, but often it is related to improvement in or alleviation of gender dysphoria.

Are there any treatments or medications for migraine I should avoid since I am on gender-affirming hormone therapy?

There are no specific studies on the traditional or newer therapies for migraine in gender-diverse patients on GAHT. However, based on our understanding of how hormones are metabolized, there are a handful of medications that you may want to consider avoiding until better data is available.

Estrogen and testosterone are metabolized through a specific pathway in the liver, and a couple of medications used to treat migraine are also metabolized through that same pathway. It has been suggested to avoid these medications as there is a possibility the medications may interact. For people on testosterone, some oral preventive medications like valproic acid and zonisamide can affect levels of testosterone so these should be used with caution. For those on estrogen, topiramate and carbamazepine/ oxcarbazepine can affect levels as well, so if you are on any of these medications, your hormone levels should be monitored regularly.

Suggested Reading

Aloisi AM, Bachiocco V, Costantino A. Cross-sex hormone administration changes pain in transsexual women and men. Pain 2007;132(suppl. 1): S60-S67.

Craft RM, Mogil JS, Aloisi AM. Sex differences in pain and analgesia: the role of gonadal hormones. Eur J Pain 2004; 8:397-411.

Hranilovich, JA, Kaiser, EA, Pace, A, Barber, M, Ziplow, J. Headache in transgender and gender-diverse patients: A narrative review. *Headache*. 2021; 61: 1040– 1050.

MacGregor EA, vanden Brink AM. Transgender and migraine. In: van den Brink AM, MacGregor EA, eds. Gender and Migraine. Cham: Springer; 2019; 113-127.

The World Professional Association for Transgender Health. Standards of Care for the Health of Transsexual, Transgender, and Gender Nonconforming People, 7th Version. 2011. Http://www.wpath.org/publications/soc

How is it Possible for one person to have so Many Different Headaches?

Roger K. Cady, MD
Kathleen Farmer-Cady, PsyD

I'm confused. How can I have so many different headaches?

At 12, my headaches began. A couple of years later, in the middle of allergy season, my headaches were interfering with my schoolwork. I visited my Primary Care doctor who pinpointed my problem as sinus headaches.

Over the next several years, after several antihistamines, desensitization shots, and steroids, I made an appointment with an ENT physician. He identified a bone spur in my nose and recommended and conducted surgery. My headaches never resolved but they improved for several months in the late Fall and Winter but worsened in the Spring and early Summer.

Later a friend whose mother was a physician suggested I seek help from a neurologist. I was diagnosed as having migraine. She prescribed a triptan which helped but warned that I should only use this medicine when I was certain I was having a migraine. She cautioned that triptans constricted blood vessels and could cause heart attacks by pinching off the blood flow in my heart. Because the medicine often produced tingling and sometimes slight chest pressure, I was careful to take it only when I really needed it. If the triptan failed to work, the headache sent me to bed for days.

At 19, I had the most severe headache of my life. I sought help at the emergency room. The doctor thought a blood vessel had broken inside my head. He ordered a CT scan and spinal tap. The studies were normal, but he diagnosed my very severe headaches as cluster headache. He explained that cluster was the worst pain a person could have and were called suicide headaches--not what I needed to hear.

From then on, I sought relief from other physicians, counselors, and psychiatrists. Each had a different message for me. I was told I was under too much stress and had depression and anxiety, bipolar disorder, fibromyalgia, and even bad bacteria in my intestines. I saw massage therapists, chiropractic doctors, nutritionists, and a holistic doctor. Lots of new diagnoses each with different solutions and all promising a cure for my headaches.

Years later, I was having headaches all the time, almost every day. Another healthcare provider (HCP) told me I had yet another kind of headache, 'chronic daily headache.' He explained that some days the headaches were tension headache but other days they were migraine. He called these 'mixed headaches' and 'tension/vascular headaches' because they involved both the muscles and blood vessels. The tension headache was due to my poor posture that resulted from holding my head still for long periods to avoid head movement when I had headaches.

A colleague at work recommended another neurologist who had helped her a lot. This neurologist diagnosed me with chronic migraine that she described as a new diagnosis that replaced the diagnosis of chronic daily headache. She suggested that instead of classifying the headaches as either migraine or tension headaches, I should think of all the headaches as being either migraine or headaches that will become migraine if I don't treat them as soon as the headache begins.

She was the first to put me on prevention medication. It was supposed to prevent headaches and also help me lose weight but all it did was made me forget people's names, so I was switched to another medicine to prevent migraine which I take daily to this day even though it doesn't seem to be helping. She suggested a new triptan and gave me high doses of an over-the-counter medicine to treat minor headaches as soon as they began. When all else failed, I was to rely on a pain killer for rescue so I could stay out of the emergency room.

Two years later, I was diagnosed as having medication overuse headache, meaning I was taking medication too often and my taking too much medication was now the cause of my headaches. That didn't make any sense to me.

I was referred to you because you are a headache specialist and I need help. I hope you will give me more than just another diagnosis.

I hope so too. I've had an opportunity to carefully review your medical history. After an examination, you and I will begin by discussing the first question you asked me, "How can I have so many different headaches?"

Thank you for the opportunity to help you manage your headache. I want to let you know from the start I don't have all the answers, but I believe if we work together from a clean slate, we'll get close to finding most of the answers you're looking for. The key for us to accomplish this is working together as partners. You are the expert of your headaches and experience. I am trained in medicine and headache diseases. Together I think we can discover solutions that help you control headaches.

Your story exemplifies the "spectrum of headache symptoms" that is often experienced over time by people with a primary headache disorder. Headaches are great masqueraders and depending on life circumstances and what might have triggered a specific headache there can be a wide range of different symptoms a person might experience. Headaches can range from being mild with slight discomfort to excruciating with confinement for days in bed and with pain being amplified by exposure to light, sound, touch or odors. These disabling headaches affect the entire body, causing nausea and sometimes vomiting, diarrhea, constipation, abdominal pain, sore muscles, brain fog, inability to sleep, anxiety, depression, even heart irregularities. In other words, "when your head hurts, the whole body suffers." In describing this variety of symptoms to a clinician, a barrage of different diagnoses often follows.

I think I have been everywhere on the 'spectrum' you just described. Why do doctors make diagnosing headaches so confusing?

Physicians are trained to focus primarily on the symptom of headache and see the primary problem as pain rather than systemic disruption of your nervous system. The various diagnoses you have been given reflect the clinician's best interpretation of symptoms you describe and then the best pharmacological match for the diagnosis they provide. So, the more diagnoses you receive the more treatment and particularly the more medication one is likely to receive.

Confusion occurs around the fact that headache is a nearly universal human experience that creates a spectrum of various symptoms and the potential for many different diagnoses. Worldwide, tension headache is the most common. Migraine occurs in about 12% of humans and cluster affects an estimated 0.5% of the population at least in the US. Of all the primary headaches, migraine is probably the best understood. What we know about migraine is used to explain the other primary headaches, like tension and cluster, so that too can be create even more confusion.

Do I have migraine?

Yes. Migraine is diagnosed when in a person's lifetime at least 5 headaches lasting 4-72 hours occur with the following characteristics: 1) moderate to severe intensity, on one side of the head, and/or throbbing; 2) nausea with/without vomiting or sensitivity to both light and sound.

But that description of migraine is only a small part of the story. The process of migraine may begin hours or sometimes days before the headache. Symptoms may include fatigue, brain fog, sensitivity to light, sound, and odors, irritability, and stiff muscles. These can continue during the headache and even after it resolves. One third of patients sometimes experience another set of warning symptoms called aura. This may develop an hour or so before the headache with flashing, scintillating lights, tingling in the hands, arms, and face, or other symptoms, such as speech problems or dizziness. Sometimes this leads to the false assumption that the individual has a serious eye disease or possibly is having a stroke. When the aura resolves, the headache is usually on its way.

Since you have been having headaches on more than 15 days per month for several years and most of these headaches meet criteria for migraine, your actual diagnosis is chronic migraine. Also, you are requiring medication to treat migraine and other headaches on more than 15 days per month – meaning you have a second diagnosis of medication overuse headache. Through a lifetime, those having frequent, uncontrolled migraine may find themselves burdened with multiple headache diagnoses while living with one of the most disabling diseases in the world--migraine.

Wow, that explains a lot. So, do I have "sinus headaches" too?

Even though you probably have nasal allergies that can be a risk factor or a trigger for migraine, treating allergies and even sinus surgery did not resolve your headaches. It is more likely that during some of your migraine attacks the brain activates nerves in the nasal and sinus structures causing symptoms that often mimic sinus disease. Studies have demonstrated that most people with self-diagnosed "sinus headaches" do in fact have migraine and generally it responds well to migraine treatment.

Okay, I think we're on a roll. Do I have cluster headache?

No. The characteristics of cluster headache include: 1) At least 5 lifetime attacks of a severe or very severe headache lasting 15 minutes to 3 hours that may strike once every other day to 8 times a day; 2) The headache occurs on one side of the head, usually around the eye or in the temple area; 3) On the same side as the headache, there is redness and tearing of the eye, sometimes swelling around the eye or a drooping eyelid with changes in the size of the pupil, nasal congestion and a runny nose; 4) The cluster period may continue for weeks to months and then spontaneously resolves only to return later. Sometimes there is no remission for over a year and then it is called chronic cluster headache.

Unfortunately, those with migraine may be given a cluster diagnosis when a very severe headache is around the eye and accompanied by eye and nasal symptoms. However, based on your history, I do not believe you have cluster headache.

Do I have tension-type headache?

That's a good question. There is a simple answer and a more complicated one. Simply, the diagnosis of tension-type headache is excluded in someone with chronic migraine because non-migraine headaches, such as tension-type headache, are already part of the chronic migraine picture.

The more complicated and perhaps more important answer is that probably you were given a diagnosis of tension headache when your migraine attacks were less frequent and at that point in time it was probably correct by current diagnostic standards. However, one thing most people with migraine realize early on is that not all migraine attacks are created equal and as we discussed they experience a spectrum of attacks ranging from those that are mild to those that are severe. So, within the spectrum of headaches, some are clearly migraine; others that are not quite migraine and labeled by clinicians as probable migraine; and there are another group that are clearly tension-type headache. Differentiating these different expressions of headache is complicated further by factoring in people's efforts to treat headaches. I hope you see diagnosis is not as black and white as many believe it to be.

Often individuals receive many headache diagnoses each with different instructions and medications on how it should be treated. Unfortunately, these treatments may simply delay the use of effective treatment to the point when they are no longer effective. If your headaches are poorly controlled the frequency may increase which then results in increased use of medication. Many individuals get caught in a vicious cycle of frequent headaches and poor response to treatment medications leading to more headaches and more medication. As it is for you, many with chronic migraine are burdened for years by medication overuse headache, severe disability, and misinformation about their diagnoses.

I suggest you think of migraine as being the underlying headache disease that we are working to manage. The origin of migraine is likely genetic, meaning that individuals like you have inherited a nervous system that is more sensitive to their internal and external environments. Changes in these environments can trigger the nervous system to express what seems to be many unique headaches. Another paradox is that a little migraine or one that is just beginning often responds better to treatment than a severe one. Early treatment is more likely to resolve the migraine completely. Late treatment may only take the edge off some symptoms, or it may not be effective at all, resulting in use of many doses of medicine before the headache resolves.

Consider it our job going forward to create a management plan specifically for you. That includes: 1) an understandable diagnosis; 2) having access to the right combination of medications that safely and effectively prevents and treats migraine attacks; 3) education about lifestyle adjustments that will sustain control of this disease for a lifetime.

Well, there is only one question left. Is my migraine caused because I don't cope well with stress?

Your question exposes a common belief among those with migraine and those that treat patients with migraine: "I am somehow causing my migraines." No, you are most emphatically not. Migraine is a genetic disease and what you eat, drink, and experience are no different than what people without migraine do in their lives. Your challenge is to organize your life going forward in such a way that migraine is not the centerpiece to how you are going to live your life.

Many individuals with migraine fear when the next episode will occur. This keeps a person on-edge with worry, which, ironically, increases the probability of another migraine. They always have medication available and frequently develop complex strategies for how and when to use each medication they have.

The key to success is to redirect one's attention to an activity that you value and look forward to, such as, swimming, writing, hiking, biking, dancing. Whatever you want to do. When you engage daily in a fun, rewarding activity, you will be less prone to migraine.

Also, identify the areas of your body that signal tension, such as, muscles in the neck or the knot in your stomach. These are warnings that you need to change direction, relax or engage in a fun activity to sooth the tightness before the headache materializes.

It's all a matter of reading and listening to your body and choosing a route of action other than passively living through another migraine. This takes practice. It's not necessarily easy. It won't work all the time but it's a beginning to engage in an activity as an alternative to standing by and waiting for the migraine to occur.

Good luck! You can do it. Perhaps you can receive support from a group of other people living with migraine who are dedicated to erasing the power of migraine from their life.

Suggested Readings

Aurora SK, Wilkinson F. The brain is hyperexcitable in migraine. *Cephalalgia*. 2007; 27(12):1442-1453.

Cady R, Schreiber C, Farmer K, Sheftell, F. Primary headaches: a convergence hypothesis. *Headache*. 2002; 42: 204-216.

Cady R, Schreiber CP. Sinus headache or migraine? Considerations in making a differential diagnosis. *Neurology*. 2002; 58 (9 suppl 6): S10-S14.

Kaniecki RG. Migraine and tension-type headache: an assessment of challenges in diagnosis. *Neurology*. 2002; 58 (9 suppl 6): S15-S20.

Lipton RB, Stewart WF, Cady R, Hall C, O'Quinn S, Gutterman D. Sumatriptan for the range of headaches in migraine sufferers: results of the Spectrum Study. *Headache*. 2000; 40 (10): 783-791.

“WHAT IS CAUSING MY MIGRAINES?”

JOHN F. ROTHROCK MD

My primary care doctor told me that migraines are vascular headaches. Is there is something wrong with my blood vessels?

For many years migraine was thought to result primarily from abnormal vascular reactivity, with arterial constriction and consequent retinal or brain ischemia producing aura symptoms and "compensatory" dilation of cranial arteries in turn causing the characteristic pulsatile, sickening pain of the disorder. This primary vascular hypothesis gradually has given way to something more complex and, frankly, more interesting. With the ascendance of a "unified" hypothesis that more effectively describes migraines biogenesis, we now think of migraine as a primary *brain* disorder that in some respects is analogous to primary epilepsy.

Although migraine and epilepsy clinically manifest themselves in very different ways, each reflects a brain that is inherently "hypersensitive”. Both in epilepsy and in migraine that hypersensitivity may be reflected on EEG, and in migraine specifically photic stimulation will provoke a disorganized EEG pattern that may include epileptiform discharges. Providing further evidence that individuals with migraine may have hypersensitivity which is especially prominent within the visual/occipital cortex are the findings elicited by visual evoked response (VER) testing: an exaggerated/high amplitude cortical wave that does not “fatigue” with repetitive stimulation. Migraine and epilepsy are bi-directionally "comorbid"; if one has migraine, he/she has an increased likelihood of having epilepsy as well…and vice versa. In the case of so-called "migralepsy", the two disorders blend together clinically such that seizure activity occurs always or nearly always in the setting of an acute migraine episode. If these two clinically distinct disorders similarly reflect inherently sensitized brain cortex, then it should not be surprising that medications which stabilize and desensitize cortex may be effective in treating both (egs, divalproex sodium and topiramate).

Along with the cerebral cortex itself, the various components of migraine's biologic "circuitry" include the brain stem (and the trigeminal nucleus caudalis of the medulla, in particular), the trigeminal nerve and the synaptic junction that lies between the trigeminal nerve endings and head pain receptors located on the meningeal vasculature. While release of vasoactive peptides at the trigeminovascular junction may produce arterial changes (including vasodilation) that contribute to the head pain of migraine, these changes typically occur as a consequence of a pain signal which arises "upstream" in the circuitry, arriving at the terminus of the migraine circuit via electrochemical transmission.

Two chemicals - protein neurotransmitters - that play major roles in modulating the transmission of head pain signal are serotonin and calcitonin gene-related peptide (CGRP). Medications which activate serotonin receptors that inhibit head pain signaling will "short-circuit the circuit". This appears to be the major mechanism by which the triptans and lasmiditan can terminate migraine episodes. The anti-CGRP monoclonal antibodies (erenumab, galcanezumab, fremanezumab, eptinezumab) and the "gepants" (ubrogepant, rimegepant, atogepant) block the receptor to CGRP or directly inactivate that protein molecule, and in doing so they desensitize the acutely or chronically sensitized migraine circuitry. The fact that these "designer drugs" for acute migraine treatment and migraine prophylaxis were synthesized to "fit" the existing hypothetical model for migraine's biogenesis and are so clinically effective reinforces the notion that this "unified" model at least approximates what is occurring at the molecular level.

But my headaches are so severe. Surely there is something wrong with my brain. Shouldn't we do some testing to find out what is causing these attacks of head pain? Maybe an MRI scan?

Even with its astounding resolution and sensitivity, it is beyond the capacity of MRI to visualize the biologic underpinnings of migraine. It appears that primary migraine is likely to be genetic in origin, either inherited or a consequence of gene mutation during embryogenesis. Approximately 50% of migraine patients evaluated in an outpatient setting will report that at least one first-degree family member also has migraine. If first-degree family members of the patient are interviewed directly, that proportion rises to 90% or more. Just under 40 million Americans actively experience migraine, and for them it is no more "wrong" to have migraine then it is to have blue eyes or red hair.

Thus the familiar constellation of symptoms that we term "migraine" appears to result from a genetically sensitized brain and, more specifically, from a genetically sensitized circuit of cortical neurons, nuclei, ganglion cells and axons that, when sufficiently stimulated, activate to produce the symptoms. As a *primary* headache disorder, your migraine is a part of you and your individual biology. Migraine is <u>not</u> a secondary headache disorder intrinsically foreign to you and indicative of an acquired neurologic or systemic disease.

<u>If</u> your history is consistent with migraine, <u>if</u> there are no "red flags" in your history to suggest that either a) something else may be mimicking migraine and causing *migrainous* headaches or b) that you have a new/acquired secondary headache superimposed upon your pre-existing migraine, and <u>if</u> your neurologic exam is normal, then the yield of brain MRI or other neurodiagnostic testing will be extremely low. There currently exists no test - even brain biopsy - that specifically can diagnose or confirm migraine. In rare variants of migraine there are genetic mutations specific for the particular variant, but genetic testing will not assist in the diagnosis of more typical migraine. To date, investigators have identified over 40 genetic mutations associated with the most common clinical types of migraine…and there may be many more. We have a long way to go before genetic testing will be helpful in diagnosing and managing migraine.

But my migraine is much worse than my twin sister's. And my mother's. Why should that be?

While your genetic predisposition to migraine may be similar or identical to that which produces the migraine experienced by your sister and mother, many factors intervene to influence how much or little that genetic predisposition will be clinically expressed. The process by which these influences promote or inhibit gene expression is termed *epigenetics*, and it's likely that although our genome itself is fixed, our *epigenome* is constantly changing as we pass through life.

The migraine circuitry is highly responsive to changes in the internal and external environments. For example, in women migraine may worsen clinically as a consequence of the natural fluctuation in the sex hormone levels that they experience during a menstrual cycle, as a consequence of pregnancy, or in the perimenopausal years. For both genders, changes in barometric pressure, sleep habits or dietary routine may influence one's migraine burden, and physical or emotional stress is a commonly cited aggravator of migraine. The migraine you experience as an adult may even reflect epigenetic changes that occurred much earlier in life; for example, the emotional nurturing you receive during early childhood appears to influence both the age at which you first begin to experience migraine and the likelihood of your eventually developing the chronic variant of migraine. There is even evidence that the epigenome may be inherited along with the genome itself. In other words, the way you feel and behave in this moment may in part reflect circumstances that affected your forebearers in the generations preceding you.

Again, no "triggers" or "aggravators", internal or external, represent the cause of your migraine. Instead, they are potentially modifiable external factors that act upon your intrinsic biogenetic predisposition to experiencing migraine. Stress may aggravate migraine, but it is not the cause of your migraine. Your migraine may routinely activate the day prior to menstrual flow onset, but this implies neither that your hormones are abnormal nor that hormonal fluctuations are the primary cause of your migraine.

Can my migraine be cured?

As evidenced by descriptions written in Mesopotamia thousands of years ago, migraine has co-existed with humankind for an awfully long time. For whatever reason, natural selection - the pruning shears of evolution - has not seen fit to eliminate migraine from our midst, and the disorder remains highly prevalent in our general population. It is, if you will, a "part of us", and to speak of "curing" migraine is much the same as seeking to "cure", say, a propensity for motion sickness.

The day may come when we can perform gene editing, identify the particular genetic permutation that is producing a given patient's migraine, intervene to "engineer" that permutation so as to silence its clinical effect and thus "cure" migraine. Until then, however, the best we can do is attempt to modify migraine's natural course in a positive manner by prescribing pharmacologic and non-pharmacologic therapies that serve to desensitize migraine's biological circuitry. Even when therapeutic intervention is wildly successful and the patient becomes headache-free or nearly so, migraine is still there, lurking beneath the surface, biologically present even if clinically quiescent, and the patient remains at risk for eventually experiencing recurrence of migraine episodes.

Why have I not responded to so many of the migraine therapies I have been prescribed?

First, did your lack of response to a medication prescribed for migraine prevention result from your failure to administer an adequate dose of that medication for an adequate amount of time? Did your lack of response to a medication prescribed for acute migraine treatment result from your administering that medication at a point in the migraine episode where it was predestined to fail?

Even when a migraine therapy is administered optimally, there is no guarantee of success. Again, there appear to exist many genetic permutations associated with migraine, and it's reasonable to presume that at the molecular level there may be variations in the structure and physiology of the migraine circuitry previously described. For example, in some migraineurs serotonin may assume a relatively minor role relative to CGRP, or vice versa. In others, neither neuropeptide may dominate, nor will glutamate, an excitatory neurotransmitter, serve as the driving force behind generating and conducting the head pain signal.

If this presumption is correct, then one should not expect any given therapeutic intervention to be 100% effective in all migraineurs, and arriving at an effective treatment strategy is typically is a matter of educated trial and error. There is a real scarcity of variables which will assist healthcare providers in predicting which migraine patient will respond to a given migraine therapy.

To make things even more complex, it's logical to assume that the molecular components of migraine's biologic circuitry are dynamic, with receptor sensitivity changing either as a consequence of migraine attack frequency, alterations induced by prophylactic therapy, epigenetic influences or simply the advance of years. To treat migraine effectively, then, one must be nimble and prepared to shift an existing treatment strategy so as to match the concurrent migraine burden.

Despite its prevalence, migraine is a complex disorder that poses a challenge to those who attempt to treat it. That's the bad news. The good news: over the course of the last three decades we have been witness to nothing less than a revolution in our understanding of "what causes migraine". With this understanding has come a veritable deluge of new therapies offering the migraineur new options for management that are safe, well-tolerated and clinically effective.

Suggested reading

Charles A. The pathophysiology of migraine: implications for clinical management. *Lancet/Neurology* 2017. http://dx.doi.org/10.1016/S1474-4422(17)30435-0.

Cutrer FM. Pathophysiology of migraine. *Seminars in Neurology* 2010; 30(2): 120-130.

Dodick D. A phase-by-phase review of migraine pathophysiology. *Headache* 2018; https://doi.org/10.1111/head.13300.

Goadsby P, Holland P, Martins-Oliveira, et al. Pathophysiology of migraine: a disorder of sensory processing. *Physiol Rev* 2017; 97:553-622.

Goadsby P, Holland P. Pathophysiology of migraine: an update. *Neurologic Clinics* 2019; 37: 651-671.

Noack H, Rothrock J. Migraine: definitions, mechanisms, and treatment. *Southern Med J* 1996; 89:762-769.

WHAT KINDS OF THINGS CAN TRIGGER MY HEADACHES?

ROBERT KANIECKI, MD

It's frustrating but I kept a log, and I can't seem to find any specific thing that triggers my headaches. Is that common?

You are certainly not alone. Many patients are frustrated by the inability to identify the "cause" of their migraines. They may believe that by avoiding their triggers or making easy changes in diet they may rid themselves of their headaches. Unfortunately, things are not so simple. Although I find that most patients can identify at least a few triggers for migraines, this is not true for everyone. Some have no triggers. Migraines can often occur randomly, without any obvious triggering mechanism. Others report that many of the things they believe would bring on a migraine "don't do it every time." The brain of a migraine person can be influenced by multiple internal factors and therefore react unpredictably to various external factors. Some people also require the accumulation of several triggers which only cause migraine when seen in combination. For example, certain women report red wine as a trigger for migraine, but only when consumed during the time of a menstrual period. Finally, more than a few migraine patients are just unfamiliar with possible triggers and simply don't know what to look for when completing their diaries. Don't get discouraged. We can review a list of the most common migraine triggers and I'll encourage you to continue keeping a headache diary for another three months.

What are the most common triggers for migraines?

The migraine brain is very sensitive to *change*. Stress is widely accepted as the most common migraine trigger, but it is the *change* in stress levels that most commonly is connected to the start of a migraine or series of migraines. An abrupt increase in stress – for example an argument with your boss - can bring on attack, but so can relaxation after a period of stress. Some get the headache the week of final exams or a funeral, while others report headaches the week afterwards. Hormonal *change* in women is quite likely the second most reliable trigger. The menstrual cycle may be associated with predictable attacks on a monthly basis (commonly known as "menstrual migraine"). Puberty, pregnancy, menopause, and various hormonal birth control options all can aggravate migraine headaches. *Changes* in sleep patterns (oversleeping or under-sleeping), *changes* in food or water intake (hunger or thirst), or *changes* in weather/barometric pressure are all common triggers. In addition to these triggers related to change, exposure of the migraine brain to excessive sensory information may also produce migraine attacks. Excessively bright or flashing lights, loud noises, strong odors, or extremes of temperature may also be linked by some patients to their migraine attacks. When considering these factors, you need to understand that not every patient has the same set of triggers. During my seventeen years of experiencing migraines, I found my triggers to be artificial sweeteners, skipped meals, and exposure to strong odors such as nail polish removers and pine cleaners. I never found stress or sleep deprivation to be factors. Most patients can identify with a few of these triggers, some have no triggers, while a very small minority will report that "just about anything" can bring on a migraine attack.

Can you explain to me how these things like bright light can actually cause a headache?

The migraine brain and nervous system are hypersensitive by nature. Many patients recognize they are sensitive to light, noise, or odors both between and especially during migraine attacks. They are more likely to report motion sensitivity from a young age, well before the age of migraines. They are more likely to have mood sensitivity (depression), nerve sensitivity (anxiety), and sleep sensitivity (issues falling or staying asleep). The gastrointestinal tract is also potentially more sensitive. Both colic in babies and irritable bowel (constipation and/or diarrhea) in adults have been shown to occur with greater prevalence among those with migraine. I like to explain to patients that they have a high performance, high maintenance nervous system. They drive the Dodge Challenger Hellcat instead of the Dodge Dart. With the proper care, this nervous system has tremendous energy and potential. It can lead to successful personal accomplishments and career successes. On the other hand, pushing this system too hard or beyond the person's individual limits – for example with too much bright light in those sensitive to light – can cause the brain's engine to overheat to the point it must shut down to cool off.

I found most of my headaches are coming on Saturdays and Sundays. What might be causing that?

"Weekend migraines" are not unusual at all. One of the most common explanations is a reduction in stress levels on the weekend following a busy week of work or school. This type of attack is commonly known as a "letdown" migraine. Such headaches develop during periods of relaxation after a time of stress, with attacks frustratingly happening on weekends and vacations. A second possible explanation involves the potential impact of sleeping in beyond the typical weekday wakeup time. Oversleeping may itself act as a migraine trigger, while the associated delays in breakfast or morning caffeine can also contribute to the likelihood of migraine developing on weekend mornings. A third potential factor might involve some patients drinking alcohol more frequently or in greater amounts on Friday or Saturday nights when compared to the week. My advice is to set your alarm early on the weekends, getting the same number of hours of sleep as you do during the week, and follow your weekday breakfast and caffeine routines. Vary the alcohol intake if the first steps are not helpful.

I love chocolate – I mean <u>really</u> love chocolate - but I read on the internet that it could be causing me more headaches? Do I need to stop?

Both clinical experience and research studies indicate that chocolate may be overly blamed for triggering migraines. The explanation partly lies in understanding the physiologic stages of migraine. There is a phase in migraine known as prodrome where one of the first symptoms of the developing migraine itself is a craving for certain foods, such as chocolate. In that situation, the patient experiences the craving, eats the chocolate, and then gets the migraine, subsequently blaming the migraine on the chocolate. However, the migraine was already in motion, and whether the person ate chocolate or a mint, the attack would have occurred. It is true that some are sensitive to chocolate and may find their migraines triggered by it, but that can only be learned through trial and error. Most patients with migraine can be happily advised to continue eating chocolate without restriction – albeit in moderation.

I know it sounds strange, but I think my headaches are sometimes related to the barometric pressure. It seems like I get more with rainy days. Am I crazy?

You are not crazy. Changes in weather, most commonly those changes associated with big drops in barometric pressure, have been linked to migraine attacks by countless patients. The more dramatic the change, the more likely it is to be linked to an individual attack. Dramatic swings in temperature associated with some of these weather fronts, such as those seen in the spring and fall seasons in many areas of the country, seem to provoke the greatest difficulties. Unfortunately, there is little to do about this trigger since it is essentially impossible to avoid - unless one moves elsewhere – and I have yet to learn of the "perfect" location for those with migraine.

I wake up with most of my migraines and I've tried more than a dozen pillows but cannot seem to find the right one. What's the best pillow for someone with migraine headaches?

Your choice in pillow is unlikely to blame. Morning migraines are extraordinarily common. One study found that 50 percent of all migraines occurring on any given day develop between 4 am and 9 am. That is half of all migraines developing in a five-hour span of time in the morning, and the other half starting during the other nineteen hours of the day. In essence there is a "hightide" for migraine attacks in those hours. It is something that has been long known about migraine, yet the actual basis is not completely understood. Most believe it may be due to some normal brain activity and chemistry changes which occur during the latter stages of sleep. In this setting of morning headache other explanations may need to be explored. Some patients may have sleep apnea, some others may grind their teeth at night, and some others may have neck issues that are aggravated during sleep. Most, however, just find that their migraines occur commonly in the morning. As for the "best migraine pillow," I have yet to hear of any consistent recommendation from my migraine patients.

I tried all kinds of diets, but I still got migraines. I eliminated dairy then gluten. I tried eliminating carbs, alcohol, cheese, sweets, and they still came five or six times per month. What's the best diet for migraine patients?

Compared to other triggers such as stress, hormone changes, scheduling changes, and excessive exposure to sensory stimuli such as light noise and odors, dietary triggers are much less common in migraine. Perhaps only 15 percent of individuals will report dietary triggers, and by the time they reach our office they often have already identified certain specific foods. Those foods should be avoided in those patients. For most patients who have no clear dietary triggers I simply recommend eating frequent small meals that minimize or eliminate additives and preservatives. I suggest reading the packaging carefully and avoiding those products with long lists of unnatural ingredients. The greater the processing required in the preparation of the food, the greater the likelihood it may trigger a migraine attack. Fresh meats, fresh fruits or vegetables, simple grains, and fish are all acceptable. Simple dietary changes may be helpful for those recognizing problems with a specific food or two, but drastic elimination diets are rarely necessary. We should also review beverages. Caffeinated beverages are permissible in limited amounts – ideally 8-12 ounces per day at the most – and artificially sweetened ones should be avoided. Certain individuals are also sensitive to alcoholic beverages, particularly red wine, so I encourage you track your alcohol intake on your headache diaries to see if you may be sensitive.

Caffeine has me confused. Sometimes it seems like I get headaches if I have too much, other times when I skip it. Since I see it is in some headache medicines, is it helpful to continue drinking three cups of coffee each day?

The pros and cons of caffeine in migraine are relatively easy to explain. The pro: caffeine helps “amplify” the effects of certain pain relievers such as acetaminophen or aspirin. That’s why it is included in certain over-the-counter headache medications. It is what we know as an “analgesic adjuvant.” The con: caffeine is a stimulant, one that could potentially agitate or overstimulate the “hypersensitive” nervous system of migraine we previously discussed. In the setting of chronic caffeine intake, both overuse of caffeine and caffeine withdrawal may trigger a migraine attack. Migraine attacks are often activated by exposing the brain to the forces of either overstimulation (too much caffeine) or change (skipped or abruptly lowered caffeine). Most headache specialists recommend limiting caffeine intake to a maximum of 100 mg per day, and if caffeine is both taken regularly and in moderation, such doses are reasonably well-tolerated by most patients with migraine.

Suggested Readings

Alstadhaug A, Salvesen R, Bekkelund S. Weekend migraine. *Cephalalgia* 2007;27: 343-346

Baldacci F, Vedovello M, Ulivi M, et al. How aware are migraineurs of their triggers? *Headache* 2013;53: 834-837

Hayne DP, Martin PR. Relating Photophobia, Visual Aura, and Visual Triggers of Headache and Migraine. *Headache* 2019;59: 430-442

Hindiyeh N, Zhang N, Farrar M, et al. The Role of Diet and Nutrition in Migraine Triggers and Treatment: A Systematic Literature Review. *Headache* 2020; 60: 1300–1316

Karsan N, Bose P, Newman J, Goadsby P. Are some patient-perceived migraine triggers simply early manifestations of the attack? *Journal of Neurology* 2021;268: 1885-1893

Maasumi K, Tepper SJ, Kriegler JS. Menstrual Migraine and Treatment Options: Review. *Headache* 2017;57: 194-208

Martin PR. Managing headache triggers: Think 'coping' not 'avoidance.' *Cephalalgia* 2010; 30:634-637

Marmura M. Triggers, Protectors, and Predictors in Episodic Migraine. *Curr Pain Headache Rep* 2018 Oct 5;22(12):81. doi: 10.1007/s11916-018-0734-0.

Nowaczewska M, Wiciński M, Kaźmierczak W. The Ambiguous Role of Caffeine in Migraine Headache: From Trigger to Treatment. *Nutrients* 2020 Aug; 12(8): 2259

Pavlovic JM, Buse DC, Sollars CM, Haut S, Lipton RB. Trigger factors and premonitory features of migraine attacks: summary of studies. *Headache* 2014;54: 1670-1679

Pellegrino ABW, Davis-Martin RE, Houle TT, Turner DP, Smitherman TA. Perceived triggers of primary headache disorders: A meta-analysis. *Cephalalgia* 2018;38: 1188-1198

Peris F, Donoghue S, Torres F, Mian A, Wöber C. Towards improved migraine management: Determining potential trigger factors in individual patients. *Cephalalgia* 2017;37: 452-463.

Spierings EL, Donoghue S, Mian A, Wöber C. Sufficiency and necessity in migraine: how do we figure out if triggers are absolute or partial and, if partial, additive or potentiating? *Curr Pain Headache Rep* 2014 Oct;18(10):455. doi: 10.1007/s11916-014-0455-y.

Turner D, Lebowitz A, Chtay I, Houle T. Headache Triggers as Surprise. *Headache* 2019;59: 495-508

Wöber C, Brannath W, Schmidt K, Kapitan M, Rudel E, Wessely P, Wöber-Bingöl C; PAMINA Study Group. Prospective analysis of factors related to migraine attacks: the PAMINA study. *Cephalalgia* 2007;27: 304-314

Zebenholzer K, Rudel E, Frantal S, et al. Migraine and weather: a prospective diary-based analysis. *Cephalalgia* 2011;31: 391-400

Is My Diet Causing My Headaches?

Shannon Babineau MD

Clinical Assistant Professor of Neurology and Pediatrics Sidney Kimmel Medical College of Thomas Jefferson University

Staff Child Neurologist Atlantic Medical Group

Are there foods that can trigger my headaches?

There are many foods that have been implicated in triggering migraine attacks. Up to 30% of migraine sufferers report that specific foods can trigger a migraine. Common foods that have been identified as migraine triggers include chocolate, nuts, citrus fruits, salami, cheese, caffeine, alcohol, foods with MSG, foods with nitrites, and artificial sweeteners. Migraine sufferers will often report that a migraine is more likely to occur on the days when these foods have been consumed. However, there has been significant difficulty in medical studies identifying true causation between a specific food and migraine occurrence. In studies where migraine sufferers track diet and headaches carefully in a diary, there is often very little, or no association found between the food and the likelihood of a migraine. In a study where participants who felt chocolate was a trigger for their migraines, they were given either chocolate or carob without knowing, and they were not more likely to get migraine after eating chocolate versus the carob.

Might there be another explanation why I might feel sensitive to certain foods?

Complicating things further, many migraine sufferers experience a prodrome with their migraines. A prodrome is a series of symptoms that come before the more widely recognized headache, nausea, vomiting, and environmental sensitivity that is part of the migraine attack. Prodromal symptoms include yawning, neck pain, fatigue, and sometimes food cravings. Chocolate craving is a commonly reported prodromal symptom.

So, for some, eating chocolate may be a craving driven by a migraine that has already started. However, because of the timing, it can be misinterpreted as a trigger.

Are food triggers all in our minds?

It's complicated; so many different foods and chemicals within food are consumed daily, habits around eating can vary significantly from day to day, all coupled with the delay that may occur between exposure to the food trigger and the migraine (up to 1-2 days) making studies in this field very difficult and self-identification in everyday life even more difficult. Most likely there are certain specific foods that can trigger a specific migraine attack, but this is likely in a small percentage of people for a small percentage of attacks. In one study specific foods were identified as a trigger in 1-7% of people with migraine, compared to fatigue and missed meals which were found in 20-30% of people. Of the studies that have looked at specific migraine triggers, the best evidence supports the role of monosodium glutamate (MSG), artificial sweeteners (aspartame), tyramine and histamine containing foods, chocolate, and nitrite containing foods as migraine triggers.

Why do certain foods trigger headaches?

There are several different mechanisms by which "trigger foods" can lead to migraine. Some of these foods can activate pathways in the brain that make the brain more pain sensitive. The chemicals may mimic the way the brain's pain activating chemicals work or they may modify how sensitive the brain is to pain signals. Some of the foods may have indirect effects by triggering inflammation, changing the way the blood vessels in the brain respond, or making the brain more "excitable" and prone to creating a migraine.

What about gluten?

People with celiac disease are more likely to have migraines than the general population and in those with both conditions (migraine and celiac), removal of gluten from the diet improves the frequency and severity of migraines. There is weaker evidence to support that those with gluten sensitivity, not celiac disease, may also find improvement in migraine frequency and severity with a gluten-free diet. However, there is no strong evidence that a gluten-free diet in the general population helps migraines. There are many people who opt for a gluten-free diet who reduce the amount of processed carbohydrates they eat, and this may be what is helping. However, you should be careful when eating gluten-free; because of the popularity of gluten-free diets, substitutes are easy to find for most foods and gluten-free does not necessarily mean healthy. Many of these substitutes are highly processed and can be higher in calories than the gluten-rich items, leading to unwanted health effects.

Are there are other dietary habits that could be contributing to my headaches?

Not eating regularly and hunger are listed among the top 5 triggers for migraine. The likelihood of migraine increases with the duration of the fast. People that skip meals or eat irregularly through the day have more frequent migraines. Many migraine sufferers need to eat at least 3-6 meals per day, or every 3 hours. An even blood sugar through the day is likely to be helpful. This would mean eating foods that take longer to digest and provide a more even release of sugar into the body. Foods that are high in protein, complex carbohydrates, and healthy fats should be added to each meal. Heavy sugar/simple carbohydrate consumption should be reduced or avoided when possible.

What about caffeine?

Caffeine is tricky for migraine suffers. Many people use caffeine to treat migraine. It has been shown to be effective on its own or in combination with other analgesics. It may even enhance the effectiveness of analgesics. However, there are people who find caffeine to be a specific trigger for a migraine attack. For those people, eating or drinking something containing caffeine, like chocolate, coffee, tea or soda, will trigger a migraine. More commonly migraine sufferers who overuse caffeine find that they get a rebound or withdrawal headache if they go too long without caffeine in their system. Often it can occur in the morning before the normal "morning coffee/tea". In those that routinely drink more than 400mg of caffeine/day, withdrawal headache can be more common. Remember some over the counter migraine treatments have caffeine in them too, so make sure to include the caffeine content in those medications in your total daily caffeine tally. There can also be caffeine in some drinks that are not typically thought of as caffeinated like certain waters or coffee shop "non-coffee" drinks. If caffeine is part of your routine, keep it as that, with a routine dose daily at amounts less than 400mg/day. Or, if possible, try to limit caffeine consumption to 2-3 days/week or less.

What about alcohol?

Alcohol has been identified as a trigger for migraines as well. In sensitive migraine sufferers, a migraine attack can be triggered within 3 hours of consuming an alcoholic beverage. Some migraine sufferers can be sensitive to very small amounts of alcohol. Many people, even non- migraine sufferers, can get headache when they have over-indulged in alcohol, part of a hangover. Those with migraine seem to be more susceptible to hangover headache the next day. It is not clear if it is the alcohol itself that is the trigger or a component of the alcoholic drinks. Components of alcoholic drinks including tyramine, phenylethylamine, histamine, sulphites and flavonoid phenols have been implicated but as with other food triggers, the studies have not panned out. Like other food triggers, there are likely many different factors at play and alcohol as a trigger may be overestimated. If there isn't a clear relationship between alcohol and migraine for you, drinking in moderation may be okay.

How can I figure out if I have food triggers?

There are a few different ways to identify food triggers. One way is to keep a food diary along with your migraine diary. If you have frequent migraines, more than two/week, every day write down the foods you eat with as much detail including the brand used or restaurant if possible. This will allow you to go back and look at the nutritional contents/additives if there is concern that food is a trigger. Once you have completed this over 6-8 weeks go back and look to see if there seem to be similar foods occurring on days you report a migraine that are not there on days without migraine. If you have less frequent migraines, 1/week or less, you can wait until you have a migraine and then write down all the foods eaten that day. If you have migraines every day or if you struggle to keep diaries, this method is not going to be helpful. In that case, I would suggest eliminating some of the higher risk migraine trigger foods from your diet: MSG, artificial sweeteners (aspartame), tyramine and histamine containing foods, chocolate, and nitrite containing foods. Note that MSG can be hard to identify because it has many names: natural flavor, kombu extract, hydrolyzed plant protein, hydrolyzed vegetable protein, and just "flavoring". Histamine can be found in some fish, cheeses, processed meats, fruits including strawberries/tomatoes, fermented foods, and alcoholic beverages. Tyramine is found in a number of foods and beverages including cheese, wine, broad beans, sausage, and yeast extracts. Nitrites are found in preserved meat like bacon, sausage, ham, and lunch meats. Remove these foods for 6-8 weeks and monitor headache frequency. If improved, you can slowly add back in these foods and monitor return of headaches, hopefully aiding in identification of which foods specifically trigger your headaches. Another way to identify food triggers is to get tested for IgG food antibodies. This can be done through a blood test ordered by your physician. These tests are often not covered by insurance, so they can be costly. I would discuss the cost benefit of doing this testing with your physician before paying for this type of testing.

Should I do an elimination diet/migraine diet to treat my migraines?

There are many different diets that have been advertised as "cures" for migraine. There is no scientific evidence that there is any one type of diet that will significantly reduce migraines. There have been many scientific trials to look for possible suggestions without consistent success. Elimination diets, which at times can severely restrict what is eaten, are not generally recommended as they are difficult to adhere to and can lead to nutritional deficiencies. In addition, I caution about using elimination diets in children/teens particularly if they are already picky eaters. I would recommend first working on having the child consume regular meals through the day as frequently as every 3 hours (particularly if they are under 10 years old) with protein, as this has much better evidence to support effectiveness than a diet that eliminates a lot of foods.

Are there any diets that can help?

There are some diets that have shown some medical evidence for help with migraines. Low fat diets, where calories from fat make up 23.5% of the total calories consumed, have been shown to help compared to a diet with normal fat content (calories from fat making up 35% or more of the total calories consumed). Diets that are high in omega 3 fats and low in omega 6 fats have also had some promising results. As mentioned above, personalized elimination diets based on IgG antibody blood tests have had success. Also, in specific populations of people, diet can be helpful, like gluten freedom in celiac disease and gluten sensitivity. For those who have signs of histamine intolerance (flushing, diarrhea, wheezing, urticaria, or rhinitis on ingestion of histamine rich foods) may find improvement in migraine with low histamine diet.

Ketogenic diets have shown some positive results as well. However, this diet can have negative health effects including high cholesterol, osteoporosis, and kidney changes. It is best to consult with your doctor before trying any type of significant dietary modification to understand the possible risks and benefits. You may also want to seek the help of a nutritionist to ensure that you are continuing to eat a healthy, nutritious diet. Nutritionists can also be helpful in teaching which foods to avoid and new ways of cooking with your new diet.

So what should I do with my diet?

Start by making sure to eat consistently throughout the day and avoid fasting. Ensure you are taking in foods that are lower in processed carbohydrates and higher in protein/healthy fats. Overall, try to avoid foods that have a lot of additives. Pay attention to caffeine consumption as well as alcohol consumption. Try to reduce daily caffeine intake to 200mg/day or less. For extra credit you can try keeping a food diary to record foods you are eating every day and whether you experience migraine on that day. Food diaries can be difficult, especially with frequent headaches, and specific food triggers for migraine are only likely in a small percentage of migraine patients. If you have symptoms of gluten intolerance or histamine sensitivity, consider speaking to your doctor about possible testing for celiac and discussion about likelihood of these conditions. Give these changes some time. It can take up to 2-3 months to see the benefits from these types of modifications. And of course, making sure to work on other lifestyle modifications as well.

If you are ready for a higher level of commitment to dietary changes to treat your migraines you can consider a personalized approach to food elimination by getting IgG food antibody testing with your doctor and then following the recommendations of foods to avoid. Or, you could consider a more generalized dietary change like higher omega 3/lower omega 6 or a lower fat diet. Ketogenic diets should only be undertaken under the supervision of a doctor given the possible risks. Consider seeing a nutritionist if you are interested in any of these diets. They can be a wealth of information and a great support when trying to make these changes.

Suggested Reading

Finkel, Alan G., Juanita A. Yerry, and J. Douglas Mann. "Dietary considerations in migraine management: does a consistent diet improve migraine?" *Current pain and headache reports* 17.11 (2013): 1-8.

Gelfand, Amy A., and Samantha L. Irwin. "Lifestyle Advice for Pediatric Migraine: Blaming the Patient, or Evidence Based?" *Seminars in neurology*. Vol. 40. No. 03. Thieme Medical Publishers, 2020.

Kelman, Leslie. "The triggers or precipitants of the acute migraine attack." *Cephalalgia* 27.5 (2007): 394-402.

Marcus, D. A., et al. "A double-blind provocative study chocolate as a trigger of headache." *Cephalalgia* 17.8 (1997): 855-862.

Martin, Vincent T., and Brinder Vij. "Diet and headache: part 1." *Headache: The Journal of Head and Face Pain* 56.9 (2016): 1543-1552.

Martin, Vincent T., and Brinder Vij. "Diet and headache: part 2." *Headache: The Journal of Head and Face Pain* 56.9 (2016): 1553-1562.

Peris, Francesc, et al. "Towards improved migraine management: Determining potential trigger factors in individual patients." *Cephalalgia* 37.5 (2017): 452-463.

Slavin, Margaret, and Jessica Ailani. "A clinical approach to addressing diet with migraine patients." *Current neurology and neuroscience reports* 17.2 (2017): 17.

When Should I go to the Emergency Room for My Headaches?

María-Carmen Wilson, MD
Associate Professor of Neurology
University of Queensland/Ochsner Medical School
Covington, Louisiana
Cristina Cabret-Aymat, MD
Neurology/ Headache and Facial Pain
Ochsner, North Shore Region
Covington, Louisiana

None of the medications that has been prescribed works, I cannot stand this migraine any longer. I am going to go the* emergency *room so they can treat my pain.

During a severe or prolonged migraine attacks when the typical medications you have been prescribed do not work, a lot of patients end up going to the emergency room. If you have an established diagnosis of migraine and in the midst of a severe attack there might be concern that what is going on is something else than migraine. We recommend going to emergency room if pain begins suddenly, if you experience the worse headache of life, or you experience new neurological symptoms like numbness, weakness, vision loss, fever, confusion, loss of consciousness or some other worrisome symptoms; then the ER is the right choice.

The ER unfortunately is not a migraine friendly place as it tends to be loud, bright, and full of strong odors where there is typically a long wait. An ER trip does not mean necessarily leaving with pain freedom as frequently either pain might continue or it returns hours later. The treatment of migraine in the ER varies by location and provider examining you. Typically, very few of the medications given are migraine specific. Commonly a combination of 2 or more medications are provided known as "migraine cocktails". A recent emergency room study compared intravenous hydromorphone, with intravenous prochlorperazine plus diphenhydramine. The results revealed that the combination of prochlorperazine (Compazine) plus diphenhydramine was more effective than hydromorphone. Going to the ER ends up being costly, more than likely, unnecessary testing, bloodwork, CT scan, and lumbar punctures are done. Our suggestion is to discuss an action plan with your specialist to include migraine specific medications for management of moderate to severe attacks. Also, to discuss rescue strategies for when your typical treatment fails you with goal of aborting attack at home. Remember to stay well hydrated, rest, and a quiet, cool, and a dark environment. If a trip to ER is inevitable, then we recommend having a plan with your specialist about medications recommended for a typical migraine that cannot wait any longer.

I have had several transient spells of visual disturbance followed by a severe headache. Should I go to the emergency room?

This is not enough information to make a good decision. It is quite possible that you are experiencing a visual migraine aura. However, it is important to characterize the episode in detail. A typical visual aura related to migraine begins gradually, is unilateral, and progresses over 4 to 5 minutes increasing in size, reaching a peak in about 15 to 20 minutes, in a "crescendo" fashion. The visual disturbance dissipates as gradually as it commences. Episodes can last from 5 minutes and up to an hour. The headache can accompany or follow the aura. There are several manifestations of visual aura which we call fortification spectra, scintillating scotoma. This manifestation consists of a C-shape zig-zag colorful lines in the periphery, that enlarges as the aura progresses encircling a dimming, darkening of spot. At the peak, the entire visual field is affected. Other forms of visual aura consist of scotomata, "black spots," visual deficits in half the visual field, or photopsias which consist of bright spots and flashes of light. The gradual onset and resolution of the visual aura is typical of migraine and not of other neurological conditions. An example of a visual disturbance requiring an immediate evaluation is the sudden loss of vision in one eye, this is called "amaurosis fugax" and may be an indication of clots in the carotid artery which can lead to stroke. This tends to be painless and not followed by a headache. This is important to keep details on what occurs so that you can discuss with your primary care physician or neurologist to decide next step in action. If you have episode of visual loss or other quick onset of neurological symptoms, then we do suggest you being evaluated emergently.

I get very frequent, severe headaches associated with nausea and vomiting; the attacks are very disabling. Every time this happens, I panic and go to the emergency room.

If you have a diagnosis of migraine, the presence of nausea and vomiting can be as disabling as the head pain. Nausea and vomiting can lead to dehydration and impaired absorption of oral medications due to migraine associated gastroparesis. Migraine associated gastroparesis is delayed gastric emptying which leads to poor absorption of oral medications. The best approach to manage your migraine attacks is to develop a plan with your specialist that includes a comprehensive approach that addresses the different symptoms associated with migraine. Treatment of the attacks should include migraine specific medications, in your case, antinausea medication as well.

We have a lot of weapons in our armamentarium to prevent the attacks and to optimize acute treatment. In your case, using a non-oral route would be more effective. Intranasal or injectable medications are approved and would be indicated for these attacks. Non-oral formulations of triptans, NSAIDs, antinausea medication, and dihydroergotamine are medications options. Additionally, there is a lot of fear and anxiety associated with migraine attacks; thus, it's important to practice mindfulness exercises that can help complement the medication to avoid these significant stress and panic situations. An addition to medications, there are nonpharmacological neuromodulation devices that can aid an acute attack. These FDA cleared external devices have been shown to be effective at aborting acute attacks. These devices target pain transmitted fibers implicated in migraine mechanism. The neuromodulation devices include transcutaneous supraorbital neurostimulator (Cefaly), Remote electrical neuromodulation (Nerivio), transcutaneous vagus nerve stimulator (Gammacore), and dual trigeminal and occipital external neurostimulator (Relivion). The transcutaneous supraorbital neurostimulator (Cefaly) is an electrical stimulator applied to the forehead via a self-adhesive electrode which stimulates upper branches of the trigeminal nerve which transmits some of the pain associated with migraine. The transcutaneous vagal nerve stimulator (Gammacore) is a handheld device that uses electrical stimulation targeting the vagus nerve in the neck. The remote electrical neuromodulation device (REN) Nerivio is a smartphone-controlled wearable that is worn in upper arm, in which upper arm peripheral nerves are stimulated to inhibit pain from migraine. The dual trigeminal/occipital stimulator (Relivion) is worn as a headset and targets multiple nerves (supraorbital and occipital) on the head has been shown to reduce pain and other migraine related symptoms like light and sound sensitivities. We have a lot of options to offer and tailor to each individual patient and attack.

I do not normally get headache, but I suddenly developed extreme head pain, I vomited profusely and have blurred vision. What should I do?

These symptoms are worrisome and should prompt an immediate visit to the ED. This is what we call a "thunderclap" headache. The extreme intensity of the pain along with the profuse vomiting and blurred vision cold be indicative of increased intracranial pressure. This is a medical emergency, the cause could be related to a variety of serious conditions like intracranial bleed (subarachnoid hemorrhage from ruptured aneurysm or intracranial hemorrhage), meningitis, intracranial pressure changes or a clot in the veins of the brain, amongst other. This type of headache has to be evaluated by a physician emergently and emergent neuroimaging and other studies are needed to find a cause and treat appropriately. All of the causes of thunderclap headache are not serious, but that can only be determined after testing.

I have a new onset of headache, much worse when I am up and worsening through the day and significantly improves when I lay down. I have a cold and cannot stop coughing. Is this an emergency?

Any new onset of headache, particularly in patients without previous history of headache or a change in the habitual pattern should be investigated. This does not necessarily mean that it is an emergency, but prompt investigation leads to quicker treatment and decreased suffering. In this case, the positional component of the head pain, worse when in the upright position and better when laying down, coupled with the history of frequent coughing could be indicative of a low-pressure headache. Low pressure headache is usually due to cerebrospinal fluid (CSF) leak. Underlying arthritis can contribute to wear and tear of the meninges. Once integrity is lost, CSF leaks. As the brain is floating in CSF, the decrease in the normal amount of fluid causes the brain to "sag" and pull on pain sensitive structures leading to pain when upright. This headache needs prompt neuroimaging with MRI brain with and without contrast. If findings and history are suggestive of low-pressure headache then early management of this which can include procedure such as epidural blood patch and often CT myelogram to identify the location of the leak.

I suffer from migraine, but I have a new headache in the back of my head and neck. I am having problems with balance and have blurred vision. Otherwise, I am a healthy, I exercise and lift weights. Should I be concerned?

A new headache is always considered a "red flag." Blurred vision and problems with balance along with a new posterior head and neck pain should be investigated. The fact that you have a primary headache diagnosis such as migraine, does not mean that other causes of headache cannot occur. Unexplained vision disturbance warrants emergent evaluation. Information regarding the onset of the episode is important and the activities prior to the onset of the new symptoms. Weight lifting maybe a risk factor along with movements that hyperextend the neck such as roller coaster, beauty salon hair washing, chiropractic manipulation, among others. The constellation of symptoms including posterior head and neck pain, difficulty with balance and blurred vision may be indicative of posterior circulation problem. This could be due to vertebral artery dissection. In this case, you should go to the ED for evaluation.

I am a 65 y/o man with new onset of headaches gradually getting worse. I am concerned that I may have a brain tumor. Should I go the Emergency room?

It is quite common, particularly for non-headache sufferers, to be concerned about the dreaded brain tumor in the presence of a new onset of headache. While new onset of headache after the age of 50 is worrisome, gradual onset without any acute neurological symptoms permits evaluation in the outpatient setting. You will need a detailed history, medication review, and neurological examination. Workup will likely include blood work and neuroimaging studies to investigate for secondary causes of headache. As for other conditions, age is a risk factor for tumors. A new onset of headache gradually getting worse should be evaluated. However, progressive headache as an isolated symptom should be evaluated in the outpatient setting. Furthermore, headache is not always a presenting symptom of a brain tumor. Seizures, visual disturbance, numbness, weakness, vertigo, imbalance and other symptoms may be the first manifestation.

My elderly mother has a new headache in the left temple, she has not been feeling well, running a low-grade fever, weight loss. Could this be serious?

When people over the age of 50 develop progressive headache in the temporal region along with symptoms of malaise and low-grade fever, the first diagnosis that comes to mind is giant cell arteritis. Like in every headache case, the history is of paramount importance. Abrupt onset of visual disturbance, like transient monocular vision loss, is worrisome. The history will include information regarding the presence of other possible symptoms like claudication of the jaw (pain with sustained chewing). In the examination, there will be evaluation for fever, tender palpable, nodular, "ropy" temporal artery, and local hair loss, and dry cough. Blood work is very helpful guiding future testing. An elevated erythrocyte sedimentation rate (ESR) and C-reactive protein (CRP), are simple blood tests, that indicate further investigation. It is clear that this patient must be evaluated, but not necessarily in the ED. We do recommend evaluation at ER if the patient has had an episode of visual loss or neurological deficits. Otherwise, the patient should be seen promptly in the outpatient setting as immediate treatment is necessary to prevent ominous consequences. This is an example of a classic secondary headache that can be seen in those above age of 50. There are other headaches that are common in seniors. Evaluation in the ED is indicated in the presence of new and acute headache, change in habitual headache pattern if preexisting headaches or the presence of sudden onset of neurological symptoms.

My wife, a breast cancer survivor, complains of a persistent headache, double vision, ringing in the ears. Lately, she seems confused and has been falling. Do we need to go to the emergency room?

Yes, this constellation of neurological symptoms is very worrisome and should prompt immediate investigations for a space occupying lesion like brain metastasis. A history of cancer in a patient with new onset or worsening headache is concerning for secondary headache. Headache is rarely the only presentation of brain tumor. The incidence of headache in populations of patients affected by brain tumor is from 32% to 71%. Typically, patients do have additional symptoms indicating involvement of various intracranial structures. These for example could be personality changes, confusion, signs of intracranial hypertension (such as nausea, vomiting, blurry vision, double vision), worse headache in morning, worsening with Valsalva maneuvers, balance problems, weakness, numbness, or seizure. These should prompt quick evaluation for detailed history, examination and further workup with neuroimaging techniques.

Last night during sexual activity, I suffered an extreme, throbbing headache starting in the back of the head, rapidly affecting the entire head, throbbing, nausea and vomiting, sensitivity to light, sound, and motion. I wonder if I should go to the ER or if this is going to go away by itself?

Headaches associated with sexual activity usually have a benign etiology but can have a very serious cause. In this situation, we recommend going to the ED where proper investigations will be conducted promptly to exclude a variety of conditions. The diagnosis always requires exclusion of intracranial causes such as hemorrhage or structural causes. The conditions that need to be excluded are subarachnoid hemorrhage due to vascular malformation, arterial dissection, reversible cerebral vasoconstriction syndrome (RCVS), cerebral venous thrombosis, headache due to spontaneous intracranial hypotension, intracranial infection, among other serious causes. Sexual activity headache can also be due to primary headache disorder. It is important that this headache is investigated emergently with neuroimaging typically brain and arterial imaging of head/neck and at times also lumbar puncture is indicated in the acute case. Once a serious cause has been excluded, there is no need to go to the ED every time it happens, rather, the neurologist or headache specialist will treat accordingly. For primary sexual activity headache 75% of patients report single or single bouts of attacks and a chronic course would be seen by 25% of patients. Among patients with chronic course of sexual headache at baseline the remission rate at three years is 69%.

Suggested Reading

Ailani J, et al.; Board of Directors of the American Headache Society. The American Headache Society Consensus Statement: Update on integrating new migraine treatments into clinical practice. Headache. 2021 Jun 23.

Charles A. The Migraine Aura. Continuum (Minneap Minn). 2018 Aug;24(4, Headache):1009-1022.

Evans RW and Mokri B. Headache in cervical artery dissections. Headache 2002; 42: 1061–1063.

Frese A, Rahmann A, Gregor N, Biehl K, Husstedt IW, Evers S. Headache associated with sexual activity: prognosis and treatment options. Cephalalgia. 2007 Nov;27(11):1265-70.

Friedman BW, et al. Randomized study of IV prochlorperazine plus diphenhydramine vs IV hydromorphone for migraine. Neurology. 2017 Nov 14;89(20):2075-2082.

Kaniecki RG, Levin AD. Headache in the elderly. Handb Clin Neurol. 2019; 167: 511-528.

Kim JG, et al. Headache characteristics of uncomplicated intracranial vertebral artery dissection and validation of ICHD-3 beta diagnostic criteria for headache attributed to intracranial artery dissection. Cephalalgia 2015; 35: 516–526

Láinez MJ, García-Casado A, Gascón F. Optimal management of severe nausea and vomiting in migraine: improving patient outcomes. Patient Relat Outcome Meas. 2013 Oct 11; 4:61-73.

Mokri B. Spontaneous Intracranial Hypotension. Continuum (Minneap Minn). 2015 Aug;21(4 Headache):1086-108.

Nahas SJ. Headache and temporal arteritis: when to suspect and how to manage. Curr Pain Headache Rep. 2012 Aug;16(4):371-8.

Orr SL et al. (2014). Canadian Headache Society systematic review and recommendations on the treatment of migraine pain in emergency settings. Cephalalgia, 0(0): 1-14.

Palmieri A, Valentinis L, Zanchin G. Update on headache and brain tumors. *Cephalalgia*. 2021;41(4):431-437.

Pfund Z, Szapáry L, Jászberényi O, Nagy F, Czopf J. Headache in intracranial tumors. Cephalalgia. 1999 Nov;19(9):787-90; discussion 765.

Sharma TL. Common Primary and Secondary Causes of Headache in the Elderly. Headache. 2018 Mar;58(3):479-484.

Starling AJ. Diagnosis and Management of Headache in Older Adults. Mayo Clin Proc. 2018 Feb; 93(2):252-262.

Viana M, Tronvik EA, Do TP, Zecca C, Hougaard A. Clinical features of visual migraine aura: a systematic review. J Headache Pain. 2019 May 30;20(1):64.

Yeh Y-C, Fuh J-L, Chen S-P, Wang S-J. Clinical features, imaging findings and outcomes of headache associated with sexual activity. *Cephalalgia*. 2010; 30(11):1329-1335.

Exploding Head Syndrome

Mohamed Elshorafa, MD
Assistant Professor of Headache Medicine
and Child Neurology
Department of Neurology
The Icahn School of Medicine at Mt. Sinai
New York City

My first headache felt like an explosion, what's that about?

There are a number of reasons for headaches to feel like an "explosion" and it is important to get more information about where, when, how long and in what physical situation you were in when it occurred. That being said, most of the common presenting descriptions of primary headache disorders are not quite described in that fashion. So when physicians hear that word we tend to think of some of the more severe intracranial disorders leading to a secondary headache.

Well, that doesn't sound good, what are some of these other disorders?

Before we even get into that discussion, the details of the headache presentation and your history of headaches will be important to review. When did you experience this headache? How long did it last? How fast did it come on? Where did you feel it? How bad was the pain? Did it happen just once or multiple times? What were you doing when that pain came on? Were there any associated symptoms including visual, sensory or motor changes?

It happened once when I was asleep, I felt it all over my head, it lasted for a few seconds and I woke up feeling really scared for some reason. You know, like breathing heavily and my heart was racing. I'm not sure I actually felt any pain to be honest. The "sensation" was there and then disappeared just as quickly.

Did you notice an inability to move your muscles for a brief period during this time too?

YES! That's exactly what happened. What is that?

What you're describing is a very unique presentation of something we call Exploding Head Syndrome (EHS). A scary sounding, but actually benign diagnosis, that tends to occur in older age people during the wake-sleep transition or even during sleep. The American Academy of Sleep Medicine classifies it as a "sensory parasomnia" with the following diagnostic criteria: an experience of sudden loud noise or sense of explosion occurring at the wake-sleep transition or during sleep, followed by immediate arousal often with a sense of fright, and without significant pain. Did you ever have any headaches or a primary headache disorder in the past?

Not really. I had headaches here and there but never really paid much attention to them.

How often is "here and there" and when did they start?

A couple times a month since I was young, I'm not too sure exactly when though.

Where did you feel them the most? How long would those last? Was there any associated nausea/vomiting or light and sound sensitivity? Any visual or sensory changes beforehand?

My vision was never an issue nor were there any sensory changes I can remember. The pain could be on the left or right side of my head, lasting almost the whole day, sometimes with nausea but no vomiting and I wouldn't say I'd be sensitive to light or sound.

Would you have some fatigue and prefer to lay down in a quiet/dark space?

Yeah. I would usually take some over-the-counter pain medications and really want to go to bed, but because I work full-time and have a family I just push through until it goes away the next day.

Sounds like you probably also had migraines without aura that were low frequency and luckily never seemed to significantly impact your daily life or work. This is also a very common co-morbid condition with EHS.

Ok so that means I've always had headache problems? What about those severe disorders you alluded to earlier?

First off, the chances of those are very low but are important to discuss. The primary concern falls into either of two categories, vascular or non-vascular. Each of these should be looked into with neuroimaging which should initially start with a CT scan of the head to confirm no active bleeding is occuring, then followed up with an MRI with and without contrast to rule out any anatomical pathologies. It would also be prudent to obtain blood vessel imaging in your head/neck with either CTA or MRA/MRV.

So, you're saying there's a potential I have a serious bleed or cancer in my head right now?

Potentially? Yes. Probability? Very low. There are a lot of key differences between what you are describing and those more serious intracranial complications I mentioned. For instance, one vascular cause of "explosive" type headaches is a subarachnoid hemorrhage. Patients with that diagnosis are not likely to be in the conversational shape--meaning without any pain--that you are in while talking to me right now. They are usually not doing too well by the time they get to the hospital or clinic. The headaches are described in the literature as "thunderclap headaches" with patients often complaining of "the worst headache of their life" and continues to get worse with some brief periods of minor improvement. People also tend to experience other symptoms like vomiting and neck pain/stiffness in addition to any persistent neurological symptoms. Another example, known as" reversible cerebral vasoconstriction syndrome (RCVS) often recurs over days to weeks, is associated with exertional activities, drugs, or exposure to extreme temperatures. None of these above symptoms are consistent with what you've described.

What about cancer? Am I dying?

Potentially? Yes, you could have a tumor. Probability? Again, very low. That's why we need to get an MRI which can show us if there are any lesions in your brain. Because intracranial tumors can present in a multitude of fashions, we can't definitively rule it out without getting these scans. I would at the very least tell you that this is very rare and not something I would expect to see in your case.

Ok. So, what if I don't have a brain bleed or a tumor, where did this come from and what can we do about it? You mentioned something about this being "benign"?

Yes, it is benign. Though this can certainly be jarring and the name sounds scary, it does not cause any neurologic damage both short or long-term. It's found almost equally in women and men with a ratio of about 1.5:1. There is no concrete evidence as to the origins of this headache syndrome, but research suggests it could be a sensory variant of a hypnic jerk.

In English, please.

Well, you've probably experienced something similar to this before: a sudden muscle jerk when you're in that transitional period from wakefulness to sleep? That's essentially the same thing but in this case, it's more of an abnormal "sensation" that your brain experiences causing the symptoms that you described earlier. This probably also explains the heavy breathing and fast heart beat given how unusual the feeling must have been to your body. One thing we have seen as a common trend, however, is that these episodes tend to occur in the setting of increased stress. As far as what you can do about it? Well, there have been no clinical trials investigating treatment options as most cases tend to resolve without any intervention. Given the association with stress, though, relaxation techniques are an effective initial approach. For more refractory cases, there have been anecdotal reports of treatments including benzodiazepines (clonazepam, clobazam, and others) and tricyclic antidepressants (amitriptyline and others) that have been successful. But again, since the symptoms are extremely brief and benign, treatment with medications is probably unnecessary and side effects should be weighed against the potential benefits.

So, this won't affect my brain now, but does it mean I'll be at risk for other things later?

No. There is no known scientific evidence to suggest that having EHS increases risks for any other medical disorders including stroke, cognitive impairment or sleep disorders.

Well, speaking of sleep, is this going to happen again every time I sleep? If so, what can I do to prevent it? Are there any triggers I should look out for?

That's a good question and the majority of people who experience EHS will likely not have another episode. Even if they do recur, there is a good chance that they will get better and go away with time. Some reviews suggest an association with insomnia and if present, should be evaluated further by a sleep medicine specialist. Apart from stress, there are no other known triggers. If it does occur, though, just remember that it's benign and try to use any form of relaxation techniques such as deep breathing or brief mindful meditation, as the symptoms are only temporary and will rapidly resolve. Again, stress relief and maintaining good sleep hygiene are the best ways to manage EHS. That having all been said, just because EHS doesn't confer any risk of developing other medical problems, I still would suggest that you should pay attention if certain symptoms persist, such as increasing severity of the headache, speech difficulties, vision changes, weakness or abnormal sensory changes in your arms and legs. If you notice any of those then you should certainly call 911 to be evaluated immediately as they may be signs of a stroke or other cerebrovascular emergency.

I take medications for my blood pressure and diabetes. Can any of those be causing this?

Not likely. There isn't any known link between any medications and EHS.

Is there anything I can change with my diet or are there any supplements I can use to help?

With regards to treatment tailored towards EHS, no dietary supplement has been studied well enough to show any benefits at this time. That being said, as with all types of primary headache diagnosis, there are generally five main day to day things to work on in order to prevent recurrence:

1. Sleep Hygiene - maintaining good sleep of 7-8 hours a night, no late meals or caffeine after 2-3pm, no TV/phone/computers in bed
2. Mood - there is a strong link with headaches and improved mood can lead to better headache control and vice versa
3. Hydration - at least 2 liters of non-caffeinated beverages per day
4. Diet - eating regular meals at consistent times and avoid skipping meals, if possible, but can snack in between
5. Exercise - For example, aerobic exercise for at least 30 minutes three times a week will help reduce frequency or severity of migraine.

Remember, your brain may be more prone to getting these headaches, but that doesn't mean your life needs to suffer as a result of it.

References

American Academy of Sleep Medicine. International classification of sleep disorders. 3rd ed. Darien: American Academy of Sleep Medicine; 2014. Diagnostic criteria for EHS.

Ceriani, C.E.J., Nahas, S.J. Exploding Head Syndrome: a Review. Curr Pain Headache Rep 22, 63 (2018).

Frese A, Summ O, Evers S. Exploding head syndrome: six new cases and review of the literature. Cephalgia. 2014;34(10):823–7. A review of all cases reported in the literature through (2014).

Gillis K, Ng MC. Exploding head syndrome in the epilepsy monitoring unit: case report and literature review. Neurodiagn J. 2017;57(2):133–8.

Green MW. The exploding head syndrome. Curr Pain Headache Rep. 2001; 5:279–80.

Salih F, Klingbiel R, Zschenderlein R, Grosse P. Acoustic sleep starts with sleep-onset insomnia related to a brainstem lesion. Neurol. 2008; 70:1935–7.

"You Say I Have Migraine. Can't You Do a Scan to Prove That? Can You Rule Out a Brain Tumor?"

Stephanie J. Nahas, MD, MSEd

How are you so sure I just have migraine?

Migraine is a very complex neurobiological disease which results in unpredictable attacks of head pain and other symptoms. We make the diagnosis based on the symptoms someone describes and by making sure that there isn't some other reason for the symptoms. Usually, we just need to get a clear story consistent with migraine, and make sure a physical and neurological exam reveals no unexpected findings. That is enough to diagnose someone with migraine, and no other testing is needed to make that diagnosis. There is no "migraine test" or "migraine scan." We make the diagnosis "clinically," that is to say, based on what we, as clinicians, can hear, see, and feel from your story and your exam. We only order tests when we suspect that something else is going on.

So how do you know that I have migraine, though?

You described to me that you have experienced many attacks over the course of your life. They started when you were a teenager, which is fairly typical, but in reality, migraine attacks can start at any age. You say that your attacks are all pretty similar, though some are definitely worse than others. This also is typical. You can tell you might get an attack that day or the next day, because you start to feel a little "off," perhaps more tired than usual, or craving foods you don't normally eat a lot, or urinating more often, or having mild mood changes, or feeling some stiffness in your neck. We call this the prodrome of the attack, or the warning signs. Then, when the attack actually starts, you feel increasing pain in your head, usually on one side or the other, which becomes moderate to severe and starts to throb. You have to limit your physical activity, otherwise it gets worse. You also notice that lights and noises bother you more than usual, and you might feel nauseated or even throw up. This goes on for several hours unless you take something for it. That is a very typical description of a migraine attack, and in fact, it meets every characteristic feature in the official definition of a migraine attack. You also have noted that sometimes certain things can trigger these attacks, like too much stress, too little sleep, or eating or drinking too much of the wrong things, like processed foods, caffeine, or alcohol. All of that is also very typical for migraine. I've also asked you about other symptoms during and between attacks to make sure I don't think you have a different headache disorder or some other problem causing your attacks. For example, you don't have weakness on one side of your body, vertigo, or complete loss of vision with attacks, which could mean a different kind of migraine disease. You don't get symptoms like a red, puffy, watery eye, or a runny nose on one side, or a full feeling in your ear, which could mean a headache disorder different from migraine. You don't always have attacks first thing in the morning, so I don't think you have something like sleep apnea, teeth grinding overnight, or caffeine withdrawal in the morning to explain the problem. You don't have any symptoms or findings that suggest it's from another medical issue, like high blood pressure or a thyroid problem. Your neurologic exam is completely normal, which means it's unlikely that you have any kind of concerning lesion in the brain.

But what if you just scan my brain to be sure? Especially if I'm having an attack at the time? You said migraine is a brain disease, right?

Yes, migraine is a brain disease, and we can pretty reliably link the symptoms of migraine to actual changes within the brain. This is based on centuries of experience and research. Remember that prodrome you told me about? That's happening because of changes in a part of the brain called your hypothalamus, a small cluster of groups of neurons that helps to regulate things like sleep, hormones, hunger, mood, and a lot of other things. Also, there are changes in dopamine levels and dopamine sensitivity during the prodrome, which probably explains the tiredness, cravings, urination, and mood changes you get. For some people, this can also cause yawning, nausea, restlessness, and other symptoms. When all this starts happening, there are connections to the nerves that run between your neck and your brain that start to get activated, and you can begin to feel neck pain. There are more connections between your head structures and your brain, also connected to the neck-brain circuits, and these all start get activated also. Once they're activated enough, they connect to and activate other parts of the brain too, and you start to feel the pain and other symptoms of the attack. But, a scan can't "see" any of this. Scans only look at how the brain and everything around it are *built*, but they don't show what the brain is actually *doing*. Only special experimental scans can do that, and you have to be in a scientific study to get one.

But what if I actually do have a brain tumor?

Brain tumors generally don't cause headaches like yours, and in fact, they often don't even cause headaches at all, especially when they are benign. When a brain tumor is the reason for headache, usually the attacks are increasing over time with no other reasonable explanation. Also, there tends to be constant, or near constant pain, from increasing pressure in the head due to the tumor. We can see signs of high pressure in the head by looking at the back of your eyes for swelling. Also, when pressure inside the head is high, someone experiences spots of vision loss and pulsing noises in their ears. Tumors also usually cause someone to have seizures, as well as weakness, loss of sensation, loss of vision, or language problems that are persistent, depending on where the tumor is located, how big it is, and how fast it's growing.

What if I have something else wrong in there? Like an aneurysm or MS?

In your case, it's unlikely we would discover those things, or anything else. When an aneurysm causes headaches, it's typically from them growing rapidly, leaking, or bursting. When there is headache because of that, it's either progressive over time or very sudden and explosive. Aneurysms are uncommon, and the biggest risks for them are high blood pressure, smoking, a rare kind of kidney disease, and having a close family member with an aneurysm – none of that applies to you. People with MS get headaches, but usually not from their MS. They have MS *plus* migraine or some other headache disorder. MS causes other neurologic symptoms that come on fairly suddenly, persist for days to months, and then start to fade, in most cases. This happens over and over again, and eventually, the symptoms persist. MS can cause a different kind of headache problem called trigeminal neuralgia, which is very different from migraine. Headache resembling migraine is not something MS typically causes.

Can't you just check anyway? I'm really anxious about this.

Generally speaking, we don't order any test just out of curiosity or worry. We have to be concerned about something specific in order to justify the use of resources, and to be able to interpret the results correctly. We also know that there are certain minor abnormalities that can be seen in anyone but which might not be of any significance. We call these incidental findings. Sometimes when these are seen, it leads to even more testing, more worry, and possibly unnecessary treatments that could cause harm. For migraine in particular, it is fairly common to see "white spots" in the brain, and even though they can resemble small strokes or Lyme disease or even MS, we don't think they signify anything. They're just there, but we don't know why. From everything we know so far, we believe they are completely benign. It's kind of like looking at black and white pictures instead of color pictures. If we had the right technology, the white spots from migraine, strokes, Lyme disease, and MS all probably would look different on a scan, but with the tools we have available, they can all look the same. So we could check one just to set your mind at ease if it's normal like I suspect, but you also have to be prepared for a report that says you could have strokes, MS, Lyme disease, or any number of other incidental findings we aren't expecting. The radiologist has to report everything he or she sees, even if it's benign or incidental, and sometimes the radiologist is overly cautious and lists every scary possibility, even if the chances of something scary are very low. It's very rare for us to do a brain scan for migraine and discover something serious and unexpected.

Ok, well, where do we go from here? How will you or I know if I do ever need a scan?

Like with any other case, we're going to follow your symptoms and response to treatment closely. We're going to be on the lookout for unexpected changes in your attack patterns. We're going to watch out for new symptoms, particularly neurologic ones, which could mean something is going wrong inside your brain. We call things like these "red flags." There are other red flags as well. If you, heaven forbid, develop some kind of cancer, we will be very concerned that a change in your attacks could mean spread of the cancer to your brain, and we will check for that. If your immune system becomes compromised for any reason, we will be mindful that you could be more susceptible to a brain infection. If you get explosive headaches, we will need to investigate further. And of course, as you get older, you will be at risk for other things that can happen, so we will be vigilant about that, especially if your headaches are changing unexpectedly.

So if my symptoms don't improve in the next few weeks, we'll get a scan?

No, probably not. Treatment usually takes time to work, and it's a process of trial and error. I know what medications and other treatments work *in general* for migraine, but I really have no way of predicting what's going to work best *for you*. It can take months, sometimes more than a year, or even longer, to come up with the best plan for an individual. And even with the best plans, we rarely get rid of migraine completely. We just change it from a problem that can run and ruin your life with chaos and suffering, to a problem that you can control to minimize the interruption of your day-to-day routine and to help you live your best life.

You're really sure?

Nothing is ever 100% certain, of course, but I'm as certain as I can be about this. And I promise, you and I are going to work together for as long as it takes to get you better. And the entire time, we will be checking in with each other about red flags or other worries that would mean we need to take another look.

Suggested readings

Demarquay G, Moisset X, Lantéri-Minet M, et al. Revised guidelines of the french headache society for the diagnosis and management of migraine in adults. part 1: Diagnosis and assessment. *Rev Neurol* 2021; 177(7):725-33.

Eigenbrodt AK, Ashina H, Khan S, et al. Diagnosis and management of migraine in ten steps. *Nat Rev Neurol* 2021; 17(8):501-14.

Loder E, Weizenbaum E, Frishberg B, Silberstein S. Choosing wisely in headache medicine: The American Headache Society's list of five things physicians and patients should question. *Headache* 2013; 53(10):1651-9.

Robbins MS, Dodick DW. Diagnosing secondary and primary headache disorders. *CONTINUUM Lifelong Learn Neurol* 2021;27(3):572-85.

Whitehead MT, Cardenas AM, Corey AS, et al. ACR appropriateness criteria® headache. *J Am Coll Radiol* 2019; 16(11): S364-77.

"IS THERE SOMETHING I CAN TAKE WHEN I GET A HEADACHE?"

OLIVIA BEGASSE DE DHAEM, MD, FAHS
DIRECTOR OF NEUROLOGY MENTORSHIP AND COMMUNITY ENGAGEMENT
ASSISTANT NEUROLOGY PROGRAM DIRECTOR
WESTCHESTER MEDICAL CENTER
HAWTHORNE, NEW YORK, USA
SAIT ASHINA, MD
ASSISTANT PROFESSOR OF NEUROLOGY AND ANESTHESIA
HARVARD MEDICAL SCHOOL
BETH ISRAEL DEACONESS MEDICAL CENTER
BOSTON, MASSACHUSETTS, USA

I have bad headache and lights bother me. Can I take a combination analgesic Excedrin Tension Headache for my headache?

Depending on other accompanying symptoms such as nausea, a severe headache with light sensitivity may be a migraine attack. Tension headaches, also called "tension-type" headaches, have a mild to moderate pain intensity. There is no downside in trying a combination analgesic containing acetaminophen and caffeine with or without aspirin, and in taking it in moderation if it has helped you with similar migraine attacks in the past. However, there are other options that may be better for severe migraine. Those with headache disorders can have different attacks with different severity and symptoms. Generally, we recommend taking acetaminophen, a nonsteroidal anti-inflammatory drug (NSAID) such as ibuprofen, or combination analgesics medication containing acetaminophen and caffeine with or without aspirin for the milder attacks of migraine or tension headaches. But we recommend using more migraine-specific medications, such as triptans, for moderate or severe attacks of migraine. One commonly prescribed triptan is called "sumatriptan." Triptans work best when taken as early as possible in the beginning of a migraine attack. Even if the caffeine in combination analgesics is meant to potentiate the effect of its other components such as acetaminophen, it is important to be mindful of your total daily caffeine consumption. Caffeine is a double-edge sword: it can help with a headache, but when daily consumption of caffeine exceeds 200 mg per day, it can lead to more headaches, known as "caffeine-withdrawal" headaches.

I saw a television commercial about new headache medication last night. Is it something I can take for my headache?

A new class of medications, the gepants, can be used to treat migraine attack. Ubrogepant was approved by the FDA in December 2019 for the acute treatment of migraine. Rimegepant received FDA approval for acute treatment as well as the prevention of migraine. Unlike other acute medications such as acetaminophen, NSAIDs, combination analgesics or triptans, gepants are not thought to cause so-called "rebound" or "medication overuse" headache, meaning that frequently taking gepants may not put you at risk of the headache worsening. The efficacy and tolerability of triptans and gepants have not been directly compared in so-called head-to-head in trials, but it seems that gepants have lesser efficacy but fewer side effects than triptans. That being said, research results are averages of predefined endpoints or outcomes. People have different primary goals: pain relief, regain of function, improvement in other symptoms, etc. Everyone has a different experience and responds to different medications in different ways. Some medications can work wonders for some people, and not others. Hence, it may be worth trying a gepant. Gepants are currently approved by the FDA to treat migraine in adults, not children, and the use of gepants is currently not recommended during pregnancy or breastfeeding. Of note is that orally disintegrating rimegepant works best when taken on an empty stomach. It is important to give your doctor the full list of medications you are taking, as some medications interact with gepants. The use of gepants is appropriate when triptans are contraindicated, when triptans led to intolerable side effects, or when at least two different triptans did not provide adequate migraine attack relief. Contraindications to triptans include cardiovascular disease such as a history of stroke, transient ischemic attack (TIA), coronary artery disease, uncontrolled high blood pressure; severe liver disease; and specific migraine types (hemiplegic migraine and migraine with brainstem aura, formerly known as "basilar migraine").

Ibuprofen does not help me anymore. Could you prescribe something for my migraine?

There are many other options that might help. It is important to know that there are migraine-specific acute medications, such as triptans, which when taken as needed may be more effective in treatment of moderate-to-severe migraine attacks. Unless there are contraindications, the first line treatment of migraine attack can be a triptan. If there are contraindications, inadequate relief from triptans, or burdensome side effects with triptans, other options include ditans, gepants or dihydroergotamine, also known as "DHE".

We all want your headaches to be under control and these medications are good options. However, before jumping to prescriptions, it is important to first discuss with your provider the problems you are experiencing. Is ibuprofen not helping anymore because your headaches worsened? Do you have a new type of headache? Have you had any other changes in your health and/or life? Have your headaches been so frequent that you had to take ibuprofen almost every day (your only treatment option so far) and now your brain got used to ibuprofen and is not responding to it as a treatment anymore? Depending on the answers to those questions, you may need further workup and/or a preventive medication (a medication you take regularly regardless of whether you have a migraine attack that day, to help decrease the frequency and severity of your headaches).

I take acetaminophen every day for my headache. I feel pressure in my headache.

It seems counterintuitive, but sometimes taking acute medications frequently to alleviate a headache attack leads to more or chronic or almost daily headaches in the long-run. The migraine brain can get used to certain substances like caffeine or medications such as NSAIDs, triptans, or combination analgesics such as butalbital/acetaminophen/caffeine. As the brain gets used to these substances or medications, you can develop headaches when they wear off, which leads to more headaches and increased use of these substances and medications. It is not your fault. You have a headache, so you try to treat it with the tools you have. People with headache disorders sometimes also think it is "normal" to have headaches, because that is what they know. Things can be different. It is important to discuss your headaches with your provider in order to develop an optimal plan to deal with your headaches. You may need both acute treatment options you take as needed when you have a headache and preventive or "prophylactic" treatment that you take regularly to help decrease the frequency and severity of your headaches.

I've tried everything. Nothing works for my headache. What can I do now?

The first step is re-evaluation and making sure the diagnosis is correct. Further workup may be needed in case of refractory or treatment resistant migraine. Once the diagnosis is confirmed and the workup is completed, it is good to sit down and go over all the potential treatment options: acute, preventive, rescue, pharmacologic, and non-pharmacologic. Medications that did not work 20 years ago can sometimes work when tried again. Once there are an inadequate response, side effects, or contraindications to the first, second, third line medications, devices, and non-pharmacologic options, your provider will have to think outside of the box and may want to also talk with peers to come up with other ideas. There are lots of options though. It can also be helpful to check in with your provider from time to time too as other ideas may arise and new medications may come to the market. For example, within the last two years, lasmiditan, ubrogepant, rimegepant, and a new more efficient method of nasal spray delivery of dihydroergotamine (DHE) came on the market for the acute treatment of migraine. Devices can also be helpful such as the transcutaneous supraorbital nerve stimulator, single pulse transcutaneous magnetic stimulator, remote electrical neuromodulation, or non-invasive vagus nerve stimulator. Combining acute medications together such as an NSAIDs with a triptan and with an anti-nausea medication, or different routes of administration such as the self-injection of ketorolac may provide more relief. Having refractory migraine can be socially, financially, emotionally, and physically very difficult and isolating. Getting in touch with patient organizations can also provide you with new ideas or connect you with other providers, support groups, or virtual group session with pain psychologists. There is hope; it is about connecting with the people who may help find what works for you.

I have severe migraine attacks, but I am very sensitive to medications. What can I do?

If you feel comfortable trying medications, an option is to try a very low dose at home on a quiet day for the first time. The dose may be too low to treat the attack, but it would give you a sense whether you can tolerate the medication.

There are also non-medication options that you can use when needed for migraine attacks such as devices (as mentioned above: transcutaneous supraorbital nerve stimulator, single pulse transcutaneous magnetic stimulator, remote electrical neuromodulation, or non-invasive vagus nerve stimulator). Behavioral approaches that can help reduce the frequency and severity of migraine attacks and hence reduce the need for acute medications to take as needed. Please make sure you drink enough water and eat regular meals with slow absorbed carbohydrates. Increasing the omega-3 fats (found in cold-water fish, flaxseeds, chia seeds, walnuts, leafy vegetables, legumes, some algae) and limiting the omega-6 fats (fried and processed foods) in your diet may help too. The migraine brain does not like changes, keeping a regular schedule with regular meals and sleep helps. Regular exercise may help too, if possible. Some vitamins and supplements may help such as riboflavin, coenzyme Q10, magnesium, and ginger. Behavioral interventions that have been proven to work for migraine prevention include biofeedback, relaxation training, and cognitive behavioral therapy.

My insurance lets me fill 9 triptans per month, but I have 12 migraine days per month. What do I take the other 3 days per month?

You can take aspirin, NSAIDs, or combination analgesics such as acetaminophen/aspirin/caffeine for the mild-to-moderate attacks. You can save the triptans for the more severe attacks. That being said, triptans work best when taken as early as possible and it is sometimes very difficult to know early on if this will become a severe attack. Hence, this stratified strategy can be logistically tricky. Adding anti-emetic medications can help increase the effect of the other acute medications. There is also the potential to be creative coming up with additional acute treatment options, such as adding a low dose tizanidine (a muscle relaxant), low dose amitriptyline as needed, or intramuscular ketorolac as examples.

Now looking at the big picture, 12 migraine days per month is a lot and sounds disabling. It would be good to discuss preventive therapy or adding to the current preventive regimen with your provider.

What are acute medications that don't have to be taken by mouth? I cannot take medications by mouth because of the nausea, sometimes vomiting or difficulty swallowing when I have a headache. I have delayed gastric emptying, which delays the absorption of medications and may decrease their efficacy.

Regarding the nausea, anti-nausea medications can help with both the nausea and the migraine attack. The trick would be to have a sense of when the migraine attack is going to hit, so you can take the anti-nausea medication before you get too nauseated to be able to actually absorb. Of note, the anti-nausea medication prochlorperazine exists in suppository form, so you don't need to worry about keeping it down if you used that route of administration. If you have issues swallowing, some medications come in the form of orally disintegrating tablets such as rizatriptan, rimegepant, and ondansetron.

Regarding acute migraine medications that don't have to be taken by mouth, other options include triptans in the form of a nasal spray or self-injection under the skin, DHE or lidocaine nasal sprays. A gepant nasal spray, vazegepant, should come on the market soon too.

Triptans work for my migraine attacks, but they knock me out. Is there another medication I could take and still be able to work?

It is always good to try several triptans as some may be better tolerated than others, and we cannot predict in advance which ones will work best for you. Lasmiditan has a warning for drowsiness; people cannot drive nor operate heavy machinery for 8 hours after taking it. Gepants and NSAIDs may be your best bets. Some NSAIDs work faster than others such as a prescription the medicine diclofenac power that is dissolved.

In addition to medications, try to drink enough water, lower the lights, try to take breaks when you can lay down, if possible, at work. Other non-medication options that may help include a light with a specific wavelength of green light or devices such as the remote electrical neuromodulation that can be discretely worn on your upper arm. There is a light that uses a specific and pure wavelength of green light, the wavelength that is the least irritating to the migraine brain. It is free of side effects, and may help during an attack and/or prevent attacks. Green light has been shown to reduce pain intensity of ongoing migraine headache.

I am pregnant. What can I take when I have a migraine attack?

The good news is that most women see an improvement in their migraine attacks during pregnancy. If you develop different, new, or severe headaches in pregnancy, please contact your doctor or medical provider. The first line acute treatment for migraine attacks in pregnancy is acetaminophen, with or without metoclopramide, an anti-nausea medication. Diphenhydramine can also be used. The second line is sumatriptan. Sumatriptan use in pregnancy has not been associated with adverse outcomes of pregnancy nor major congenital malformations in two large observational studies. Studies did not show any evidence of birth defects or adverse outcomes of pregnancy with the use of the transcutaneous supraorbital nerve stimulator device during pregnancy. NSAIDs should be avoided during the first and third trimester of pregnancy due to increased risk of miscarriage and premature closure of the ductus arteriosus, opening between the two major blood vessels leading from the heart in the fetus. Gepants and ditans should also be avoided in pregnancy; more studies will be needed to recommend these treatments during pregnancy or breastfeeding. Butalbital-containing medications should be avoided in pregnancy due to their association with increased risk of fetal heart defects and withdrawal seizures. Butalbital-containing medications are not recommended for the acute treatment of headaches outside of pregnancy anyway.

Suggested reading

Ailani J, Burch RC, Robbins MS; Board of Directors of the American Headache Society. The American Headache Society Consensus Statement: Update on integrating new migraine treatments into clinical practice. *Headache*. 2021;61(7):1021-1039.

Ashina M. Migraine. N Engl J Med. 2020 Nov 5;383(19):1866-1876

Ashina M, Buse DC, Ashina H, Pozo-Rosich P, Peres MFP, Lee MJ, Terwindt GM, Halker Singh R, Tassorelli C, Do TP, Mitsikostas DD, Dodick DW. Migraine: integrated approaches to clinical management and emerging treatments. Lancet. 2021 Apr 17;397(10283):1505-1518.

Ashina S, Mitsikostas DD, Lee MJ, Yamani N, Wang SJ, Messina R, Ashina H, Buse DC, Pozo-Rosich P, Jensen RH, Diener HC, Lipton RB. Tension-type headache. Nat Rev Dis Primers. 2021 Mar 25;7(1):24.

Burch R. Headache in Pregnancy and the Puerperium. *Neurol Clin*. 2019; 37(1):31-51.

Lipton RB, Stewart WF, Stone AM, Láinez MJA, Sawyer JPC. Stratified Care vs Step Care Strategies for Migraine: The Disability in Strategies of Care (DISC) Study: A Randomized Trial *JAMA.* 2000; 284(20): 2599–2605.

Pérez-Muñoz A, Buse DC, Andrasik F. Behavioral Interventions for Migraine. *Neurol Clin.* 2019;37(4):789-813

Tepper D. Gepants. *Headache*. 2020; 60(5):1037-1039.

Do I Need Prevention?

Olga Fermo, MD
Senior Associate Consultant
Department of Neurology
Mayo Clinic Florida
Jacksonville, Florida
USA

"How do I know I need prevention for my migraines?"

A preventive or prophylactic treatment, is one that you take daily, monthly, or quarterly with the intention of improving your migraines in the long-run. The goal is to over time reduce the frequency of your headaches by at least half, or at minimum improve headache severity and/or the response to as-needed treatments, as well as reducing the chance of migraines progressing. While slightly more than one-third of people with migraine *need* a preventive treatment, fewer than 13% are using one.

The need for a preventive treatment is determined by how many headaches you have, how well they respond to as-needed treatment, how disabling they are, and your personal preference. People with chronic migraine, meaning those who experience 15 or more headache days per month, should always be offered a preventive treatment simply based on how often they have headaches. People with fewer than 4 migraines per month who do not experience any impairment related to the migraines generally do not need a preventive. People who have infrequent migraines, but find them difficult to treat, or find the as-needed medications difficult to tolerate or cannot use them for medical reasons, should be offered prevention. People with significant headache-related impairment, for example, those needing bed rest or at the extreme those with temporarily paralysis during the migraine called "hemiplegic migraines" should be offered prevention even if these attacks are infrequent. Studies have shown that having more migraines, taking more as-needed medication, and having a poor response to as-needed medication promotes more migraines to occur in the future. For this reason, people with frequent migraines, for example 6 per month, and certainly more than 10 per month, should be offered prevention regardless of how disabling the migraines are.

"How long does it take to know that a preventive regimen is working?"

You have numerous options for prevention. The specific regimen you choose depends on your previous treatment history, your medical history and current medications, which side-effects you *want* to have, and which side-effects you want to avoid. Except for the most recent additions to the armamentarium, called "CGRP antagonists", every other treatment used for migraine prevention is "borrowed" for another pharmacologic class but is used because it happens to work on the nervous system pathways implicated in migraine. *The specific choice of preventive is probably less important to your outcome then is the sufficient dose and duration of treatment.* All treatments described in this chapter need to be used regularly for several months, unless you develop intolerable side effects or an allergic reaction. In other words, each treatment needs to be trialed at a therapeutic dose for a sufficient period before it is deemed a treatment "failure." For most oral medications, a sufficient trial represents 8-12 weeks of daily use. OnabotulinumtoxinA should be administered at least 2 to 3 times at intervals of 12 weeks to judge response, and along similar lines, the large molecule CGRP antagonist injections need to be used for several months before effect is seen. It is possible to see results earlier, but you should not prematurely discontinue the treatments if the response is not seen right away.

"I've been on preventive regimens in the past, but they never worked - I had to keep taking analgesics daily. Why is that?"

As described above, treatment can be "failed" because it is stopped prematurely but there is another important roadblock to be aware of, and that is the impact of medication overuse. Medication overuse refers to using as-needed medications frequently enough that it leads to the development of medication overuse headache (MOH). MOH is a separate headache disorder that migraineurs are prone to, regardless of what they take the as-needed medication for (headache or non-headache pain). In general it occurs when triptans, dihydroergotamine, opiates, and other prescription or over-the-counter combination preparations containing caffeine are used more often than 10 days per month; non-steroidal anti-inflammatory drugs (NSAIDs) are used more than 15 days per month, or the combination of different classes of medications totals more than 10 days per month

(ICDH3). Despite this official definition, the development of MOH has been shown to occur with even less opiate use (8 days per month) and butalbital use (5 days per month). When MOH develops, there are actual structural and functional changes that occur in the brain that promote pain and are separate from those occurring in migraine. *The majority of preventive treatments will not work to reduce migraines, regardless of dosage and length or treatment, when MOH is active.* In other words, ongoing medication overuse renders even the best preventive treatments ineffective. The only way to stop MOH is to detoxify from the overused medication, though this will trigger an uncomfortable withdrawal period (with worse headaches). This, in combination with the expected lag of improvement from preventives, necessitates the use of a bridging treatment. Bridging treatments provide a head start to relief. Specific bridging treatments are beyond the scope of this chapter, but briefly, include defined courses of oral medications, intravenous infusions, or nerve blocks. A bridge may be necessary to jump start your relief when first starting prevention.

"What types of preventives are available?"

Preventive agents fall into classes of oral medications, injectable monoclonal antibodies to CGRP, onabotulinumtoxinA, and neuromodulation devices. The specific classes and agents will be discussed further below. Out of the choices to be described, only a few are FDA (U.S. Food and Drug Administration) approved in the United States for the purpose of preventing migraine. The only oral medications with the approval for preventing episodic migraine are propranolol, timolol, divalproex, topiramate, and rimegepant. There are no oral medications FDA approved in the US for prevention of chronic migraine. All the monoclonal antibodies to be discussed are approved for the prevention of both episodic and chronic migraine. OnabotulinumtoxinA and the 4 injectable CGRP monoclonal antibodies are the only approved medications for the prevention of chronic migraine. There are two stimulation devices available on the market for prevention. The Cefaly device is cleared for the prevention of episodic migraine, and the SpringTMS device is cleared for the prevention of both episodic and chronic migraine. Some patients and prescribing providers will prefer to start with the treatments which carry FDA approval, because these have been studied to show more benefit then harm for the intended purpose. However, it is important to recognize that off-label (meaning, approved the by FDA but only for uses other than migraine) choices are very common, especially after first-line treatments have been ineffective, and these do have proven efficacy in research studies. The specific treatments will be discussed next.

"I've never been prescribed anything to prevent my migraines, before, what are my first-line options?"

Most patients starting out with prevention are offered an oral medication first line. Most oral medications belong to classes whose original purpose was something other than migraine prevention, specifically – antiepileptics (medicine for seizure prevention), antihypertensives (medicine for high blood pressure or pulse), antidepressants (medicine to treat depression), and antihistamine (medicine to treat allergies).

Antiepileptics

Topiramate

Topiramate is well established as a highly efficacious choice for the prevention of episodic migraine. It is approved for migraine prevention in patients 12 years of age and older. While its original purpose was for the treatment of epilepsy, it acts on a number of targets in the brain that together reduce the brain's excitability, raising the threshold for developing migraine. The recommended starting dose for adolescents and adults is 25mg in the evening, raising the daily dosage by weekly intervals of 25mg until 50mg twice a day is reached. While the maximum dose for migraine prevention is 200mg per day, multiple studies showed that, in general, higher dosing was no more effective then 100mg per day. Topiramate comes with a number of treatment-related adverse effects. The most common side effect is paresthesia, or a numbness/tingling sensation, typically around the mouth and in the fingertips and toes, occurring in about half of patients. Despite its presence, it rarely leads to drug discontinuation. It is dose dependent and can easily be mitigated with potassium supplementation or increased intake of potassium rich foods or beverages. Around one in five patients treated with topiramate will experience cognitive problems, including word-finding problems, difficulty concentrating, and problems with memory. When present, these are more likely to lead to drug discontinuation and are reversible once the drug is stopped. There are two extended release topiramate formulations on the market, and studies support that use of these rather than the immediate-release form may mitigate the cognitive side effects. Topiramate is notable for being the only preventive agent to induce a modest weight loss during therapy, or at the minimum, is expected to be weight neutral. This is in the context of all other oral agents being either weight-neutral or more commonly, promoting weight gain. There are several situations in which topiramate should not be used, or used with caution. It should not be used during pregnancy, or by women planning pregnancy in the close future, as it can cause cleft lip and/or cleft palate in the fetus. Topiramate can lower the effectiveness of estrogen containing oral contraceptives at doses greater than 200mg per day. Caution should be used when prescribing topiramate to patients with history of mood disorders, as it can increase the risk of suicidal ideation. Caution should also be used with a history of kidney stones and glaucoma as it can promote both conditions. All antiepileptics should be withdrawn gradually if the plan is to stop as to avoid precipitating a seizure. Topiramate is an excellent first-choice preventive, especially when you need a weight-neutral treatment, but you should understand the possible side effects before starting this medication.

Divalproex sodium

Multiple placebo-controlled studies have found divalproex sodium to be highly effective at reducing migraines. The exact mechanism by which it prevents migraine is unknown, but may relate to the promotion of inhibitory activity in the brain. You will find several formulations of divalproex sodium on the market, including a twice or three times a day enteric coated/delayed release formulation and a once a day extended release formulation. The extended release formulation may be more convenient to use and can be better tolerated. The recommended starting dose is 250-500mg at bedtime with gradual increase to 1000-1500mg per day as tolerated. The dose that is sufficient for migraine prevention is often lower than that needed for seizure control. The most common side effects are gastrointestinal, including nausea, vomiting and diarrhea and these are likely to subside with time. Weight gain with divalproex sodium is common, and a small proportion of patients can develop tremor and hair loss with prolonged use. The hair loss may be temporary even if the medication is continued and it may respond to zinc and selenium supplementation. Divalproex sodium is generally not associated with any cognitive side effects. It can cause problems with the liver, pancreas and with blood cell counts, so it should not be started if you have pre-existing liver or bleeding disorders. The risk for serious liver problems is greatest for children, those taking multiple anti-seizure drugs, and those with congenital problems with metabolism. Your healthcare provider will typically obtain or review blood work prior to initiating or changing the dose of divalproex sodium and will need to monitor blood work if periodically if staying on this medicine long-term. Divalproex sodium should not be used concurrently with topiramate because of a rare but serious potential interaction. It should not be used for migraine prevention by women who are pregnant, planning to conceive, or sexually active without a reliable form of contraception because it can cause serious birth defects. Divalproex is most useful if you have epilepsy or a mood disorder (mania or anxiety) as it can treat multiple concurrent problems, but for most patients, especially women of child-bearing age, the long-term side effect profile limits routine use. However, you may be offered divalproex as a short-term agent (for example – 2-3 months) to quickly induce a remission of headaches, while preparing to start a treatment that takes longer to work (for example onabotulinumtoxinA).

Zonisamide

Zonisamide is an antiseizure drug that is similar in mechanism to topiramate, with additional action on calcium channels. Several small studies have shown it to be effective in reducing headache days when compared either to placebo or topiramate. It has the rare potential of causing a serious and life threating skin reaction called "Stevens-Johnson Syndrome" or toxic epidermal necrolysis, like several other antiseizure medications, when titrated upward too quickly. When the medication is introduced at a low dose and gradually titrated to effect it is well-tolerated. You can begin zonisamide at 100mg daily and raise it in weekly 100mg intervals until 400mg daily or so is reached, though some people need to start 25mg or 50mg daily and raise it more gradually in 25mg or 50mg increments. It can cause fetal harm and should not be used for migraine prevention in women who are pregnant or planning to conceive. Like topiramate, zonisamide may cause decreased appetite and mild weight reduction, or at least be weight neutral. Zonisamide is particularly appropriate if you had a good headache response to topiramate, but the side effects of topiramate precluded further use.

Gabapentin and Pregabalin

In the United States, gabapentin is indicated for the treatment of postherpetic neuralgia in adults and the management of certain seizure disorders in patients 3 years of age and older. However, it is common to use gabapentin for a variety of off-label conditions, including headaches, because it is considered a very "low risk" medication. The official guidelines state there is insufficient quality evidence to support or refute the use of gabapentin for migraine prevention and a 2016 Cochrane review on the same subject concluded gabapentin is not efficacious for the prevention of episodic migraine. Gabapentin changes the transmission of pain signals between nerves in the brain and spinal cord by interfering with calcium channels though it may have additional, less studied, mechanisms pertinent to migraine. The maximum dose of gabapentin for adults with normal kidney function is 3600mg per day, generally divided into three doses per day. Doses ranging from 900-2400mg per day have been studied for migraine prevention. Since people with migraine are often more sensitive to medication side-effects and may see relief at a lower dose compared to the treatment of other conditions (i.e. epilepsy), a low and slow approach should be considered with gabapentin. This may mean starting with 100-300mg before bed and raising in weekly intervals of 100-300mg until therapeutic effect is seen or tolerance is exhausted, as opposed to the suggested daily titration in 300mg intervals in post-herpetic neuralgia. The most common side effects of gabapentin to be aware of, include dizziness, fatigue, nausea and somnolence. While the literature clearly does not support the use of gabapentin as a first-line choice in the prevention of migraine, it is well-tolerated and has an excellent drug-interaction profile, making it a reasonable choice after highly efficacious drugs have been exhausted especially due to poor tolerance, and for those patients on several prescription drugs, for whom drug-drug interactions are a concern.

Pregabalin is an antiepileptic closely related to gabapentin. In the United States it is approved for the treatment of neuropathic pain associated with diabetic neuropathy, postherpetic neuralgia, certain types of seizures, fibromyalgia, and neuropathic pain associated with spinal cord injury. Its mechanism of action is like that of gabapentin, that is described above. At the time of the 2016 Cochrane review examining the efficacy of pregabalin as a migraine preventive, there are insufficient (prospective, placebo-controlled) trials on the subject. The most common side effects of pregabalin include dizziness, somnolence, dry mouth, swelling, blurred vision, weight gain, and thinking abnormalities While pregabalin is not an evidence-based first line choice for the prevention of migraine, it may be a good choice if your migraines co-exist with fibromyalgia, postherpetic neuralgia, diabetic neuropathy, or spinal cord injury.

Antihypertensives

Beta-blockers

The beta-adrenergic receptor antagonists, commonly referred to as “beta-blockers”, are medications that block the stress hormones epinephrine and norepinephrine from working. Beta-blockers are normally prescribed to treat high blood pressure, heart arrhythmias, and chest pain but are also used for several non-cardiac purposes including the treatment of migraine, anxiety, some types of tremor, some problems associated with cirrhosis, and some types of thyroid conditions. You do not need to have high blood pressure in order to benefit from this class of medications, though your health care provider will generally avoid this class if your blood pressure and pulse are low to begin with. The mechanism in which they help migraine is not fully understood, but may involve interactions with several pain-controlling centers in the brainstem, reduced excitability of brain regions involved in vision and hearing, and through action on the thalamus, an area in the brain that traffics all sensory information. There are many beta-blockers on the market, but not all of them are used for migraine prevention. There is ample evidence to support propranolol, metoprolol, and timolol as effective and atenolol and nadolol as probably effective for episodic migraine prevention. Propranolol and timolol, however, are the only beta-blockers that are FDA approved for the purpose of migraine prevention. Dosing depends on the medication and formulation (immediate release versus extended release) chosen. Beta-blockers should be avoided for migraine prevention if there is low blood pressure, fatigue, impotence, or unstable depression at baseline as these problems can be increased by beta-blockers. Caution is advised if you are diabetic because beta-blockers may mask some of the symptoms of low blood sugar. Beta blockers should not be used if have asthma, a slow heart rate, and/or heart failure. They may cause exercise intolerance but conversely can be useful if your migraines are precipitated by exercise. While nonpharmacologic measures are encouraged first line during pregnancy, if pharmacologic migraine prevention is necessary, the beta-blockers propranolol or metoprolol are the preferred choices but should be paused shortly before delivery for obstetrical reasons. They may also be used during breastfeeding. In summary, beta-blockers are appropriate highly efficacious first-line choices for migraine prevention for most patients without contraindications, but in particular are appropriate when migraine coexists with high blood pressure, angina, anxiety, or essential tremor or in women who are trying to conceive or are already pregnant.

Verapamil

Verapamil is a calcium channel blocker belonging to the antihypertensive class of medications. There is insufficient evidence in the research literature to support or refute the routine use of verapamil for migraine prevention. While some consider it a low efficacy treatment for migraines, it has a good side effect profile and thus may be useful if you normally have a hard time tolerating medications. There is frequent anecdotal use of verapamil for the prevention of migraine aura – meaning a fully reversible stroke-like event that occurs with or without headache. Verapamil is actually more useful for the management of other, non-migraine headache disorders. It is the treatment of choice for prevention of cluster headaches and may be considered second line for the treatment of other trigeminal autonomic cephalalgias, the family to which cluster headaches belong. When used for this purpose, a dose as high as 480-720mg divided in two or three doses may be needed, and the immediate-release formulation is preferred. Verapamil affects the electricity of the heart, so it is customary to check an electrocardiogram (ECG) prior to first use, after dose changes, and routinely afterwards if therapy is maintained particularly at high doses. Common side effects include constipation and low blood pressure. In summary, verapamil is best reserved for the prevention of cluster headaches, migraines if they coexist with cluster headaches, migraines with aura, or situations in which the diagnosis is unclear (if the diagnosis is cluster or migraine).

Lisinopril and Candesartan

Lisinopril and candesartan are antihypertensives that each act on the renin-angiotensin system (RAS), a hormonal pathway that regulates blood pressure, but in different ways. Lisinopril is referred to as an "angiotensin converting enzyme" (ACE) inhibitor and candesartan is referred to as an "angiotensin receptor blocker" (ARB). Both have been used for migraine prevention and are currently recommended as only second or third line agents for episodic migraine prevention. It is unclear how lisinopril and candesartan help migraine. Several possible mechanisms for lisinopril include action on a brain-specific RAS pathway, changes to how blood vessels react to stress hormones, breakdown of pain promoting transmitters in the nervous system, and changes to the body's endorphin system. Less is known about the potential role that candesartan plays in migraine, though it may have a role as an antioxidant. Candesartan is thought to be more effective at preventing migraines compared to other members of the ARB class because its chemical properties may allow it to readily enter the brain. The recommended effective doses for range from 10mg to 40mg for lisinopril and 16mg for candesartan. Both are overall very well-tolerated medications. The main limiting side effect of lisinopril is cough, necessitating discontinuation or change over to an ARB. Candesartan may cause abnormal skin sensations called "paresthesias" (pins and needles sensations), these are reversible if the medication is stopped. Both medications can be considered as early choices for migraine prevention in people who have coexisting high blood pressure. Along similar lines, if you are already prescribed an ACE inhibitor or ARB for the management of high blood pressure, it may make the most sense to switch you to lisinopril or candesartan to gain some additional migraine control. Otherwise, low dose lisinopril and candesartan are great choices for people looking for a regimen with an excellent side effect profile, as long as the baseline blood pressure is in the normal range.

Antidepressants

Antidepressants are very effective choices for prevention, regardless whether you have depression/anxiety or not. The two classes of antidepressants effective for the prevention of headache disorders are called the "tricyclic antidepressants" (TCAs) and the "selective serotonin and norepinephrine reuptake inhibitors" (SNRIs). The TCAs, most notably amitriptyline, change the way multiple neurotransmitters including serotonin, norepinephrine, acetylcholine, histamine, and dopamine work in the brain ultimately increasing the threshold for migraine to develop. They are also effective for the prevention of chronic tension-type headaches, as well as other non-headache chronic pain conditions such as fibromyalgia or neuropathy. Amitriptyline is the prototype of this class, acting on the most neurotransmitters which may result in better pain relief but also more adverse effects. For this reason, some people may tolerate the metabolite of amitriptyline, called nortriptyline, better. Protriptyline and doxepin are additional members of the TCA class that can be used for migraine prevention but have little data in the literature to support their use. The dosing of TCAs depends on the indication and the specific drug choice. Since all but protriptyline are sedating, they should be used before bed, ideally 8-10 hours before waking. This author recommends starting amitriptyline at 10mg, raising in weekly 10mg intervals until the lowest therapeutic or highest tolerated dose is reached, whichever comes first. For patients who are particularly sensitive to sedating medications, nortriptyline is available in a liquid formulation and thus allows for doses lower than 10mg to be used. The doses of TCAs used for pain control are often significantly lower than the doses required to treat depression or anxiety, though in patients who have both, higher doses may be needed. Side effects with TCAs are fairly common and limit their use, despite good efficacy for a variety of pain conditions. These include fatigue, dry mouth, nausea, dizziness, weight gain, fast heart rate, blurred vision, orthostatic intolerance, and urinary retention. Elderly patients can be in particular prone to develop adverse effects so caution is advised in this population. The SNRI class can be offered to take advantage of the beneficial aspects of the TCAs with fewer side effects. Venlafaxine, in particular, is recommended as a second-line choice for migraine prevention, and like the TCAs, is also effective against tension-type headache and non-headache musculoskeletal or nerve pain. As opposed to the TCAs which are almost all sedating medications, thus may be useful in treating coexisting insomnia, venlafaxine is considered an energizing medication similar to a stimulant and should be used in the morning. For the same reason, some people will be too jittery on venlafaxine, and some can develop high blood pressure, especially if there is already that tendency. At introductory doses below 150mg per day, venlafaxine does not act on the norepinephrine system which is necessary for pain relief. Thus, this author recommends starting venlafaxine XR at 37.5mg for one week, doubling to 75mg for the second week, and reaching the 150mg dose the third week and beyond. Venlafaxine can cause an uncomfortable (but not dangerous) withdrawal syndrome if stopped abruptly, and for some patients can occur as soon as the daily dose is delayed. Duloxetine can serve as an alternative SNRI for people who cannot take venlafaxine. While duloxetine is not officially indicated by the FDA for the prevention of headaches, it is approved for the treatment of diabetic peripheral neuropathy, fibromyalgia, and chronic musculoskeletal pain. Duloxetine should be started at 20-30mg daily, this author recommends morning dosage unless the medication is found to be sedating, and gradually raised in 20-30mg intervals until at least 60mg daily is reached. Antidepressants have many roles making them good choices for migraine or tension-type headache prevention when these coexist with other disorders, including disorders outside of anxiety and depression. The choice of specific antidepressant depends on which side effects are desirable to treat coexisting conditions. Both TCAs and SNRIs can be used to treat headaches along with nerve pain (i.e. diabetic neuropathy) and musculoskeletal pain (i.e. chronic neck pain, fibromyalgia). Most TCAs are sedating thus can be offered to also treat insomnia but should not be offered when fatigue is already a problem. On the contrary, the SNRIs, in particular venlafaxine, are energizing and can be offered when daytime fatigue is a problem.

"My main symptoms are not headache and pain. My doctor diagnosed me with a migraine variant, what do I do to prevent that?"

There are several special situations in migraine in which certain preventive options may be better than others.

The migraine aura is a (usually) short lasting, fully reversible neurological event that accompanies or is followed by a migraine headache within one hour. Most of these events involve changes to vision or sensation (numbness, tingling) but come people can experience difficulties with expressing language or speech. There are several rare subsets of migraine with aura and these include migraine with brainstem aura when it consists of vertigo, changes to hearing, balance, and consciousness; hemiplegic migraine, when the aura causes weakness to one side of the body, and retinal migraine when the aura consists of vision changes occurring in just one eye. Auras can even occur in isolation, without an accompanying headache at all. It is universally accepted that the migraine aura is caused by an electrical event in the brain called "cortical spreading depression". This may be related to the fact that people who experience auras have been found to have brains that are more easily excitable, even between migraine attacks. This is most likely an inherited trait, as the risk of having migraine with aura is twice as high (as compared to migraine without aura) if a first-degree relative also experienced auras. Since auras are thought to be generated by abnormal electrical events in the brain, it makes sense to use preventive medications which change the brain's "electrochemistry," which is determined by concentrations of electrolytes inside and outside of brain cells. Medications that can serve this purpose include magnesium, antiepileptics, and sometimes calcium channel blockers. After reassurance has been given, most auras will not need specific prevention as they are short lasting and benign, but some people experience prolonged and/or frequent auras, or ones with severe symptoms like paralysis. Those are the cases in which prevention aimed specifically at auras should always be offered. For routine auras, it is this author's opinion that this can most easily be accomplished with the addition of daily oral magnesium to the existing regimen. Magnesium glycinate works particularly well. Animal models in the laboratory have shown that magnesium can play an important role in the process of aura, and case reports show have shown intravenous magnesium to be successful in terminating prolonged auras in the hospital. When a stronger treatment is needed, this author chooses to offer lamotrigine. Lamotrigine is an antiepileptic that has little to no effect on the headache aspect of migraine but has long been regarded as an excellent and well-tolerated preventive of auras. In situations where there is a need for both headache and aura prevention however, it would be preferable to use the high efficacy antiepileptics topiramate or divalproex sodium, or perhaps the calcium channel blocker verapamil. Flunarizine, a calcium channel blocker, that is not available in the United States, has been considered as the most effective preventive for migraine with brainstem aura and hemiplegic migraine. Verapamil, a calcium channel blocker, has been used anecdotally in lieu in countries where flunarizine is not available, in addition to topiramate, valproate, lamotrigine, acetazolamide, and candesartan.

Vestibular migraine is a variant of migraine in which recurrent sensations of vertigo or dizziness are accompanied by at least one typical symptom of migraine including headache, light or noise sensitivity, or visual aura. It is clearly recognized as a very common cause of vertigo, yet little is known about the changes that take place in the brain during an attack. Preventive treatment is the mainstay of therapy especially since effective as-needed treatments for individual attacks are lacking. While it is clear that vestibular migraines can improve with preventive treatment, there are no evidence-based guidelines for treatment as there are for episodic migraine. Most oral agents described earlier have been used for prevention of vestibular migraine including topiramate, valproic acid, lamotrigine, propranolol, amitriptyline, nortriptyline, venlafaxine, flunarizine, but also medications not typically used in migraine prevention including acetazolamide, paroxetine, and cinnarizine. While many of these have shown improvement in small studies, no drug has proven to be superior. It is thus recommended to treat vestibular migraine according to the same principles described earlier in which the regimen is tailored to the desired side effects and coexisting conditions.

Oral calcitonin gene-related peptide (CGRP) antagonists

Rimegepant, an oral medication initially developed for as-needed treatment of migraine, also received FDA approval for prevention of episodic migraine in the United States in May 2021. Rimegepant blocks the receptor for CGRP, a molecule that is key to the migraine signaling pathway. Rimegepant is taken as one dose per day, every other day. This is a well-tolerated treatment with a side effect profile like placebo in research studies. Atogepant is a similar medication for the prevention of migraine.

"I have tried several oral medications for prevention in the past, and although they all worked pretty well, I could not tolerate taking them in the long run. Plus I have a hard time remembering to take my treatments every day. Are there any options for me?"

It is customary that after several types of oral preventives have been tried, and failed either due to intolerable side effects, or lack of efficacy after 2-3 months of use, the injectable migraine preventives can be offered. These treatments include monthly or quarterly monoclonal antibodies, or in-office quarterly onabotulinumtoxinA injections. These are especially useful for people who have difficulty taking treatments every day – for example someone who works different shifts throughout the week and cannot always take a sedating medication at the same time each day.

Anti-CGRP Monoclonal Antibodies

The four available monoclonal antibodies (mAbs) targeting the CGRP molecule or CGRP receptor were the first migraine-specific preventive treatments to be developed. The first three treatments to be available on the market, erenumab, galcanezumab, and fremanezumab are subcutaneous injections meant to be injected at home, whereas the most recent treatment, eptinezumab, is a quarterly intravenous infusion administered in a clinical setting. Erenumab is administered in either a 70mg or 140mg monthly dose. There is evidence that the 140 dose is more effective in the most refractory cases. Galcanezumab is administered as a loading dose of two 120mg injections the first month, followed by a single 120mg dose monthly thereafter. Fremanezumab may be injected either 225mg monthly or 675mg quarterly. Eptinezumab is a 100mg or 300mg intravenous infusion every 12 weeks. The advantages of using the mAbs especially in comparison to earlier oral preventive medications, include relative fast onset of action, easier adherence (since it does not need to be remembered every day), potential to work even in the presence of medication overuse headache, minimal potential for drug interactions since these treatments are not metabolized through the liver and kidneys, and low “brain” side effect profile (drowsiness, cognitive impairment, dizziness) since these medications are too large to enter the brain. The side effects most encountered include injection site reactions. Woman who are using the mAbs should be using adequate contraception for pregnancy prevention. The molecule that the mAbs act on, CGRP, plays a role in normal blood flow to the placenta. In early pregnancy, it is unlikely that the mAbs could cross the placenta, but this is possible after 20-22 weeks gestation and the effects of changing CGRP function in the fetus is unknown. The mAbs should be stopped prior to planning pregnancy. This author recommends stopping the medication 5 or 6 months before conception to allow it to fully clear from the body. In summary, the mAbs are appropriate treatments for patients who previously had difficulty adhering to, or tolerating oral preventive medications, or who need a treatment with little potential for drug-drug interactions. Pregnancy planning should be taken into consideration prior to start mAbs, since these injections need to be stopped well before pregnancy occurs.

OnabotulinumtoxinA

OnabotulinumtoxinA has several FDA approved medical uses, one of which is the prevention of chronic migraine in adults older that age 18. OnabotulinumtoxinA works to help migraine through a process called "chemical denervation." It changes how pain-transmitting nerve endings work, so that over time they have fewer pain-signals (including CGRP) to release. It is administered as a 31-injection protocol targeting 5 standard areas of the scalp and neck (forehead, each temple, back of the head, upper neck, and shoulders). Other injection paradigms are being studied. While an early response to the injections is possible, it is actually normally not to see any benefit right away, because the process of chemical denervation takes several sessions to take effect (around 2 to 3). Notably, the protocol continues to improve headaches over time, only reaching a plateau around the 30-month (of treatment) mark. OnabotulinumtoxinA has been extensively studied for medical purposes over a time span of 30 years. Multiple studies speak to the safety and the tolerability of the treatment over time. The most common side effect of onabotulinumtoxinA injected for chronic migraine prevention is temporary neck pain and a droopy eye lid. These improve over time and are less likely to occur with repeated injections. This treatment should be avoided or used with caution in patients with underlying neuromuscular disorders (or example, myasthenia gravis). It is common practice to withhold onabotulinumtoxinA injections for chronic migraine during pregnancy, though a 24-year-review of a safety database supports no higher risk of fetal defects in mothers exposed to onabotulinumtoxinA during pregnancy, than the general population. if you choose to begin onabotulinumtoxinA injections for your migraines, it is important to let your provider know of any other botulinum toxin injections you are receiving (medical or cosmetic). It is possible and safe to receive injections in multiple areas at the same time, but the dose and timing need to be coordinated. The standard onabotulinumtoxinA protocol for prevention of chronic migraine is an excellent choice for the majority of patients suffering from chronic migraine, especially when medication safety is a concern. It is important to be mindful of pregnancy planning when initiating this regimen.

"Once I start a preventive regimen, will I have to be taking it for the rest of my life?"

Prevention should certainly be stopped (and changed to a different agent) when intolerable side effects or allergic reactions develop. The treatment should be changed if the intended result (50% improvement in headache frequency or severity) is not shown after a sufficient treatment trial. It is acceptable to attempt a slow wean off the prevention agents after the headaches have been in remission for at least 6 months.

References

1. Silberstein S, Holland FS, Freitag F, Dodick DD, Argoff C, Ashman E. *Evidence-Based Guideline Update: Pharmacologic Treatment for Episodic Migraine Prevention in Adults Report of the Quality Standards Subcommittee of the American Academy of Neurology and the American Headache Society*.; 2012. www.neurology.org
2. Parikh SK, Silberstein SD. Preventive Treatment for Episodic Migraine. *Neurol Clin*. 2019;37(4):753-770. doi:10.1016/j.ncl.2019.07.004
3. Lipton RB, Bigal ; M E, Diamond ; M, Freitag ; F, Reed ML, Stewart WF. *Migraine Prevalence, Disease Burden, and the Need for Preventive Therapy*.; 2007.
4. Olesen J. The International Classification of Headache Disorders, 3rd edition. *Cephalagia*. 2013;33(9):629-808. doi:10.1177/0333102413485658
5. Bigal ME, Serrano D, Buse D, Scher A, Stewart WF, Lipton RB. Acute migraine medications and evolution from episodic to chronic migraine: A longitudinal population-based study. *Headache*. 2008;48(8):1157-1168. doi:10.1111/j.1526-4610.2008.01217.x
6. Lipton RB. *Tracing Transformation Chronic Migraine Classification, Progression, and Epidemiology*.; 2009.
7. Silberstein S. Preventive treatment of migraine: an overview. *Cephalagia*. 1997;17:67-72.
8. SD S. Preventive Migraine Treatment. *Continuum (Minneap Minn)*. 2015;21(4 Headache):973-989. doi:10.1212/CON.0000000000000199
9. Tepper SJ. Medication-Overuse Headache. doi:10.1111/j.1526-4610.1994.hed3401001.x/pdf
10. Silberstein SD. Topiramate in Migraine Prevention: A 2016 Perspective. *Headache*. 2017;57(1):165-178. doi:10.1111/head.12997
11. Aurora SK, Brin MF. Chronic Migraine: An Update on Physiology, Imaging, and the Mechanism of Action of Two Available Pharmacologic Therapies. *Headache*. 2017;57(1):109-125. doi:10.1111/head.12999
12. Jansenn Pharmaceutics I. Topamax: HIGHLIGHTS OF PRESCRIBING INFORMATION. Published online 2020. Accessed July 30, 2021. www.fda.gov/medwatch.
13. Linde M, Mulleners WM, Chronicle EP, Mccrory DC. Valproate (valproic acid or sodium valproate or a combination of the two) for the prophylaxis of episodic migraine in adults. *Cochrane Database Syst Rev*. 2013;2013(6). doi:10.1002/14651858.CD010611
14. AbbVie Inc. Deapkote delayed-release tablets: HIGHLIGHTS OF

PRESCRIBING INFORMATION. Published online 2021. Accessed July 30, 2021. www.fda.gov/medwatch.
15. AbbVie Inc. Depakote ER: HIGHLIGHTS OF PRESCRIBING INFORMATION. Published online 2021. Accessed July 30, 2021. www.fda.gov/medwatch.
16. Freitag F, Collins S, Carlson H, et al. *A Randomized Trial of Divalproex Sodium Extended-Release Tablets in Migraine Prophylaxis*.; 2002.
17. Silberstein SD. *Divalproex Sodium in Headache: Literature Review and Clinical Guidelines*.; 1996.
18. Parikh SK, Silberstein SD. Current Status of Antiepileptic Drugs as Preventive Migraine Therapy. *Curr Treat Options Neurol*. 2019;21(4). doi:10.1007/s11940-019-0558-1
19. Pfizer. Neurontin: HIGHLIGHTS OF PRESCRIBING INFORMATION. Published online 2021. Accessed July 30, 2021. www.fda.gov/medwatch.
20. Perloff MD, Berlin RK, Gillette M, Petersile MJ, Kurowski D. Gabapentin in headache disorders: What is the evidence? *Pain Med (United States)*. 2016;17(1):162-171. doi:10.1111/pme.12931
21. Linde M, Mulleners WM, Chronicle EP, Mccrory DC. Gabapentin or pregabalin for the prophylaxis of episodic migraine in adults. *Cochrane Database Syst Rev*. 2013;2013(6). doi:10.1002/14651858.CD010609
22. Pfizer. Lyrica: HIGHLIGHTS OF PRESCRIBING INFORMATION. Published online 2017. Accessed July 30, 2021. www.fda.gov/medwatch.
23. Barry JD, Williams SR. Beta Adrenergic Blocking Agents. *ECG Emerg Med Acute Care*. Published online June 3, 2018:260-262. Accessed July 30, 2021. https://www.ncbi.nlm.nih.gov/books/NBK548127/
24. Galletti F, Cupini LM, Corbelli I, Calabresi P, Sarchielli P. Pathophysiological basis of migraine prophylaxis. *Prog Neurobiol*. 2009;89(2):176-192. doi:10.1016/j.pneurobio.2009.07.005
25. Akrimax Pharmaceuticals I. Inderal ® (propranolol hydrochloride) Tablets Rx only. Published online 2010. Accessed July 30, 2021. www.wyeth.com
26. Brandes JL. Migraine in women. *Contin Lifelong Learn Neurol*. 2012;18(4):835-852. doi:10.1212/01.CON.0000418646.70149.71
27. Yu W, Horowitz SH. *Treatment of Sporadic Hemiplegic Migraine with Calcium-Channel Blocker Verapamil*.; 2003.
28. Burish M. *Cluster Headache and Other Trigeminal Autonomic Cephalalgias*.; 2018. https://journals.lww.com/continuum
29. Dorosch T, Ganzer CA, Lin M, Seifan A. Efficacy of Angiotensin-Converting Enzyme Inhibitors and Angiotensin Receptor Blockers in

the Preventative Treatment of Episodic Migraine in Adults. *Curr Pain Headache Rep*. 2019;23(11). doi:10.1007/s11916-019-0823-8
30. RG K. Tension-type headache. *Continuum (Minneap Minn)*. 2012;18(4):823-834. doi:10.1212/01.CON.0000418645.32032.32
31. Hornig-Rohan M, Amsterdam JD. Venlafaxine versus stimulant therapy in patients with dual diagnosis ADD and depression. *Prog Neuro-Psychopharmacology Biol Psychiatry*. 2002;26(3):585-589. doi:10.1016/S0278-5846(01)00312-8
32. Eli Lilly. Cymbalta: HIGHLIGHTS OF PRESCRIBING INFORMATION. Published online 2020. Accessed July 30, 2021. www.fda.gov/medwatch.
33. Charles A. *The Migraine Aura*.; 2018. https://journals.lww.com/continuum
34. Datta R, Aguirre GK, Hu S, Detre JA, Cucchiara B. Interictal cortical hyperresponsiveness in migraine is directly related to the presence of aura. *Cephalalgia*. 2013;33(6):365-374. doi:10.1177/0333102412474503
35. Chen SP, Ayata C. Novel Therapeutic Targets Against Spreading Depression. *Headache*. 2017;57(9):1340-1358. doi:10.1111/head.13154
36. Evans RW, Lay CL. A persistent migraine aura. *Headache*. 2000;40(8):696-698. doi:10.1046/j.1526-4610.2000.040008696.x
37. Rozen TD. *Brief Communication Aborting a Prolonged Migrainous Aura With Intravenous Prochlorperazine and Magnesium Sulfate*.; 2003.
38. Pascual J, Caminero AB, Mateos V, et al. *Brief Communication Preventing Disturbing Migraine Aura With Lamotrigine: An Open Study*.; 2004.
39. Buch D, Chabriat H. Lamotrigine in the Prevention of Migraine With Aura: A Narrative Review. *Headache*. 2019;59(8):1187-1197. doi:10.1111/head.13615
40. Peer Mohamed B, Goadsby PJ, Prabhakar P. Safety and efficacy of flunarizine in childhood migraine: 11 years' experience, with emphasis on its effect in hemiplegic migraine. *Dev Med Child Neurol*. 2012;54(3):274-277. doi:10.1111/j.1469-8749.2011.04154.x
41. N P, AH S, J H, MD F, GM T. Familial and sporadic hemiplegic migraine: diagnosis and treatment. *Curr Treat Options Neurol*. 2013;15(1):13-27. doi:10.1007/S11940-012-0208-3
42. Bisdorff AR. Management of vestibular migraine. *Ther Adv Neurol Disord*. 2011;4(3):183-191. doi:10.1177/1756285611401647
43. Byun YJ, Levy DA, Nguyen SA, Brennan E, Rizk HG. Treatment of Vestibular Migraine: A Systematic Review and Meta-analysis.

Laryngoscope. Published online 2020. doi:10.1002/lary.28546
44. Salmito MC, Duarte JA, Morganti LOG, et al. Tratamento profilático da migrânea vestibular. *Braz J Otorhinolaryngol*. 2017;83(4):404-410. doi:10.1016/j.bjorl.2016.04.022
45. Lauritsen CG, Marmura MJ. Current Treatment Options: Vestibular Migraine. *Curr Treat Options Neurol*. 2017;19(11). doi:10.1007/s11940-017-0476-z
46. Croop R, Lipton RB, Kudrow D, et al. Oral rimegepant for preventive treatment of migraine: a phase 2/3, randomised, double-blind, placebo-controlled trial. *Lancet*. 2021;397(10268):51-60. doi:10.1016/S0140-6736(20)32544-7
47. PJ G, DW D, J A, et al. Safety, tolerability, and efficacy of orally administered atogepant for the prevention of episodic migraine in adults: a double-blind, randomised phase 2b/3 trial. *Lancet Neurol*. 2020;19(9):727-737. doi:10.1016/S1474-4422(20)30234-9
48. Dodick DW. CGRP ligand and receptor monoclonal antibodies for migraine prevention: Evidence review and clinical implications: *https://doi.org/101177/0333102418821662*. 2019;39(3):445-458. doi:10.1177/0333102418821662
49. Allergan. Botox (onabotulinumtoxinA): HIGHLIGHTS OF PRESCRIBING INFORMATION. Published online 2021. Accessed July 30, 2021. www.fda.gov/medwatch.
50. Winner PK, Blumenfeld AM, Eross EJ, et al. Long-Term Safety and Tolerability of OnabotulinumtoxinA Treatment in Patients with Chronic Migraine: Results of the COMPEL Study. *Drug Saf*. 2019;42(8):1013-1024. doi:10.1007/s40264-019-00824-3
51. Dodick DW, Silberstein SD, Lipton RB, DeGryse RE, Adams AM, Diener HC. Early onset of effect of onabotulinumtoxinA for chronic migraine treatment: Analysis of PREEMPT data. *Cephalalgia*. 2019;39(8):945-956. doi:10.1177/0333102418825382
52. Santoro A, Copetti M, Miscio AM, Leone MA, Fontana A. Chronic migraine long-term regular treatment with onabotulinumtoxinA: a retrospective real-life observational study up to 4 years of therapy. *Neurol Sci 2020 417*. 2020;41(7):1809-1820. doi:10.1007/S10072-020-04283-Y
53. MF B, RS K, A S, et al. Pregnancy outcomes following exposure to onabotulinumtoxinA. *Pharmacoepidemiol Drug Saf*. 2016;25(2):179-187. doi:10.1002/PDS.3920

How Important are Vitamins in Headache?

Georgia Kane, MD
Director of Headache Center of Excellence at the Tampa VA
Assistant Professor
University of South Florida, College of Medicine
Tampa, Florida

What are the most common supplements used in headache?

It has been known for years that high dose riboflavin (vitamin B2), at 400mg daily can be beneficial in treating migraine headaches. Generally speaking, it is nerve irritation that underlies migraine and therefore many treatments are geared to nerve "stabilization" which is what riboflavin does. This is something that is used for prevention, so using it daily is necessary. It is a great option since it is very well tolerated, the most common side effect being diarrhea and polyuria (needing to urinate more than usual).

Magnesium is commonly used as well, especially in migraine with aura. In studies, low magnesium did correlate with higher changes of getting a migraine (please note that it is ionized magnesium and as such is not the typical magnesium level you would get with your blood work). It can and should be added as a daily supplement. When headaches are severe or long-lasting, they may benefit from IV infusion of magnesium as well. It is a safe option, the most common side effect being diarrhea.

Vitamin D is a prevention option and its deficiency has been shown to be associated with headaches as well as dizziness and vertigo. It too is considered a nerve stabilizer although its mechanism of action is not completely understood. This is one test that can be measured in the lab and supplementation is easy and well-tolerated. It has more recently been acknowledged (albeit somewhat controversial) that it might have some value in the prevention and management of COVID 19.

What about Vitamin A? Treatments for acne?

We have been talking thus far about vitamin deficiencies, but there is one that is worse if you take too much of it – that is vitamin A, but also vitamin E and several prescription drugs. It is found in many foods and is needed for organs to work normally. However, an excess can cause headaches, nausea, dizziness, and rarely coma and death. Pseudotumor cerebri (called this because it acts like a tumor in that it increases pressure in the brain, much like a tumor would) is a condition that causes headache. This is most likely to occur in obese women of childbearing age. It basically is an increase in intracranial pressure that can lead to blindness and shouldn't be ignored. Other than eating the liver of a polar bear (this can be swiftly lethal due to the high vitamin A content), eating liver regularly (called "liver lover's headache") and taking too much in the form of supplements are sources of this toxicity. A question that comes up commonly is if retinoids, a close relative of vitamin A (commonly found in skin care ointments) can contribute to it this. Although retinoids are derivatives of vitamin A and the main component of many anti-aging topical preparations, they alone are not commonly associated with pseudotumor. However, if taken with doxycycline there is a higher chance of this occurring and thus is not recommended to take simultaneously. Medications used for acne such as isotretinoin (in the recent past known as Accutane) is an ingested form of a retinoid and can cause this (due to higher vitamin A). The recommended dose of vitamin A per day is 700-900mcg which is easily eaten in our daily diets, supplementation is generally not needed. If pregnant or planning to become pregnant, definitely don't take it since it has been associated with serious birth defects.

What about a vitamin that when taken in normal doses can cause headaches?

You probably didn't guess it! It's niacin (vitamin B3, also known as nicotinamide). It has wonderful cholesterol lowering properties, but can cause flushing and headaches that are not dangerous, just annoying! It lasts about 20 minutes and can be very itchy as well. It is best to take at night and sleep through those side effects.

Other important considerations are high folate diets, low fat diets, and high omega3 fatty acid with low omega 6 fatty acid diets as well as turmeric/ curcumin spices all are believed to help decrease the frequency of headache. This is not strongly supported as of yet but is likely related to the decrease in inflammation that these diets are associated with and as such would only contribute to feeling better.

Suggested Readings

Bigal, ME, Borini CA, Tepper SJ, Speciali JG. Intravenous magnesium sulphate in the acute treatment of migraine without aura and migraine with aura. A randomized, double-blind, placebo-controlled study Cephalagia, 2002 Jun;22(5):345-53

Ebadi M, Montano-Loza AJ Perspective: improving vitamin D status in the management of COVID-19 Eur J Clin Nutr, 2020 Jun;74(6):856-859

Ghorbani Z, Togha M, Rafiee P, Ahmadi ZS, Rasekh Magham R, Haghighi S, Razeghi Jahromi S, Mahmoudi M. Vitamin D in migraine headache: a comprehensive review on literature. Neurol Sci. 2019 Dec; 40(12): 2459-247

Knutsen KV, Brekke M, Gjelstad S, Lagerløv P. Vitamin D status in patients with musculoskeletal pain, fatigue and headache: a cross-sectional descriptive study in a multi-ethnic general practice in Norway. Scand J Prim Health Care. 2010 Sep;28(3):166-71

Nattagh-Eshtivani E, Sani MA, Dahri M, Ghalichi F, Ghavami A, Arjang P, Tarighat-Esfanjani A. The role of nutrients in the pathogenesis and treatment of migraine headaches: Review. Biomed Pharmacother. 2018 Jun; 102:317-325

Nowaczewska M, Wiciński M, Osiński S, Kaźmierczak H. The Role of Vitamin D in Primary Headache-from Potential Mechanism to Treatment. Nutrients. 2020 Jan 17;12(1):243

Nowaczewska M, Wicinski M, Osiniski S, Kazmierczak H The role of Vitamin D in primary Headache-from potential mechanism to treatment Nutrients 2020, 12(1) 243

Schoene J, Jacquy J, Lenaerts M Effectiveness of high-dose riboflavin in migraine prophylaxis A randomized controlled trial Neurology Feb 1998, 50 (2) 466-470

Starling J, Koo J Evidence based or theoretical concern? Pseudotumor cerebri and depression as acitretin side effects Journal of drugs in Dermatology: JDD, 01 Nov 2005, 4(6):690-696

"WILL EXERCISE HELP MY HEADACHES?"

LAUREN R. NATBONY, MD

My neurologist keeps telling me that exercise will help my headaches. Is this true?

Yes, it is. In particular, aerobic exercise (or utilizing large muscle groups repetitively and maintaining an increased heart rate for a sustained period of time) is beneficial for reducing migraine frequency, possibly migraine intensity, and should be considered a preventive treatment of migraine. When exercising, the body releases endorphins, which are the body's natural pain relievers. Exercise can boost mood and well-being, decrease anxiety, promote a healthy sleep pattern, and lower stress levels. Thus, exercise can have a significant impact on the headache itself and other associated comorbidities.

One study found that physical exercise, regular relaxation exercise, and the use of topiramate were equally effective in reducing the rate of migraine. Those participants in the exercise group exercised for 40 minutes three times a week. Another study found that the combination of aerobic exercise and amitriptyline reduced the number of migraine days significantly more than amitriptyline alone. A recent study showed that, among patients with episodic migraine who used prophylactic medication, those who exercised with moderate to vigorous intensity at least three times per week had fewer monthly headaches. Therefore, exercise can be an effective intervention in the preventive treatment of migraine.

Which individuals benefit the most from exercise?

Exercise can benefit many primary headache disorders, including episodic and chronic migraine, episodic and chronic tension-type headache, and cervicogenic headache. Exercise is an effective preventative measure whether used alone or in combination with medication and may be especially beneficial in those with co-morbid neck pain. Exercise is also an essential part of recovery from post-traumatic headache. Performing aerobic exercise at an intensity below that which exacerbates symptoms has been shown to aid in concussion recovery.

Is there an ideal intensity, frequency, or duration of exercise?

An ideal exercise program should be individualized to a person's level of fitness and goals. It should incorporate cardiovascular exercise (brisk walking, running, cycling or elliptical work, swimming, rowing) and muscle-strengthening activities (weight lifting, stretching, yoga, tai chi, pilates). The intensity, frequency, and duration of exercise should be tolerable and not cause undue pain or disability. Warm-up and cool-down elements are essential in any exercise program. The planned exercise should be started at a lower intensity and speed for 5-10 minutes to allow the body to prepare for more vigorous activity. An insufficient warm-up period can trigger a headache attack. Likewise, a cool-down for 5-10 minutes after strenuous exercise can aid in recovery.

It is recommended to start with moderate-intensity exercise. If headaches worsen, exercise intensity should be further reduced. The intensity of exercise can be gauged via the "talk test." During moderate-intensity exercise, a person is too winded to sing but can talk. For vigorous-intensity activity, a person has trouble maintaining a conversation.

Clinical trials of aerobic exercise suggest that the frequency of exercise should be three to five times per week, with each exercise session ranging from 40 to 50 minutes (150 to 300 minutes a week of moderate-intensity, or 75 to 150 minutes a week of vigorous-intensity exercise). The total weekly time required for aerobic exercise can be broken down into three or more days. Spreading the weekly time across several days, and even in 10-minute bouts of exercise, provide similar benefits.

Is there a specific type of exercise that is most beneficial for headache?

Overall there are no clear data pointing to one specific type of exercise that is more effective in migraine prevention than another. However, there is some data that high-intensity interval training (HIT) may be more beneficial than moderate-intensity continuous exercise to reduce migraine frequency. HIT involves intermittent, usually regularly timed bouts of high-intensity activity alternating with brief periods of rest or low-intensity activity.

There are no specific studies evaluating strength training or stretching for migraine. However, since shoulder and neck pain are common migraine symptoms, a cervical strengthening program should be considered. For tension-type and cervicogenic headaches, low-load endurance craniocervical and cervicoscapular exercise is recommended. There should also be a strong focus on core strengthening to improve posture and reduce neck pain. For general muscular fitness, it is recommended to resistance train each major muscle group (chest, shoulders, upper and lower back, abdomen, hips, legs) 2-3 days per week. Strength training can be achieved with free weights, resistance machines, or resistance bands.

When I exercise, it causes me to have a headache. Why?

There are various causes of exercise-induced headaches. For those with migraine, intense exercise can trigger debilitating attacks. In one study, 38 percent of participants experienced migraine attacks due to or in association with exercise. Of those more than half stopped participating in their chosen sport or exercise to reduce or eliminate their migraines.

Primary exercise headache is a rare headache type that is distinct from exercise-induced migraine. The headache is brought on by and occurs only during or after strenuous physical exercise. There is no headache at other times. It is commonly described as pain on both sides of the head with a pulsating quality lasting five minutes to 48 hours. Primary exercise headache is not dangerous and tends to be self-limiting. Headaches can be managed by extending the warm-up before exercising and/or reducing the intensity of exercise. If these changes are not successful, medications can be used.

Importantly, anyone with a new or never-evaluated exercise headache should see their doctor to rule out more dangerous issues like subarachnoid hemorrhage, reversible cerebral vasoconstriction syndrome, and arterial dissection.

Are there certain types of exercise that are more likely to trigger headaches?

Exercise headaches are more commonly associated with very strenuous and high-intensity exercises such as running, tennis, swimming, rowing, weightlifting, and many contact sports. Powerlifting, for example, can trigger a migraine and is often referred to as "weightlifters' headache." It is thought that when a person with migraine lifts heavy weights, they often hold their breath, increasing the pressure on the structures around the brain.

This leads to irritation of nerves in the neck and scalp, resulting in a migraine. Likewise, strenuous exercise can impact blood flow to the brain and dilate the blood vessels, translating into pain for some.

In addition to the type of exercise performed, location and temperature are important factors. We know that headaches are more likely to be triggered when exercising in hot environments or in those with high humidity, and at high altitudes.

What can I do to prevent triggering a headache with exercise?

The first step is to modify your pre- and post-workout routine. Have a balanced snack with protein, fat, and carbohydrates about 60-90 minutes before exercising to stabilize blood sugar. Stay hydrated before, during, and after a workout. Consume at least 16oz of water for every half hour of exercise. It is important to warm up for at least 5-10 minutes to ease your body into exercise. After a workout, make sure to cool down for at least 5-10 minutes with gentle stretches to help lower your heart rate. Exercise in a cool, temperature-controlled environment if possible. Becoming overheated can trigger a migraine. Also, try to avoid exercising in high humidity and at high altitudes.

If you have neck pain, be mindful of the positioning of your head and neck, as well as your posture, during exercise. It may be helpful to avoid exercising at a time you are exposed to other known triggering factors. Migraine attacks are more likely to happen when two or more triggers occur together.

If medication is needed, naproxen or indomethacin taken 30-60 minutes before exercise may prevent headaches in some cases. However, with indomethacin and naproxen, treatment should be monitored to avoid stomach irritation. Beta-blockers such as nadolol and propranolol have also been reported to help prevent exercise-induced headaches. They are reasonable options for people who cannot take naproxen or indomethacin or for those who exercise frequently.

I have chronic migraine and get a migraine every time I try to do aerobic exercise. What am I supposed to do?

Low-impact and non-aerobic exercise can still afford benefits for migraine prevention. Some low-impact aerobic activities like cycling and walking are better for chronic migraine than muscle-strengthening exercises such as bicep curls with weights. Non-aerobic exercises such as yoga, pilates, and tai chi have also been shown to help with migraine control and may be less likely to trigger an attack.

I haven't exercised before and don't know how to start. What do you recommend?

First, set a realistic goal. People tend to start with so much enthusiasm and ambition and with a big goal. If you try to go from zero exercise to running 30 minutes every day, it will not be sustainable for very long, and you risk injury.

The key is to start with a short duration of light to moderate activity. Say 5-10 minutes to start. An increase in time per session of 5–10 min every 1–2 weeks over the first 4–6 weeks is reasonable for the average adult. After that, both intensity and duration can be gradually increased.

Exercise is as much about the activity as preparing for it, including intention, motivation, scheduling, and making time for yourself. Set a time where you're most likely to stick with exercise. It can be morning, noon, or night; however, consistency is key. If you don't set a time, you're more likely to put it off until you have more time or energy or even into the next day. Schedule exercise as an appointment on your calendar so you don't forget.

I started exercising but haven't seen any improvement in my headaches yet. How long does it take?

It takes time for the effects of exercise to appear. Most studies examine the impact of exercise after 6-12 weeks of initiation. The good news is that as you exercise more and build up your strength and endurance, headache frequency will decrease. Thus, you should continue to exercise even if there is an initial lack of improvement.

Suggested Reading

Barber M, Pace A. Exercise and Migraine Prevention: a Review of the Literature. *Curr Pain Headache Rep* 2020 Jun 11;24(8):39.

Hagan KK, Li W, Mostofsky E, Bertisch SM, et al. Prospective cohort study of routine exercise and headache outcomes among adults with episodic migraine. *Headache* 2021 Mar;61(3):493-499.

Lemmens J, De Pauw J, Van Soom T, et al. The effect of aerobic exercise on the number of migraine days, duration and pain intensity in migraine: a systematic literature review and meta-analysis. *J Headache Pain* 2019 Feb 14;20(1):16.

Machado-Oliveira L, da Silva Gauto YO, de Santana Neto FJ, et al. Effects of Different Exercise Intensities on Headache: A Systematic Review. *Am J Phys Med Rehabil* 2020 May;99(5):390-396.

Song TJ, Chu MK. Exercise in Treatment of Migraine Including Chronic Migraine. *Curr Pain Headache Rep* 2021 Feb 25;25(3):14.

Varkey E, Cider A, Carlsson J, Linde M. Exercise as migraine prophylaxis: a randomized study using relaxation and topiramate as controls. *Cephalalgia* 2011 Oct;31(14):1428-38.

Everyone Says I am Taking too Many Triptans. If I Don't, the Headache Gets Out of Control

Alan M. Rapoport, M.D.

Professor of Neurology
The David Geffen School of Medicine at UCLA
Los Angeles, California

Q: Why can't I take my triptan more than 2 days a week?

A: When patients take almost any acute care medication for migraine more often than that, they have an increased chance of developing medication overuse headache (MOH).

Q: I have heard about rebound headaches for over 20 years, but no one has used the term MOH.

A: We used to call it "rebound headache", as when the patient stopped taking the medication they were using too frequently, they got much worse for a while. We now know they can get worse just from taking it regularly and they do not have to stop it to get worse. So, we say medication overuse headache.

Q: I don't overuse it, I just take it because if I don't, my headache gets out of control and can be severe for 10 days or more. Why do you say overuse?

A: It is not the best name, as it sounds like we are blaming you for using it frequently. We know you are doing that just to feel better, but you are using it more than you should to help your headache problem. So that is the name that international headache experts gave it.

Q: I know years ago that I should not take Excedrin more than 2-3 days per week. But now you are saying triptans too?

A: Actually, almost every medicine that you take to stop a headache in progress that is becoming severe, should not be taken too often. The categories include triptans, ergotamine or dihydroergotamine, opioids, barbiturate containing medications like Fiorinal and Fioricet, aspirin, acetaminophen (Tylenol), NSAIDs (Advil, Aleve, etc.), over-the-counter pain relievers like Excedrin that also contain caffeine or any combination of these medications.

Q: But my previous doctor told me I should never be without my triptan and to take it at the very start of my migraine attack.

A: That is true, unless you are doing that more than 2 days per week. That is 8 days per month, and if you have that many headache days, we need to get you on an effective preventive medication that will decrease the number of headache days you have per month, and maybe also decrease the duration and intensity of the pain. It may also make your body more responsive to the medicine you take to stop a headache. Maybe also getting better sleep and getting rid of some of your triggers will help as well.

Q: Are you saying that there are no medicines for migraine that I can take more frequently?

A: Up until early in 2020, that would have been true. There is a new class of medicines named “gepants” that can be taken more often without causing MOH. They are named ubrogepant (Ubrelvy) and rimegepant (Nurtec) and so far, they do not seem to cause MOH. Actually, one of them has been approved by the FDA and can be used as a migraine preventive given once every other day. It decreases rather than increases headache when used over time.

Q: I have tried 3 or 4 preventive medications over the years, and they have either not worked or cause bad side effects like slow heart rate, trouble exercising, drowsiness, weight gain, trouble with memory. I guess if they were very helpful, I could tolerate one of the medicines. But there must be a better way.

A: In the last few years, 4 new preventive treatments for migraine that work to block CGRP (calcitonin gene-related peptide) have been brought to market for migraine patients. They are monoclonal antibodies against CGRP (MABs). They are injections once per month or every 3 months and one is an intravenous infusion given every 3 months. The first 3 are self-injected with an auto-injector at home. In general, they work better than the older medicine and they have fewer side effects. Although they are much more expensive, they are usually covered by insurance and Medicare. Most medical insurance companies require that you have failed 2 or 3 categories of the older preventives before they will cover them.

Q: How well do they work?

A: They usually decrease the number of headache days per month by 40 to 50% and sometimes more. In some patients, they can stop headache completely. If the older, less expensive medicine have not worked or cause some side effects, you should strongly consider trying one of these newer antibodies. Many of my patients stay on them for 1-2 years or even longer as they do so well without side effects. Once in a while one does not work or causes side effects, so we usually switch to another.

Q: How long have doctors known about MOH?

A: About 60 years ago they were found to be cause by ergots like ergotamine tartrate (Cafergot or Wigraine) when used too often. Then about 40 years ago pain meds were also found to cause MOH and now we know that any acute care medicine can cause MOH except the new gepants.

Q: What causes MOH?

A: We know a lot more about it today than we used to, but not the final answer. It seems to be caused by the results of decreasing serotonin in the brain. This prevents the body's own mechanism to rid you of pain. Also an increase in CGRP levels causes an increase in the pain of migraine, so we try to use the medicines that reverse that problem. Inflammation of the brain may also be involved.

Q: How did you treat MOH in the past? I know when I tried to stop my sumatriptan, I got so much worse.

A: For over 40 years, we had a 3-pronged approach to treat MOH. We detoxified the patient, meaning we gradually had them decrease and stop the offending medicines, and they often got worse for a short period of time, from 3 days to 2 weeks. This process can work smoothly; but there is often a worsening of pain, which almost always gets better if you stick with it. We also started a preventive medicine, which used to be in pill form and could cause several side effects and sometimes did not work very well. It took 1 to 2 months to build these medicines up to the right dose. We offered medicine to help the patients get through the withdrawal phase more easily. In some cases, patients needed to be hospitalized, which gave us the opportunity to use stronger intravenous medicine which worked better.

Q: This does not sound good to me and I would be afraid to do this.

A: The good news is, we now start patients on of these injectable antibody treatments and within a month or so, without a difficult withdrawal period, they seem to improve better than in the old days. Not everybody can get coverage for these MABs, but headache specialists can often arrange it.

Q: So, does these mean I don't have to go through a strict withdrawal, and I can keep taking my triptan or other acute medications?

A: Actually, yes. The MABs often work well enough to reduce your headaches even when you are taking acute care medicines. Then when you have fewer headaches, you won't need so many of those medicines. We encourage you to not even take them if you have a mild headache, as they often will not escalate to a more severe one, like they used to.

Q: Do you ever try patients on the new gepants medicines now that they are available?

A: That is not usually necessary, but it would be a reasonable way to treat.

Q: So, it sounds like there will be fewer patients with MOH in the future.

A: I think there will still be many patients with MOH, but the treatment is getting easier for me to prescribe and educate about and better for the patient. The monoclonal antibodies against CGRP and the newer gepants, have been effective additions to our treatment possibilities.

Q: Will the older preventive medicines still be used for treating MOH?

A: I think they will still be used as preventive medications, whether or not MOH is present. They can work in MOH, and they are much less expensive. At present, the insurance companies will not let me prescribe an injectable MAB unless the patient has had not help from, or has significant side effects from 2 or more categories of the older preventive medications?

Q: What are those categories of preventive medicines?

A: They usually include some beta blockers, epilepsy medicines, antidepressants, some blood pressure lowering medicines and a few others.

Q. Well I tried 3 different categories and sometimes more that one in each. Does that mean I would be covered if you prescribed one of the antibody treatments?

A. Probably yes, but we usually need to obtain prior authorization and that should not take too long to do.

Q. It certainly sounds like headache treatment has come a long way in the 25 years I have been dealing with my migraine. I am thankful for that and appreciate all the information you have given me.

A. Yes, compared to what I could offer a patient for migraine treatment when I first went into practice, I have so many more and better treatment options now. The medicines work better and often have fewer side effects. There are also several devices that have fewer side effects that can be effective. You are most welcome for the update. You should always be aware of the best treatments that are available.

References

1. *CNS Drugs*
   https://doi.org/10.1007/s40263-021-00818-9
   REVIEW ARTICLE
   The Evolution of Medication Overuse Headache: History, Pathophysiology and Clinical Update
   Christina Sun-Edelstein1. Alan M. Rapoport2. Wanakorn Rattanawong3. Anan Srikiatkhachorn4
   Accepted: 15 April 2021

© The Author(s), under exclusive license to Springer Nature Switzerland AG 2021
2. Bigal ME, Lipton RB. Overuse of acute migraine medications and migraine chronification. *Curr Pain Headache Rep.* 2009; 13:301–7.
3. Bigal ME, Serrano D, Buse D, Scher A, Stewart WF, Lipton RB. Acute migraine medications and evolution from episodic to chronic migraine: a longitudinal population-based study. *Headache.* 2008; 48:1157–68.

My Doctor says I am taking too Much Medication. What am I Supposed to Do for All of my Headaches?

Britany Klenofsky, MD

As needed pain relievers can certainly help reduce or eliminate the pain of a headache. However, there is such a thing as too much! While not wanting to take a daily prescription to prevent migraine is understandable, it is important to realize that as needed medications can be harmful if taken too often. Even if a medication is available over the counter, without prescription, it is still a medication. Let's not forget, you can reach a point where you want to get ahead of the headaches and be proactive, not just reactive.

What is medication overuse headache?

Medication overuse headache (MOH) refers to an increase or chronification of headache due to frequent and excessive use of medications that treat headache pain. It occurs when those with a known headache history regularly take medication to relieve headache more than 2 separate days a week or 10 separate days a month. Certain pain relievers can result in overuse with as few as 6 separate days a month (often combination analgesics and medications including barbiturates or opioids). Those with migraine are more likely to develop MOH compared to other headache disorders. While some previously denied its existence, MOH is a real problem and research has found changes (metabolic, functional, and structural) in the brains of affected patients on functional magnetic resonance imaging (fMRI).

What do I do to get rid of medication overuse headache?

The best thing to do for medication overuse headache is to stop taking the as needed pain reliever---remember either prescription or non-prescription medications can cause it. If you use the pain reliever too much, you are essentially tricking your brain into expecting the medication and giving yourself more headache days overall. Please talk to your healthcare provider and consider seeking a neurologist or Headache specialist. You should come up with a step-by-step plan with your doctor. Some of these medications, like barbiturates and opioids, may need to be slowly discontinued. Do not abruptly stop these medications due to the risk of withdrawal symptoms and other detrimental effects. On the other hand, studies have shown that triptans and simple analgesics (i.e., acetaminophen) can be abruptly discontinued for resolution of MOH. Data suggests that those who discontinue overused triptans improve over 7-10 days and those who discontinue overused simple analgesics over 2-3 weeks.

OK, I see your point. I can't do that, though, because my headaches are just way too debilitating and happen way too frequently. What should I do?

We understand that your headaches are very bad and need to be treated to avoid interrupting your life. However, it is likely that you are having extra headache days or more severe headache days due to the overuse of the analgesics. While it may be difficult in the beginning, headaches should eventually improve when medication overuse is eliminated. Data is supportive of fewer headache days with resolution of MOH. There is a "light at the end of the tunnel."

Should I start medication to prevent my headaches?

Since you are having more than 4 headache days a month and suffering from medication overuse headache, you should talk to your doctor about starting a daily medication to prevent headaches. There are quite a few medications that we prescribe daily to reduce overall headache frequency. As the headache frequency decreases, we may then re-introduce as needed analgesics to use on those occasional days – with a limitation of using them no more frequently than 10 days per month.

Recently, newer medications that influence calcitonin gene-related peptide (CGRP) have been introduced for migraine. Calcitonin gene-related peptide appears to be involved in the pathophysiology of migraine and brain receptors for CGRP are negatively affected by frequent analgesic use. Blocking CGRP has been shown to be beneficial in migraine prevention, does not worsen MOH, and in fact may help to prevent and/or treat MOH. Monthly injectables that inhibit CGRP can be used for the prevention of migraine in those with MOH.

Additionally, oral medications referred to as gepants (small molecule calcitonin gene-related peptide antagonists) are available. These medications can be used on an as needed basis to relieve an acute migraine without causing or worsening MOH. Some have also been shown to effectively prevent migraine when given daily or every other day. The headache community is seeing a great influx of prescription treatment options. Now is the time to have a conversation with your doctor, even if you thought there were no options for you in the past. Please do not be afraid that you will need to take a migraine preventive medication forever. Oftentimes, controlling headaches leads to better outcomes, and you can eventually reduce your prevention in the future.

Will the process be extra painful?

It may be difficult to transition from your medication overuse headache and the frequent desire to use a pain abortive drug. This makes it especially important to talk to a Headache specialist or neurologist as you can develop a plan to help you through the process. Not only may you need to taper the analgesic you are now taking, but you can also find alternative medications or treatment options to help with breakthrough pain in the interim. Topiramate and botulinum toxin have been known to be effective for migraine prevention specifically in patients with MOH. For those uncomfortable with newer medications, these are great options.

Is there anything else that I can do for my headaches?

Headaches can occur for numerous reasons and adjustments to lifestyle can have a significant impact on your headaches. Make sure that you are drinking lots of water to keep hydrated. Remember, coffee can dehydrate you and soda does not count as hydration! Also, start your day with a protein filled breakfast and find an exercise routine that is fun for you and fits your lifestyle.

Devices are available to wear on your forehead or arm that can prevent and/or treat migraines without having to take a pill. The supraorbital nerve stimulator is worn on the forehead via adhesive electrode pads to stimulate the trigeminal nerve (integral in the process of migraine) by sending electrical impulses. The device vibrates on your forehead and can be worn for 20 minutes a day to prevent migraines and 1 hour to abort an active migraine. The remote electronic neuromodulator device is attached to the arm at the earliest signs of a migraine. Via stimulation of nerves in the arm, neurotransmitters are released in the brain to inhibit pain signals. Other devices are also available and can be discussed with your doctor.

Remember, there is hope and there are options. Commit to helping yourself in the long term and you can see a world of difference shortly!

Suggested Reading

Ashina H, Dodick DW. Medication-overuse headache in patients with secondary headache disorders: Need for revision? Headache 2021;61:790-791.

Diener HC, Holle D, Solbach K, Gaul C. Medication-overuse headache: risk factors, pathophysiology, and management. Nat Rev Neurol 2016;12:575-83.

Green MW. Medication overuse headache. Curr Opin Neurol 2021;34:378-383.

Sun-Edelstein C, Rapoport AM, Rattanawong W, Srikiatkhachorn A. The Evolution of Medication Overuse Headache: History, Pathophysiology and Clinical Update. CNS Drugs 2021;35:545-565.

Wakerley BR. Medication-overuse headache. Pract Neurol 2019;19::399-403.

Non-invasive Neuromodulation Devices for Headache Treatment

Stewart J. Tepper, MD, FAHS

I hear that there are devices cleared by the FDA that can treat migraine. Can you tell me more?

The US Food and Drug Administration (FDA) clears devices for use in headaches based on overall evidence for effectiveness, safety, and tolerability. Devices for the treatment of headache can be physically implanted for a condition, but no device that requires surgery has been cleared by the FDA for headache management.

Instead, all the currently FDA cleared devices are portable, and people rest them on their head, neck, or arm to activate them. They are all classified by the FDA as "non-significant risk," meaning that unlike most medications they do not have significant side effects.

The devices that are available have different ways of working in headaches, and some are cleared for different types of headaches. A few of them are cleared to prevent headaches, a few to treat an individual headache attack, and a few have both acute and preventive programs and use.

What are the FDA cleared devices, and what are they used for, how are they used, and what are the side effects?

1. The first device FDA cleared is now called an External Trigeminal Stimulator or eTNS. It is also known as the "Cefaly Dual Enhanced" device. This device is FDA cleared for both acute and preventive migraine treatment. A sticky electrode is placed on the forehead, and the device is held onto the electrode with a magnet.

   The device be turned on with one push of a button for a one-hour treatment of an acute migraine attack. This can be done as often as desired to reduce migraine intensity and symptoms. A recent study showed that repeating the dose for another hour may add additional acute benefit.

To prevent migraine, the device is placed on the forehead in the evening, the button is pressed twice, which turns on the prevention program. The intensity of stimulation of the forehead slowly increases over 20 minutes and then automatically shuts off. Prevention requires dosing 20 minutes daily over at least 3 months to see reduction in migraine days. Side effects include odd buzzing sensations on the forehead or paresthesias. Some people feel relaxed after treating with the prevention program.

2. The second FDA-cleared device is the Single Pulse Transcranial Magnetic Stimulator, sTMS, also called the “sTMS mini”. This is a device the shape of a shoe box, about 10 inches long, that can be charged, and which when activated discharges a magnet at the back of the head. It is also FDA cleared for acute treatment of a migraine attack with 2-4 pulses of the magnet, and for prevention of migraine with 4 pulses twice daily. Patients can use up to 17 pulses in a day.

   Side effects are generally only a snapping sensation when the magnet pulses at the back of the head.

3. The non-invasive vagal nerve stimulator (nVNS or “gammaCore”) is a device that looks like an electric razor. After applying gel, the device is placed on the neck over the vagus nerve and activated for a 2-minute cycle. It can be placed on either side of the neck. For acute treatment of migraine, the device is cycled twice, 2 minutes each time, and if the migraine is not better, another 2 cycles can be applied in 20 minutes. Again, if the migraine needs additional treatment, 2 cycles are applied 2 hours later. For prevention of migraine, the device is cycled twice for 2 minutes 3 times daily.

   The nVNS device is the only device cleared for treatment of cluster headache. For acute treatment of episodic cluster headache, the device is cycled three times for 2 minutes each, and if the cluster attack is not resolved, again for 3 cycles after a 3-minute wait. It is not cleared for acute use in chronic cluster, only episodic cluster. The device did not work for acute treatment of chronic cluster headache attacks.

The device is also cleared for prevention of cluster headache, as an add-on adjunctive to medicine treatment. This requires three 2-minute cycles to be given twice daily every day on top of pharmaceutical prophylaxis such as verapamil or galcanezumab.

Side effects are twitching of the lip on the side of the stimulator, and sometimes throat or neck soreness or mild skin reactions on that side.

4. The Remote Electrical Neurostimulator (REN), called “Nerivio”, is FDA cleared for acute treatment of migraine in adults and adolescents. This is a device that is held on the arm by a wrap that goes around the upper arm. Once in place, the device is activated for 45 minutes with a smart phone app to treat migraine acutely. There is only a buzzing sensation on the arm, almost no side effects at all.

5. The Combined Occipital-Trigeminal Nerve Stimulator, called “Relivion”, is FDA cleared for acute treatment of migraine in adults. It sits on the head as a lightweight circular crown and stimulates the forehead and the back of the head at the same time for one hour to treat a migraine acutely. Again, paresthesias are mild as a side effect. The device should become available for patients with a prescription in late 2021.

How do these devices work in headache?

1. eTNS works by inhibiting two nerves in the forehead, the supraorbital and supratrochlear nerves that feed into the trigeminal nerve and down into the brainstem to the trigeminal cervical complex. This inhibition can stop a migraine, reduce the pain of a migraine, or, over time, prevent migraine.

2. sTMS works by pulsing the magnetic charge into the thalamus. This can stop a migraine acutely, and daily use over months can prevent migraine. The magnet also can interrupt a migraine aura by stopping cortical spreading depolarization (CSD).

3. nVNS inhibits vagal afferents to the thalamus, to stop a migraine attack or to slowly prevent migraine after months of daily use. It probably works similarly in cluster headache. nVNS can also stop migraine aura by inhibiting CSD.

4. REN uses a reflex called conditioned pain modulation. This reflex sends a signal from the arm to the lower brain to turn off a migraine. The device was created specifically to activate this reflex to stop a migraine attack. eTNS, sTMS, nVNS, and REN all work better acutely when taken early in a migraine attack, preferably turned on within 30-60 minutes of the start of a migraine.

5. The combined occipital trigeminal stimulation device works comparably to the eTNS device over the supraorbital and supratrochlear nerves but adds an inhibition of migraine through the cervically-derived Greater Occipital nerves. The hope is that adding cervical to trigeminal inhibition will increase the effectiveness of this device in stopping a migraine attack.

Who should consider using non-invasive neuromodulation?

These devices are appropriate for many people with headaches:

- Young people, early on in their migraine disorder, who want to avoid taking medications
- People who have tried numerous medications and have found them ineffective or disliked the side effects. Sometimes devices work quite well in this setting
- People with other medical conditions that prohibit certain medications or for whom medications are not a good idea
- Women planning to get pregnant who understandably do not want to use medications
- As an addition to medication to maximize therapeutic benefit

How does one get these devices? How much do they cost?

Obtaining the devices is often challenging, as most payers do not cover them. The Veterans Health Administration (VA) covers most of them, so veterans should seek VA care to access these devices.

1. eTNS is available now without a prescription. People can order the Dual Enhanced device at cefaly.com, and it costs between $400-550 one time and then $25 for 3 electrodes, each of which lasts about a month, so re-ordering the electrodes is necessary around every 3 months. There is an option for a monthly payment to pay off the device over time.

2. sTMS requires a prescription sent to the company and is rented for $350/month. It cannot be purchased.

3. nVNS requires a prescription sent to the company and costs about $600/month. The device is included for this cost, as is the gel.

4. REN requires a prescription sent to a specialty pharmacy. Each REN device is loaded to treat 12 times. The first device costs $10 to try for the 12 treatments, then $99 per device after that.

5. The combined occipital-trigeminal stimulator will be available late in 2021 with a prescription, and cost is not yet established as of July of 2021.

Any last words on devices?

Non-invasive neuromodulation devices are not used enough, and they offer effective anti-headache treatment without significant side effects. They should be considered for many headache treatment plans. They don't always terminate attacks, but they reduce headaches and can really help, so they are worth trying!

References

eTNS

Acute Treatment of Migraine

Chou et al. Acute migraine therapy with external trigeminal neurostimulation (ACME): A randomized controlled trial. *Cephalalgia.* 2019; 39(1):3-14.

Kuruvilla et al. A phase 3 randomized, double-blind, sham-controlled trial of e-TNS for the acute treatment of migraine (TEAM). *Headache* 2021;61 (Supplement 1): 99 (abstract IOR-02).

Preventive Treatment of Migraine

Schoenen et al. Migraine prevention with a supraorbital transcutaneous stimulator: a randomized controlled trial. *Neurology.* 2013; 80(8):697-704.

sTMS

Acute Treatment of Migraine

Lipton et al. Single-pulse transcranial magnetic stimulation for acute treatment of migraine with aura: a randomised, double-blind, parallel-group, sham-controlled trial. *Lancet Neurol.* 2010; 9(4):373-80.

Preventive Treatment of Migraine

Starling et al. A multicenter, prospective, single arm, open label, observational study of sTMS for migraine prevention (ESPOUSE Study). *Cephalalgia.* 2018; 38(6):1038-1048.

nVNS, Migraine

Acute Treatment of Migraine

Tassorelli et al. Noninvasive vagus nerve stimulation as acute therapy for migraine: The randomized PRESTO study. *Neurology.* 2018; 91(4):e364-e373.

Preventive Treatment of Migraine

Diener et al. Non-invasive vagus nerve stimulation (nVNS) for the preventive treatment of episodic migraine: The multicentre, double-blind, randomised, sham-controlled PREMIUM trial. *Cephalalgia.* 2019; 39(12):1475-1487.

nVNS, Cluster

Acute Treatment of Cluster

Goadsby et al. ACT2 Study Group. Non-invasive vagus nerve stimulation for the acute treatment of episodic and chronic cluster headache: A randomized, double-blind, sham-controlled ACT2 study. *Cephalalgia.* 2018; 38(5):959-969.

Preventive Treatment of Cluster

Gaul et al. Non-invasive vagus nerve stimulation for PREVention and Acute treatment of chronic cluster headache (PREVA): A randomised controlled study. *Cephalalgia.* 2016;36(6):534-46.

REN

Yarnitsky et al. Remote Electrical Neuromodulation (REN) Relieves Acute Migraine: A Randomized, Double-Blind, Placebo-Controlled, Multicenter Trial. *Headache.* 2019; 59(8):1240-1252.

Combined Occipital- Trigeminal Nerve Stimulator

Daniel O, Sharon R, Tepper SJ. A device review of Relivion®: an external combined occipital and trigeminal neurostimulation (eCOT-NS) system for self-administered treatment of migraine and major depressive disorder. *Expert Rev Med Devices.* 2021;18:333-342.

Issues for Young People

Jack Gladstein, MD

Professor of Pediatrics and Neurology
U of Maryland School of Medicine

I was surprised when you told me that kids get migraines too.

Yes, in fact there are two peak ages for first migraine in kids. The first is age 6 and the next is age 12. Before puberty boys and girls have equal chances of developing migraine. After puberty, most new migraine happens in girls. For those with first migraine before onset of puberty, 50 percent will outgrow their migraines by age 18. However, if first migraine occurs after puberty, headaches will usually last during your 20's through 50's.

I always thought of migraine as a disease of young adults. Are there subgroups of kids who have migraine real early in life?

There are migraine equivalents that present early. Children with these conditions often become regular migraine patients when they get older. When getting a migraine history in an adult, ask about infant colic. Work done in UCSF by my colleague Amy Gelfand suggest that colic may be early migraine. Infants can present with acute paroxysmal torticollis. In this condition, the infant is pale, refuses the breast or the bottle, and has her head stuck for hours to days. Work up is negative. It can recur. Similarly, a toddler who is fine, suddenly is dizzy and grabs on to a parents leg. He is mentally clear, but has vertigo. This is called acute paroxysmal vertigo. Again this can recur. 4 year olds can get recurrent bouts of severe vomiting. After a negative work up we call it "Cyclic Vomiting Syndrome". Older children can have recurrent bouts of severe abdominal pain with pallor and light sensitivity. This is called "abdominal migraine". In all these conditions, the children grow to be people who suffer with migraine.

What precautions should I suggest if I suspect my youngster has migraine?

Keep meals regular. This means that your teen needs to wake up 5 minutes earlier to eat breakfast. Keep sleep regular. All sleepovers must end at midnight (nothing good ever happens after midnight).

Keep exercise regular. Exercise in kids means get sweaty for 20 minutes. Walking the dog is helpful to parents, but does not count

Don't get dehydrated: Write a note for teacher to allow water at the desk

Identify stressors and act: Be particular to look for bullying or learning issues

No reading or texting in the car. Kids with migraine are often car sick. Eyes should be trained forward on the road. Some kids legitimately need the front passenger seat.

How are kid migraines different than those typically seen in adults?

Children's migraines are more often on both sides of the head, and last for a shorter period of time when untreated. Since teens are poor at describing pain, they may not use words like throbbing or pulsatile. These words often help pin down diagnosis, so when absent it is harder to clinch the diagnosis. A good approach is to establish the pattern with days (weeks) of normalcy in between attacks. Then establish the presence of autonomic symptoms. These would include nausea, light and sound sensitivity. During a migraine it is impossible to fight through it, so behaviorally, children try to withdraw to a dark quiet place. Even if the kids are poor describers of their pain, ask them to draw a picture.

How are the basics of migraine care different in children and adolescents?

Children and adolescents do not have freedom to access medications while in school without permission. We teach that early intervention makes migraines go away quickly. Parents of school aged children need to advocate with schools to allow immediate access to medicine for their children in the school setting.

Learning disabilities, bullying and behavioral issues play out in the school setting. The more stressed the youngster is, the harder it will be to control the headaches. Identifying triggers in school will help design interventions to settle down headache frequency.

Middle school is often fraught with problems for youngsters with migraine. As their bodies change, medicine adjustments may need to happen. Physical and cyber bullying peak during this time. So does new onset of headaches.

I am an adult who was prescribed new and exciting medications. Why can't I get them for my children?

Clinical trials for kids are hard to do. Placebo rates are as high as 68 percent in some pediatric triptan trials. In order to show that a drug is better that placebo one would have to enroll a very large cohort to show a difference. Newer trials often give everyone placebo first, and then eliminate placebo responders. Obtaining proper informed consent is difficult. Kids need to understand that not responding to a placebo is still helpful information. Since kids' headache are shorter in duration, kids on placebo may get better quickly, so different endpoints for measured success are in order. Frequent visits can be onerous for parents to take time off work, take their child out of school and come in for a research visit. For these reasons there is often a lag of a few years between the release of a new migraine drug in adults and their approval for adolescents, then ultimately children.

What should I tell my teen when (s)he goes off to college?

In some ways it will be easier to take care of your headaches and in some ways it will be harder. You will no longer have to get up early for school if you don't get enough sleep, because you can manage your class schedule in your favor. You can keep your medicines on you at all times, and not need to go through your teacher and school nurse. If you are a little quirky, it will be easier to find people with your interests without judgement. On the other hand, it is harder to handle routine bedtime and meals while away at college. Peer pressure to "party" will make it hard to do proper migraine hygiene. When deciding about college choice, you should consider meeting with the disability office to judge their flexibility to accommodate your migraine needs. With telemedicine it might be possible to meet with migraine experts even while away, so your good doctor patient relationships can be maintained.

There are many new medications that you might be eligible once you turn 18. Please discuss these before you leave for college, so that you have more choices of what to do both to treat and prevent your migraines. Bottom line, you have more control of your life once on your own. Make sure to keep regular meals exercise and sleep as part of your routine.

Suggested Reading

Leonardi M, Grazzi L, D'Amico D et. Al. Global Burden of Headache Disorders in Children and Adolescents 2007-2017. *Int J Environ Res pub health* 18:250; 2021

Kaperski J, Kabbouche MA, O'Brien HL Weberding JL. The optimal management of headache in children and adolescents. *Ther Adv Neurol Disord* 2016; 9(1)53-68

Rimsza ME, Kirk GM. Common medical problems of the college student. *Ped Clin North America* 2005; 52(1). 9-24

Gelfand AA, Buse DC, Cabana MD, Grimes B, Goadsby PJ, Allen IE. The association Between Parental Migraine and Infant Colic: A Cross-Sectional, Web-Based, U.S. Survey Study *Headache* 2019;59:988-1001

Teixeira KCS Montenegro MA Guerreiro, MM. Migraine Equivalents in Childhood *J Child Neurology* 2014, Vol. 29(10) 1366-1369

Rothner AD Wasiewski W Winner P Lewis D Stankowski J. Zolmitriptan Oral Tablet in Migraine Treatment: High Placebo Responses in Adolescents. *Headache* 2006; 46:101-109.

Diagnosis of Headache Disorders in Children and Teens

Robert H. Fryer MD PhD
Associate Professor of Neurology
Columbia University Medical Center
New York, New York

I suffer from migraines and my child has headaches. When should I take them to see a medical provider?

Headaches in childhood are very common, and in most cases have a relatively benign cause. If your child has headaches, it is always useful to start a headache diary and record the frequency of the headaches as well as the time of day the headache starts, what makes the headache go away, how often are you giving medications to treat the headache, and whether there seems to be a trigger for the headache such as activities, stress or foods. You should see a medical provider if your child's headaches:

- are increasing in frequency
- awaken them from sleep at night
- are accompanied by numbness, tingling or weakness of the face, arms or legs
- are preventing the child from participating in school or extracurricular activities
- are associated with frequent episodes of vomiting
- are requiring medications to treat the headaches once weekly or more
- are accompanied by fever

This is only a partial list, and please use your judgement as to when you should see a medical professional about your child's headaches.

My migraines did not start until I was in my 20s. Can my 8-year-old child's headaches also be migraines?

Yes, your child can be having migraines even if your migraines started much later in life. In children with migraine, we know that many of them will have a parent or sibling who also suffers from migraines. However, the age of onset of the migraines can vary greatly amongst different family members. So, the fact that your headaches started later in life does not mean that your child's headaches can't be migraines.

It is important to note that while migraine headaches are common in adults, with as many as 15-18% of the population suffering from them, they are also surprisingly common in children. Under age 10, approximately 3% of the population suffers from migraine headaches. This number may actually be higher given the difficulty in getting an accurate history from a young child.

Apart from migraine, what other types of headaches can children and teens get?

In general, headache disorders are broken down into two categories: primary headaches and secondary headaches. For most people, it is easier to understand secondary headaches so we will discuss these headaches first. Secondary headaches can be caused by another disease process in the body and the onset of these headaches typically coincides with the onset of the underlying disease process. These are called secondary headache disorders because the headache is secondary to the disease process and treatment of the disease process ameliorates the headache. One good example of this is an acute sinus infection. The headache coincides with the sinus infection and is made better once the sinus infection is treated effectively. A concussion is another example of a secondary headache. The head injury that causes the concussion brings on headaches that resolve when the concussion resolves.

Primary headaches are not caused by another underlying disease process, although they sometimes can be made worse by another disease process. With primary headaches the headache itself is the disorder, and there are usually special types of medications that we use for these types of headaches. Migraine is one of the more common primary headache disorders that we see in children; but there are other primary headache disorders that also occasionally occur at young ages. The other most common primary headache disorder is tension-type headache.

Deciding whether your child's headaches are due to a secondary cause or represent a primary headache disorder is an early step in the evaluation process by your child's medical provider. In some instances, your child's provider may order laboratory studies or imaging tests such as an MRI or head CT to help identify whether a secondary headache is present.

How can you tell the difference between different types of headaches?

With primary headache disorders such as migraine, there are symptom-based criteria that are used to help diagnose the headache. Other primary headache disorders include tension-type headaches and trigeminal autonomic cephalalgias, the latter more commonly known as variants of cluster headache. In addition, there is a fourth category that includes several rare kinds of headaches. All these types of primary headaches disorders have a set of clinical criteria that are used to make the diagnosis. It is important to note that there is no confirmatory lab test or imaging study that can confirm the diagnosis of a primary headache disorder.

To distinguish between different headache types, let me first describe the criteria for diagnosing migraines. A migraine headache is typically on one side of the head in adults or on both sides of the head in children. While a frontal localization is the most common, migraines can hurt anywhere in the head, even in the back. The pain is usually throbbing, and the headache has migrainous features such as light sensitivity (photophobia), sound sensitivity (phonophobia), nausea and vomiting. According to the diagnostic criteria, both photophobia and phonophobia or nausea or vomiting need to accompany the headache to qualify as a definite migraine. Some patients with migraine have an aura, usually near the onset of the headache, where they see spots or lines in their vision. This can last 20 minutes or so. Overall, the entire migraine headache typically lasts about 4 hours, although some people suffer from migraines that can last from 2 hours to 72 hours.

What if your headache does not have the migrainous features of photophobia and phonophobia, or nausea or vomiting? If the headache does not have these features, then it still could be a primary headache disorder. Tension-type headaches are the most common type of headache and are even more common than migraine. A tension-type headache is usually milder than a migraine and typically responds to over-the-counter medications such as acetaminophen or ibuprofen. Many patients with tension type headaches have tender muscles around the head region and the head pain is usually on both sides of the head. Photophobia or phonophobia can be present, but not both.

A third type of primary headache disorder is a trigeminal autonomic cephalalgia. Cluster headaches are probably the best-known headache in this group, although there can be other types of trigeminal autonomic cephalalgias that are distinguished by the length of the headache. Cluster headaches are associated with autonomic features, such as a droopy eyelid (ptosis), redness of the eye, nasal congestion or drainage, sweating on one side of the forehead, or tearing. The head pain is described as severe and only on one side of the head.

The fourth category of primary headache disorders include a mixed bag of different kinds of headaches. These include headaches brought on by cough or exercise, sexual activity, and many others. For each of these there is a defined set of criteria that need to be met for the diagnosis to be applied.

Occasionally, secondary headache disorders can fulfill clinical criteria for a primary headache disorder such as migraine, and it may take an astute clinician to realize that the headache disorder is secondary.

How is a headache disorder diagnosed?

In order to diagnose a headache disorder, the medical professional needs to take a comprehensive history of the headache disorder, including information about the onset of the headaches, the location and duration of the headaches, symptoms such as nausea or photophobia, and any aggravating features. They will typically also ask questions about medications used to treat the headaches and their effectiveness. In most cases, the history of the headache disorder is the most important part of the evaluation process, so it is helpful to provide as much information as possible. A comprehensive physical and neurological examination will be performed. Sometimes, this is all that is needed to make a diagnosis. Medical providers typically use a set of criteria to decide whether further workup is needed to exclude a secondary headache disorder. These tests can include laboratory tests or brain imaging. Based on the results of this comprehensive evaluation, and applying the diagnostic criteria, a diagnosis will be reached.

My head hurts all the time, what could cause this?

There are several different kinds of primary headache disorders that can give you a constant headache that does not go away. Some children can develop a headache that starts on a specific day and becomes constant within a few days. In many cases, they never suffered from significant headaches in the past. If they can recall the day that the headache starts, then the headache may be "new daily persistent headache." If they did have headaches prior to the constant headache, then it could be chronic migraine or chronic tension-type headache, depending on the features associated with the headache. Finally, hemicrania continua can cause a constant headache that does not seem to go away. This headache is usually only on one side and associated with ptosis, redness to the eye, nasal congestion, forehead sweating and other symptoms.

The MRI is normal. Does this mean that the headache is not a migraine?

It is important to point out that the diagnosis of migraine and other primary headache disorders is entirely based upon clinical criteria. There is no test that confirms the diagnosis of migraine or excludes it. The tests are used to look for other causes of headache, and these types of headaches will be treated by addressing the underlying cause. A normal MRI means that there is no evident structural cause of the headache.

Suggested Readings

Do T.P., Remmers A., Shytz H.W., Schankin C., Nelson S.E., Obermann M., Hansen J.M., Sinclair A.J., Gantenbein A.R., and Schoonman G.G. Red and orange flags for secondary headaches in clinical practice. *Neurology* 2019, vol. 92, 134-144.

Dodick D.W. Pearls: headache. *Semin Neurol* 2010, vol. 30, 74-81.

GBD 2016 Headache Collaborators. Global, regional, and national burden of migraine and tension-type headache, 1990-2016: a systematic analysis for the Global Burden of Disease Study 2016. *Lancet Neurology* 2018, vol. 17, 954-976.

Kelly M., Strelzik J., Langdon R., DiSabella M. Pediatric headache: overview. *Curr Opin Pediatr* 2018, vol. 30, 748-754

Tepper S.J., Dahlof C.G.H., Dowson A., Newman L., Mansbach H., Jones M., Webster C., and Salonen R. Prevalence and diagnosis of migraine in patients consulting their physician with a complaint of headache: data from the landmark study. *Headache* 2004, vol. 44, 856-864.

How can I Help My Child Without using Medications?

Wilson Heredia MD

Is using a preventive medication for migraine the best and only way to manage my child's migraine headaches?

It is certainly not. In fact, lifestyle modification is the cornerstone of migraine prevention in children with migraine headaches. The largest and most recognized study in the management of pediatric headaches is the Childhood and Adolescent Migraine Prevention (CHAMP) study. In that study, placebo was compared to pharmacological preventive therapy, and there was no significant difference between the pharmacological interventions and placebo. These results support a focus on lifestyle strategies that have been proven effective in prevention of pediatric migraine headaches, rather than pharmacological interventions. Among the lifestyle modifications with high success in managing headaches we have:

Sleep regulation. Sleep is fundamental for proper body and mind function, especially in the developing brain. In children with headaches, sleep plays a role in both recovery from and preventing headaches. For optimal health and development, the American Academy of Sleep Medicine recommends 9-12 hours of sleep for children 6-12 years old and 8-10 hours for children 13-18 years of age. In children with headaches, it is not only important that they sleep enough hours, but also that their sleep occurs on a regular schedule, meaning that the bedtime and wake up time should be roughly the same, regardless of whether it is a week or weekend day. You should also monitor your child for recurrent nighttime awakenings and snoring, as many children have enlarged tonsils/adenoids that can cause obstruction of airflow during sleep, leading to inadequate sleep. If there is concern for poor sleep quality or quantity, sleep hygiene techniques can be implemented. These include avoidance of naps, restricting fluids and voiding prior to bedtime, powering off electronics one hour prior to bedtime, avoiding using the bed for anything other than sleep, and maintaining both an adequate temperature and level of darkness in the room conducive for sleep.

Increased water intake. Poor water intake can cause many problems in your children, including worsening headaches. Most children drink insufficient amounts of water, especially during summer months, and this can intensify their headaches or make their headaches more difficult to control. Increasing hydration to 8-10 cups of non-caffeinated fluids has been proven to be effective in reduction of the headache burden in adults. Though no specific studies have been done in the pediatric population, there are extensive patients reports that dehydration leads to worsening headache in children, and hydration is one of the first interventions done in the Emergency Department when children present with severe and ongoing headaches.

Regular and healthy meals. Hunger is a well-known trigger for headaches both in adults and children. Several studies have shown that skipping meals, especially breakfast, can worsen or even trigger headaches.

Low or fluctuating levels of glucose in the brain could be responsible for triggering migraine headaches in children. In a study done in Europe, researchers determined that irregular eating patterns in the morning among migraine sufferers led to a high rate of missed school days. Skipping meals can also cause an increase in the intensity of headaches. It is important that your child eats all 3 main meals a day, with snacks in between.

Avoidance of caffeinated drinks. Both the consumption of caffeine and withdrawal from it can lead to headaches. Caffeine-containing drinks are frequently consumed by children and adolescents. Coffee, soft drinks, some teas, and energy drinks or pre-workout preparations can expose children to high levels of caffeine. A study conducted on adolescents who drank colas daily found that the gradual reduction of colas resulted in complete cessation of headaches. Note that it is important to decrease the daily intake of caffeine gradually to avoid withdrawal headaches. Always check the nutritional labels to make sure that any tea or soft drink is caffeine-free.

Exercise. The benefits of exercising on the health of both body and brain cannot be overestimated. In recent years there has been a decline in physical activity by adolescents, which is believed to negatively impact their headaches. Obesity and decreased levels of activity have been linked to a significant increase in headache frequency among children that suffer from migraine headaches. Studies have shown that exercise is effective in reducing the headache burden in children and adolescents. Researchers believe that this is due to a decreased perception of pain by the child, along with improvement of comorbidities commonly associated with headaches. Therefore, I strongly recommend increasing the level of exercise, especially aerobic exercise, in your child, to an extent that is sustainable and not overwhelming.

Screen time exposure. There has been a significant increase in the amount of screen time for children and adolescents through video games, smart phones, tablets, and computers. These are all now more accessible to children and often are required for school-related activities. A study of adolescents showed a strong association (80%) between headaches and over-usage of video games. Both migraine and tension-type headaches have been related to the excessive use of electronics in the adolescent population. It is important that you limit the exposure to screens for your child with headaches, and also that you make sure they are taking breaks from the screen every 30-45 minute to avoid overstimulation.

My child is suffering from headaches, but I am afraid of using medication and potential side effects. Are there any supplements that can be helpful in managing headaches in children?

Yes, there are several supplements that can provide benefits in managing headaches in children. In recent years, there has been many discussions about the role of nutraceuticals, a food or organic substance with a medicinal benefit, in the management of headaches, especially in children.
Some of the most researched supplements are listed below:

Riboflavin (Vitamin B2). Several randomized control trials have shown benefit of riboflavin in the prevention of pediatric and adolescent migraine, including a recent study which showed that riboflavin was both safe and effective in management of migraines in children without any other comorbidities. There is also evidence of riboflavin's effectiveness in management of tension-type headaches in children.

Magnesium. Magnesium is a well-known mineral in the management of headaches Magnesium deficiency has been associated with cortical spreading depression, a phenomenon that is related to the aura in migraine headaches with aura. Magnesium may also be used in the intravenous form to halt headaches in the emergency department. However, very few studies have been conducted on using magnesium in the prevention of migraine headaches in children. Current results are mixed, but some show a reduction in the intensity and frequency of headaches compared to placebo.

Coenzyme q10. Investigators have discovered that there are low levels of coenzyme q10 in children and adolescents with migraine headaches and treating the deficiency has been shown to reduce migraine frequency. However, the supplementation seems to be more effective in the first weeks of treatment with a subsequent plateau in impact on the migraines.

Melatonin. Melatonin can be extremely helpful in children with headaches, especially those with sleep-related comorbidities. Melatonin is a hormone normally produced in the pineal gland of the brain and is crucial in the regulation of our circadian rhythm (our internal clock), which is why it is commonly used in children with difficulty falling asleep. Several studies have shown that melatonin levels are low in patients suffering from different types of primary headaches (migraine, cluster and tension-type). The usage of melatonin has been proven to be effective in migraine headaches with and without sleep-related conditions.

My child's pediatrician told me that there are relaxation techniques that can help with my child's headaches is this true?

Absolutely. In fact, Cognitive Behavioral Therapy for headaches (CBT-HA), biofeedback techniques, and mindfulness-based interventions have some of the strongest supporting evidence in the management of headaches in adolescents and children, with no perceived side effects or contraindications.

CBT-HA sessions occur on a weekly basis for several weeks and have multiple treatment components, including diaphragmatic breathing, progressive muscle relaxation, imagery, active pacing, and distraction/ pleasant activity. Relaxation techniques were reported to be helpful by children and their parents. In several large and small-scale studies, there was a reduction in frequency of headaches up to 70%, reduced disability (*e.g.*, missed school days) and intensity of headaches. This evidence is positive for both migraine and non-migraine type headaches, including tension-type headaches (TTH). It was also shown, in some studies, that aside from the improvement in the headache burden, there was improvement in anxiety and depression symptoms, both common comorbidities among children and adolescents with chronic headaches.

Biofeedback techniques use sensors or electrodes to detect changes in body functions. The techniques are meant to teach the child how to control the biological changes that occur during stressful situations, such as pain from a headache. The sensors monitor the child's heart rate, breathing rate, muscle tension, and finger temperature. The child learns to recognize the changes in these parameters and is taught how to stop them, which leads to a decrease in muscle tension and amelioration of headaches. Similar to CBT, there was a significant reduction in headache frequency - up to 70% in some studies - and intensity. In one study, there was also improvement of the scalp and neck muscle tenderness reported in some patients with TTH.

Mindfulness-based interventions/relaxation training is another technique, which aims to relax the child in order to reduce the levels of pain. It is also effective in controlling anxiety. Studies have shown a 45% improvement in children with headaches managed with these techniques.

It has been postulated that the likely benefit from these three interventions is due to both the management of pain-related behavior and neuro-physiological changes to the brain. All three techniques have proven to be at least as effective as pharmacological therapy, and the sustainability and low side effect profile makes them ideal therapies for the management of different types of headaches in children and adolescents.

It is important to note that these techniques must be carried out by a licensed therapist/psychologist who has special training in one or more of these modalities.

I've seen some devices advertised for the management of headaches, are those devices safe to be used in children?

Yes, devices can be extremely useful in the management of children's headaches. In recent years the use of neuromodulation, defined as the alteration of nerve activity through targeted stimulation via an external or internal device, is one of the fastest growing fields in neurology. Devices have been approved for the management of several neurological conditions including seizures and movement disorders. In recent years many devices have been introduced to the market for the treatment of different types of headaches, both for prevention and acute treatment. Until recently, most of these devices were only used to treat adult patients, but now some have been approved for management of headaches in the pediatric population. The ease of use, the lack of adverse effects, established efficacy, and the non-invasive nature of these neuromodulation devices make them a very helpful tool in the management of children with headaches, both as first line or as adjunctive therapy.

Single-pulse Transcranial magnetic stimulation (sTMS) is indicated for the management of chronic migraine in adolescents and adults. A pivotal study done in children over the age of 12, showed that using the device twice per day was effective in migraine prevention, with a 1/3 reduction in the number of headaches and headache-related disability. The device is kidney bean-shaped and is applied in the back of the head, delivering single magnetic pulsation without any pain or discomfort. A larger study involving over 4000 children found no significant adverse effects or alterations on the developing brain with the use of this device.

External trigeminal nerve stimulation (eTNS) is indicated for both prevention and treatment of headaches. The device is a transcutaneous stimulator that was approved in adults for migraine prevention in 2014 and for abortive therapy in 2017. The indication was extended to children 12 years and older in February 2021. The device is placed on the forehead and delivers electrical pulsations to the trigeminal nerve, the cranial nerve that plays a major role in the pain related to migraine headaches. Several models of the device are available. The latest is the Dual device, that can be used for 20 minutes every day for prevention of headaches or 60 minutes for acute treatment of headaches with an optional repeat application one hour later. It is contraindicated in patients with metallic or electronic implants such as pacemakers, defibrillators, and vagal nerve stimulators. Studies in adults have shown complete termination of headaches in 1/3 of patients within an hour, and approximately 80% experienced pain relief. An additional 17% of patients were pain-free in two hours. Approximately 40% of the patients had at least 50% reduction in the number of headaches per month when using the daily-mode setting. The application is painless and is described as a light buzzing sensation. Safety data showed no significant side effects in either the adult or pediatric populations using this device. Currently this device is available online.

The Remote electrical neuromodulation (REN) is indicated for treatment of acute episodic and chronic migraine headaches in both adolescents and adults. The device is placed on the lateral upper arm and sends electrical signals to nerves under the skin, targeting the pain fibers on the nerves. The treatments last 45 minutes. The device has an interface with the user's smartphone that allows them to control the intensity of the output current of the electrical impulses. Studies in adolescents were conducted for both episodic and chronic migraine and showed that over 1/3 of the participants were pain-free after 2 hours, and over 70% had some degree of pain relief. There was also a 70% reduction in at least one of the most disabling associated symptoms (light/noise sensitivity, nausea, or vomiting). The pain freedom achieved with a single treatment was sustained in 90% of the users after 24 hours. There was no attenuation of effectiveness with repeated usage of the device. No major adverse were reported during the trials, except for pain/discomfort on the treatment arm, which resolved after finishing the treatment.

The Non-Invasive Vagus Nerve Stimulator (nVNS) works by stimulating the vagus nerve, a cranial nerve involved in the regulation of pain. It may be helpful for the preventive treatment of migraine headaches in children 12 and older. The device is placed on the neck and sends electrical stimulation to the vagus nerve. It is contraindicated in patients with an active implantable electronic device, such as a pacemaker, hearing aid implant, or any metallic device located in the neck, such as a stent, bone plate, or bone screws. Local rash, infection, swelling, cut, sore, drug patch, or surgical scars on the neck at the treatment location are also contraindications for use. One of the few studies done in children reported that approximately 50% of the migraine attacks treated were stopped with treatment, without need for rescue medications or significant side effects.

Can acupuncture be safely used and of benefit in children with headaches?

This is a question that I get asked a lot, probably because acupuncture is one of the oldest and most widely used interventions for many conditions, in particular pain management. Acupuncture works by promoting the activation of substances in our nervous system that regulate our perception of pain, as well as suppression of pain signals in the spinal cord and brainstem, which leads to inhibition of the pain pathways and reduces overall perception of pain. Several studies have been conducted regarding the usefulness of acupuncture in the management of headaches, mostly in adults. There are data from these studies showing that acupuncture can be beneficial in the prevention of migraine headaches. In adult studies, acupuncture was found to be effective in prevention of both chronic and episodic migraine headaches, as well as tension-type headaches. In children, several studies have shown promising data, including trials that compared real acupuncture versus placebo techniques. In one trial, 40% of the participants expressed complete resolution of their headaches. Alternative forms of acupuncture have also been studied, such as laser acupuncture and auricular (earlobe) acupuncture. Both forms may result in improvement in pediatric headaches. Acupuncture is typically well-tolerated in children, with the most common adverse effect being pain at the needle site. Nausea and other minor side effects are reported infrequently. Some children might fear needles, which is a limiting factor in this age group, but with proper comforting measures by the parents this can be overcome.

Recently I saw an advertisement for blue light-blocking glasses, can these glasses help with my child's headaches?

Unfortunately, there is not a clear-cut answer to this question, as there are many variables to consider.

For years, blue light-blocking eyewear has been tested in many conditions, demonstrating benefits in the management of some types of insomnia. Improvement of sleep can favorably impact the burden of headaches in children. Few studies are available addressing the usefulness of these glasses in pediatric headaches, but in theory they should be beneficial. Light has different wavelengths that are picked up by different receptors in our retinas. Several studies have shown that people with migraine are very sensitive to blue light, and therefore blocking this light would potentially help the light sensitivity experienced by some children with migraine. In a small group study of children with migraine headaches using tinted eyewear, there was reduction in the duration, frequency, and intensity of the headaches. This reduction was found to be sustained only on the participants wearing rose-tinted eyewear. You must be careful when purchasing any of these products, as many manufacturers are often not bound to quality standards.

Suggested Reading

Andrasik F, Grazzi L, Sansone E et al. Non-pharmacological Approaches for Headaches in Young Age: An Updated Review. *Front Neurol* 2018; 9: 1009.

Athaillah A, Dimyati Y, Saing B et al. Riboflavin as migraine prophylaxis in adolescents. *Paediatr Indones* 2012;52:132-137

Börner C, Urban G, Beaulieu L et al. The bottom-up approach: Non-invasive peripheral neurostimulation methods to treat migraine: A scoping review from the child neurologist's perspective. *European Journal of Paediatric Neurology* 2021;32:16-28,

Doll E, Threlkeld B, Graff D et al. Acupuncture in Adult and Pediatric Headache: A Narrative Review. *Neuropediatrics* 2019;50:346-352

Faedda N, Natalucci G, Baglioni V et al. Therapies in headache: focus on mindfulness and cognitive behavioral therapy in children and adolescents, *Expert Review of Neurotherapeutics* 2019;19:1219-1228,

Hershey AD, Lin T, Gruper Y, Harris D, Ironi A, Berk T, Szperka CL, Berenson F. Remote electrical neuromodulation for acute treatment of migraine in adolescents. *Headache* 2021;61:310-317

Kroon Van Diest AM, Ernst MM, Vaughn L, Slater S, Powers SW. CBT for Pediatric Migraine: A Qualitative Study of Patient and Parent Experience. *Headache* 2018;58:661-675.

Orr S, Venkateswaran S. Nutraceuticals in the prophylaxis of pediatric migraine: Evidence-based review and recommendations. *Cephalalgia* 2014;34:568–583

Patterson-Gentile C, Szperka C. The Changing Landscape of Pediatric Migraine Therapy a Review. *JAMA Neurol* 2018;75:881-887.

Rajapakse T, Pringsheim T. Nutraceuticals in Migraine: A Summary of Existing Guidelines for Use. *Headache* 2016;56:808-816

Singh R, Ailani J, Robbins M. Neuromodulation for the Acute and Preventive Therapy of Migraine and Cluster Headache, *Headache* 2019; 59:33-49

"Can I Pass on Headaches to My Kids?"

Monica Chan, MD

Fellow in Headache Medicine
Icahn School of Medicine at Mt. Sinai
New York City

I had migraines when I was young and I remember my mom also has them. Will my kids also get migraines when they are older?

Headaches are very common in children, up to 60% globally, and of those, 7.7 to 9.1% have migraines (though this is likely an underestimate). Seventy-five percent of children with migraine will also likely continue to get migraines as adults.

Migraines are thought to have a strong hereditary basis, but it is more complex than simply one "migraine" gene that is passed down through families. Lifestyle and environmental factors likely also play a part in whether someone gets migraines, although this is still under investigation. Different studies have shown the strong inheritance pattern in migraines. In one study, if one parent has migraines, there can be a 50-75% chance their children get migraines too. Many genes have been found to be linked with migraines but specific genes with a clear inheritance pattern have not been determined.

In genome-wide association studies (GWAS), multiple single-nucleotide polymorphisms (SNPs) have been identified that are associated with migraines. The SNPs are found in genes involved in various pathways of migraine pathology including genes for pain sensitivity and glutamatergic neurotransmission. Research is ongoing since the pathophysiology of migraines itself is quite complex. There is a rare type of migraine called "familial hemiplegic migraine" in which specific genes have been identified for certain subtypes.

Studies have shown that 75% of people with migraines report onset before age 35. The age of onset has also been found to be related to genetics. Children of parents with migraines start getting migraines an average of 11 to 12 years earlier than their parents and earlier than children without a family history of migraines. Since you have migraines, it is likely that your child has some of these "migraine genes" and may develop migraines at an earlier age.

How can I know if my kid gets migraines? Is there anything I should look out for to see if my kid will get migraines?

Migraines in children can have different characteristics than those of adults and some of this has been accounted for in the *International Classification of Headache Disorders, Third Edition (ICHD-3)* criteria. In children, migraines can be shorter than in adults; ICHD-3 defines a minimum of 2 hours, but it can be as short as 30 min in children under 5 years old. The ICHD-3 criteria also account for the fact that most children with migraines also have bilateral pain rather than unilateral pain seen in adults with migraines.

In early childhood, migraines can also manifest as other syndromes in which there is no headache component, and only later do typical migraine headaches become prominent. These were previously termed "childhood periodic syndromes" under ICHD-2, but now, under ICHD-3, are termed "episodic syndromes" that may be associated with migraine. Like migraines, these are episodes of recurrent symptoms in which patients are completely healthy in between episodes during which headaches may or may not be present. These syndromes include benign paroxysmal torticollis (BPT), cyclical vomiting syndrome (CVS), abdominal migraine, and benign paroxysmal vertigo (BPV). These episodic syndromes are thought of as both a migraine precursor and a migraine equivalent in children, and are only diagnosed after other possible causes are ruled out. Motion sickness as a child has also been found to be associated with migraines later in life.

In BPT, the child has a head tilt and is pale, without pain or vomiting, lasting minutes to days. It is diagnosed after excluding structural abnormalities in the brain. In BPV, children ages 2-4 years old can have sudden attacks of vertigo and inability to stand for a few seconds to minutes. Abdominal migraines are acute, moderate to severe attacks of midline abdominal pain lasting hours that can be associated with nausea, vomiting, pallor, and anorexia. Headaches may be absent during abdominal migraine attacks.

CVS are recurrent episodes of severe nausea and vomiting, occurring multiple times per hour.

Though infantile colic is not listed in ICHD-3 as an episodic syndrome that may be associated with migraine, studies have shown that a baby with infantile colic has an increased likelihood of developing migraines in the future compared with infants who did not have colic. Though more investigation is needed, motion sickness has also been described as a possible migraine precursor.

Can I prevent my kids from getting migraines when they are older?

Since we still do not know the exact genetic basis of everyone's migraines, we do not know if there are ways to prevent someone from developing migraines. However, maintaining a healthy lifestyle and avoiding migraine triggers can reduce migraine attack frequency. Keeping a consistent day to day routine is important; skipped meals (particularly breakfast), irregular caffeine intake, irregular sleep cycles, and stress are common migraine triggers. For some people, certain foods which trigger migraines can be avoided although other triggers such as changes in the weather are harder, if not impossible, to avoid. Trying to prevent motion sickness such as not reading or watching a screen while in a car can also help prevent a migraine attack. A mnemonic to use for lifestyle considerations is SMART - Sleep, Meals, Activity, Relaxation, Triggers.

Of course, if your child does end up having frequent migraines, preventive treatment should be considered.

Can my kids get other kinds of headaches?

Aside from migraines, children can have other primary headache disorders including tension-type headache, trigeminal autonomic cephalgias (which includes cluster headache), and primary stabbing headache. Like adults, migraines and tension-type headaches are the most common primary headaches in children.

Tension-type headaches are typically mild to moderate headaches that are often not brought up to a doctor since they have little impact on day-to-day life. They occur in 10% to 24% of children and do not have the associated symptoms seen in migraines (such as nausea and vomiting) and are never severe.

Although trigeminal autonomic cephalalgias (TACs) are rare in children, some adult patients with cluster headaches have reported that their headaches began in childhood or adolescence. Cluster headaches present with sharp pain around the eyes on one side, lasting between 30 and 180 minutes. There are autonomic symptoms such as eyelid swelling, red eyes, tearing, and constriction of pupils on the side of the headache. Children can be restless and agitated.

Primary stabbing headache has a scary sounding name which goes along with its severe symptoms; however it is another primary headache syndrome that children may have. It can also be known as an "ice pick" headache where there is 1-3 seconds of stabbing pain. Despite the alarming name, it is almost always a primary headache and is benign.

Suggested Reading

Abu-Arafeh I, Howells R. Primary Headaches in Children Under the Age of 7 Years. *Curr Pain Headache Rep*. 2014;18(3):401.

Ashina M. Migraine. *N Engl J Med*. 2020;383(19):1866-1876.

Cuvellier J-C, Lépine A. Childhood Periodic Syndromes. *Pediatr Neurol*. 2010;42(1):1-11.

Özge A, Faedda N, Abu-Arafeh I, et al. Experts' opinion about the primary headache diagnostic criteria of the ICHD-3rd edition beta in children and adolescents. *J Headache Pain*. 2017;18(1):109.

Silberstein SD, Dodick DW. Migraine Genetics: Part II. *Headache J Head Face Pain*. 2013;53(8):1218-1229.

Szperka C. Headache in Children and Adolescents. *Contin Lifelong Learn Neurol*. 2021;27(3).

THE MIGRAINE PATIENT WITH AURA

ROBERT MYERS, DO
HEADACHE SPECIALIST
HOBOKEN, NEW JERSEY

Sometimes I see squiggly lines before my migraines. What is that all about?

What you are experiencing may be a migraine visual aura. A migraine aura *is a recurrent condition* that usually lasts between 5 to 60 minutes and almost always resolves completely. Aura usually does not get worse over time and rarely results in any permanent damage to your brain or eyes. A typical migraine aura is characterized by any combination of change in vision, speech, and/or sensation that also lasts at least 5 minutes, but no more than an hour. Often the visual symptoms occur in both eyes simultaneously then migrate from the center of your vision to the periphery or towards the center from the periphery. While aura usually occurs in both eyes simultaneously. it can occur in just one eye, and when that happens it is classified as "retinal migraine." Occasionally visual aura is associated with a blind spot or focus of blurred/distorted vision. It is not unusual for visual aura to manifest as zigzag lines, bright flashing lights, 'foggy' vision, and many others. Sometimes people describe what they see in exotic ways such as "It's like there was a psychedelic rainbow in my eyes" and "everything is covered in tv static". A particularly striking manifestation of migraine aura is known as "Alice in Wonderland Syndrome" or AIWS for short. This consists of various perceptual distortions from "everything looking wavy like a fun house mirror" to things appearing much larger or smaller than they are. How long do your visual symptoms last? Do they ever last more than an hour?

They usually last 15 minutes then go away completely, but I have had a couple that have lasted a little over an hour. I have noticed that they do occur in both eyes at the same time and usually start in the center of my vision then sort of slowly move to the outer field of my vision. Usually, my headache will start after the aura, but sometimes visual symptoms happen, and I never get a headache.

It isn't unusual for a visual aura to occur without a headache, when this happens the technical term for it is "acephalgic migraine" which is the medical way to say "migraine without headache." It may seem confusing at first because most people are only familiar with the 'headache' portion of migraine, but the physiologic process of migraine consists of more than just head pain. Headache is one of the four phases of migraine. Aura is also one of the 4 phases of migraine and tends to be the shortest, typically lasting only up to 60 minutes. You mentioned that sometimes your aura lasts more than 60 minutes. Aura has traditionally been thought to only last up to 60 minutes, but research has shown that it is not uncommon for aura to last more than 60 minutes, when this occurs, we call it "prolonged aura."

The four phases of migraine are important for you to be aware of. The phases are: prodrome, aura (which some people never experience), headache phase, and postdrome. All migraineurs usually experience any number and combination of prodromal symptoms before a headache but they may not recognize these until a physician asks about them. Prodromal symptoms can manifest as irritability, yawning, cold hands and feet, increased urination, light/sound sensitivity, difficulty concentrating, food cravings, and sleep difficulty or even other symptoms prior to headache and/or aura. This prodromal phase is much longer than the migraine aura and can last from hours to days. The migraine postdrome tends to last 24-48 hours, occurs after the severe headache has resolved and can consist of difficulty concentrating, fatigue, and/or mood changes, and often a mild headache. It is important to mention that people with poorly controlled headaches may have pro and postdromal symptoms usually, but they rarely have aura all of the time.

How can you tell if these symptoms are different from a stroke? I've heard that aura increases risk of stroke. Do I need to have an MRI?

Fortunately, a good medical history can help distinguish aura from more serious neurologic conditions such as seizure and stroke. Usually, we can tell from your description of the symptoms whether it sounds like migraine aura or if more extensive evaluation is necessary to exclude other causes. This is because the clinical manifestation of aura helps distinguish it from more concerning disorders. For instance, aura tends to gradually develop over minutes whereas seizures commonly progress over seconds and transient ischemic and stroke symptoms tend to be sudden onset without fluctuation. Though there are rare exceptions to this rule.

Overall, for every 1000 migraine aura patients, about 1 to 2 will have a stroke every year. This risk increases if you have aura, but particularly if you have poorly controlled high blood pressure, high cholesterol, and/or uncontrolled diabetes so it is important to have a primary care physician that can help you optimize these. Smoking greatly increases risk of stroke for anyone so you should avoid that. Cannabis smoke and vapor might also increase this risk, so to be safe you should probably avoid this too. Estrogen containing oral contraceptives can also increase the risk of stroke for people with migraine aura, so we recommend that female patients avoid those as well. We don't know whether treating migraine will help protect against stroke, but it might.

If a stroke or seizure isn't causing these symptoms then what is? How do we know that it isn't something more serious?

Until the 20th century there was no definitive way to distinguish migraine aura from other processes such as epilepsy and stroke. Physicians have documented the aura phenomenon for hundreds of years but despite familiarity with the condition, aura, like many other central nervous system phenomena, have been notoriously difficult to study due to the complex anatomy and physiology of the brain. The underlying mechanism responsible for the migraine aura is a complex was finally identified thanks to the invention of the electroencephalogram (EEG). EEG allows neurologists to examine the electrical activity on the outer layer of the brain known as the cortex. During an aura, a wave of activation is seen crossing a large portion of the cortex, this is followed by a wave of prolonged decreased activity. A good analogy would be a forest fire, it spreads quickly, is over fast, and it takes a while for normal forest activity to resume afterwards. This process is termed "cortical spreading depression" (CSD) and has consistently been shown to occur with the migraine aura. With the identification of CSD it was now clear that aura represents its own distinct physiologic entity separate from epilepsy and stroke. Most preventive medications to treat migraine also reduce CSD.

Is this going to get worse over time? If it becomes more frequent, I think it would start interfering with my work.

People with migraine aura live normal lifespans and the aura can often become less frequent over the years, although this is not always the case. If it does increase in frequency or begins to interfere with work, then we might want to consider starting you on a medication that can help prevent the aura. While there are no specific therapies to stop or shorten the aura once it has begun, there are several migraine medications that may help prevent the attacks. These medications are classified as some anti-epileptic medications because they were initially developed to prevent seizures, some blood pressure medications, and some anti-depressant medications. They have all been around a long time and have been well studied in migraine patients. No medications have been engineered to target the aura specifically.

A friend of mine gets terrible vertigo with her headaches, could this be aura too?

Rarely aura will manifest in more exotic ways, such as slurred speech, vertigo, ear ringing, partial hearing loss, double vision, incoordination, and/or decreased level of consciousness. When this occurs, it is classified as "brainstem aura", meaning that the brain structures involved in the migraine aura process are *thought to be located the brainstem, though this is a matter of debate*. The rarest form of aura is commonly mistaken for transient ischemic attack (TIA) or stroke and is known as "hemiplegic migraine." This involves weakness on one side that is associated with any combination of visual, speech, sensation change and/or brainstem aura. If brainstem aura or hemiplegic migraine symptoms occur, we usually need to do imaging such as MRI to rule out causes like stroke and tumors as potential causes for the symptoms. As far as we know, brainstem and hemiplegic aura do not confer any greater increased risk of stroke as compared with the typical migraine aura.

My elderly grandmother just had similar symptoms for the first time in her life. She went to her ophthalmologist but they didn't see anything. What should she do?

Lots of serious medical conditions can cause transient visual changes so she did the right thing by starting with her ophthalmologist. Depending on what occurred and her medical risk factors, she may need further work up such as blood work to check cholesterol and blood sugar, imaging of the blood vessels in her neck, evaluation of her heart to check for abnormal rhythms, and screening for high blood pressure. They may determine that she has new onset visual aura. It is not rare for late life onset of migraine aura to occur, and visual symptoms are the most common manifestation of new onset migraine aura in older patients.

Suggested reading

Demarquay, G., Ducros, A., Montavont, A., & Mauguiere, F. (2018). Migraine with brainstem aura: Why not a cortical origin? *Cephalalgia*, *38*(10), 1687-1695.

Dodick, D. W. (2018). A phase-by-phase review of migraine pathophysiology. *Headache: the journal of head and face pain*, *58*, 4-16.

Haan, J., Hollander, J., & Ferrari, M. D. (2007). Migraine in the elderly: a review. *Cephalalgia*, *27*(2), 97-106.

Sheikh, H. U., Pavlovic, J., Loder, E., & Burch, R. (2018). Risk of stroke associated with use of estrogen containing contraceptives in women with migraine: a systematic review. *Headache: The Journal of Head and Face Pain*, *58*(1), 5-21.

Viana, M., Sprenger, T., Andelova, M., & Goadsby, P. J. (2013). The typical duration of migraine aura: a systematic review. *Cephalalgia*, *33*(7), 483-490.

Viana, M., Tronvik, E.A., Do, T.P. *et al.* Clinical features of visual migraine aura: a systematic review. *J Headache Pain* 20, 64 (2019).

ALICE IN WONDERLAND

SUHAIL SIDHU AND SHEENA K AURORA

When I saw AW in clinic for the first time, she was twelve, and her mother brought her in because of a strange phenomenon that AW had experienced. AW was an avid piano player, and while playing the piano, she felt that the keys lifted from the piano, and became three times their size. She had no previous neurological problems, experienced normal developmental milestones, and did well in school. AW had recently experienced some mild headaches accompanied by nausea. Her mother was a patient in my clinic and had an episodic migraine for many years.

Why do I experience these phenomena?

This visual phenomenon is known as "Alice in Wonderland Syndrome" (AIWS) also sometimes known as Todd's syndrome or lilliputian hallucinations. You may recall in the book "Alice in Wonderland' by Lewis Carroll Alice goes through a series of visual experiences when she falls into a deep hole while following a rabbit. These illusions were just ten inches tall and acquiring different sizes after eating a cake. Alice's experiences were like those which AW reported. In neurological terms it's called macropsia and micropsia. Patients may also get episodes of pelopsia, (objects appear closer than they are), teleopsia (objects appear farther than they are), or both. In AW's case this occurred in conjunction with her onset of migraine, but this is not always the case. AIWS seems to occur more often in patients with a personal or a family history of migraine.

What is the neurological basis of Alice in Wonderland Syndrome?

The putative mechanism of migraine aura is spreading cortical depression (SCD) emanating from a hyperexcitable cortex, most commonly from the occipital cortex. Imaging studies have demonstrated that a wave of excitation starts in the occipital cortex and spreads slowly. Approximately twenty years ago our group at Henry Ford Hospital under the leadership of Dr. Michael Welch had demonstrated direct current (DC) shifts using a 162 channel whole head magnetoencephalogram (MEG). These DC shifts were captured using the classic method of inducing SCD on animal brains with potassium chloride (KCl) (potassium chloride). This activity was overlaid on a functional MRI that captured areas of activation in the occipital cortex and in some patients as far as the parietal cornices.

We used the same model of activation and studied AW using BOLD (Blood Oxygen Level Dependent)-effect fMRI and found that compared to 'controls', she had more activation in the parietal areas. Although this is a single case report however it provides support the prevailing theory of hyperexcitability in migraine. Perhaps this phenomenon occurs when more eloquent areas of the occipital cortex become activated.

How is Alice in Wonderland Diagnosed?

The diagnosis is made from the history and a normal neurological and neuro-ophthalmological examination. It may be reasonable to get an MRI particularly if the phenomenon is prolonged, or there is no family history of migraine. The yield for any findings will probably be low. Whether MRA scans of the brain and neck provide additional diagnostic information is unknown from published cases. Internal carotid or vertebral artery dissection can mimic migraine with aura with visual aura only or a march of symptoms associated with a migraine-like headache.

How is Alice in Wonderland Treated?

For most patients this phenomenon lasts only a few minutes and does not seem to impair their activities of daily living. Since the original case series was published, I have had a slew of inquiries. Most patients have had a personal or a family history of migraine and were more just fascinated with the diagnosis. Some were relieved to hear that there were others that had similar experiences and wanted/needed solace and reassurance. Since this is a rare phenomenon, no medications will probably be shown to be effective in a double-blind, placebo-controlled studies therefore the selection of treatment is empirical and anecdotal. If patients start experiencing multiple events, such as some perhaps triggered by stress, I usually recommend magnesium supplementation. If they experience debilitating migraine along with this form of aura, certain medications may be helpful. Valproate, topiramate and memantine may be of particular interest since they appear to target brain hyperexcitability. Other health care practitioners have reported benefit from using calcium channel blockers and beta-blockers.

Suggested Reading

Blom, JD. Alice in Wonderland Syndrome: A Systematic Review. Neurology. Clinical Practice, Lippincott Williams & Wilkins, June 2016, www.ncbi.nlm.nih.gov/pmc/articles/PMC4909520/.

ElTarhouni AH, Beer L, Mouthon M, et al. The right thalamic ventral posterolateral nucleus seems to be determinant for macrosomatognosia: a case report. BMC Neurol 2020 Oct 28;20(1):393.

Hossain MM. Alice in Wonderland syndrome (AIWS): a research overview AIMS Neurosci. 2020 Oct 19;7(4):389-400.

Lanska DJ, Lanska JR. The Alice-in-Wonderland Syndrome. Front Neurol Neurosci 2018;42:142-150..

Sometimes I have Vision Changes that are Like My Migraine Auras, but I do Not have a Headache, are These Still Migraines?

Terrence Tian, DO, MPH

Sometimes I have vision changes that are like my migraine auras, but I do not have a headache. Are these still migraines?

They absolutely can be. You do not always have to have a headache with an aura. A migraine aura can occur before, during or even without a headache. There is something called "typical aura without headache" that is a subtype of migraine. It used to be called "acephalgic migraine." It is possible that you have this subtype of migraine depending on what symptoms you have. 38% of people with migraine with aura have experienced typical aura without headache, and vision change is the most common presentation of typical aura without headache. It is quite common for the elderly to have auras without headache, particularly older men, but they can occur in any group.

How do we know there isn't something else wrong? Are there official definitions for typical aura without headache?

We have a reference book that defines different headache types. Based on the third edition of the International Classification of Headache Disorders (ICHD-3), a typical aura without headache is a migraine with aura in which the aura is neither accompanied nor followed by a headache. It should first fulfill criteria for migraine with typical aura, which means the aura consists of visual, sensory, and/or speech/language symptoms, but without motor weakness. It is characterized by gradual development, duration of each symptom lasting no longer than one hour, and be completely reversible.

So, people do not have to ever have had a headache to have this?

It is certainly possible that some people never experience headaches in their life, but just auras. Others experience migraine headache with aura early in life, followed by a decrease in headaches later in life while they continue to have auras. Some even forget that they had migraine headaches when they were young.

Why is it that some people have a headache while others just have an aura?

The short answer is we don't know. We do not know the exact mechanism of auras and migraines and various explanations have been hypothesized in previous years. To better answer this question, we need to discuss a phenomenon called "cortical spreading depression," which we think leads to migraines and aura formation. In cortical spreading depression, a wave of intense activation of nerves spreads across the brain and is followed by a zone of suppressed of activity. This is thought to modify the local blood flow and metabolism of certain parts of the brain (brainstem and cerebral cortex) resulting in the symptoms of migraine aura, especially visual aura. This wave of neuronal depression spreads across the brain at a rate of 3 to 5mm per minute. The type of aura you experience is based on the location of the brain that is affected by the cortical spreading depression. With that said, it is thought that some auras are not accompanied by a headache because the cortical spreading depression is strong enough to trigger an aura but was not strong enough to trigger a headache.

How common is typical aura without headache?

This type of migraine accounts for about 4% of all migraines, and just like migraines in general, it is more common in females than males (3% vs 1%).

Is there an age we typically experience this?

These auras tend to occur later in life. However, one study showed perhaps there are two peak age ranges between 20 to 39 years and 60 to 69 years.

What are the usual visual auras people experience?

There is a variety of visual symptoms people can experience. Visual symptoms typically include flashes of light (photopsia), dark or blurry spot like a blind spot (scotoma) that can flicker between light and dark (scintillating scotoma), loss of vision in half of the visual field (hemianopia), double vision (diplopia), distortion of straight lines to look wavy (metamorphopsia), and transient blindness in one eye. These are not "eye" problems; these occur in the part of the brain that controls vision.

The visual aura usually begins in the center of the visual field and then progress to the outside. Less commonly it may start in the periphery and work its way into the center of vision. This usually affects both eyes and typically lasts 15-30 minutes. Duration should be between 5 and 60 minutes. Visual auras can be separated into positive and negative features. Positive features are most common and occur in 90% of people. These include bright objects (bright lights or dots, white spots, flashing lights), colored lights (multicolored zigzag patterns), and moving objects (dancing or waving lines) and result from that activation of nerves that we spoke about. Negative features are less common but still occur in 50% of people. These include things associated with some loss of vision, such as black spots, blind spots, transient vision loss, blurred vision, visual field cuts, tunnel vision, and blindness that result from the nerves being "depressed" and not firing.

Should I be concerned if I have multiple auras in a day?

Not necessarily. The visual aura can occur multiple times a day. You can also have different appearing visual auras.

Can the auras change over time?

It is also important to note that auras can change over time, so don't be alarmed by some changes in your aura. For example, one case involved a 41-year-old woman who first experienced recurrent vision changes at the age of 33 while pregnant. She described seeing gray wavy lines in her superior visual field of both eyes that lasted 5 to 30 minutes. The vision changes occurred multiple times a day and she did not have an accompanying headache. These happened during each of her pregnancies. Then at the age of 40, she experienced a different visual disturbance while driving. She saw a small silvery geometric shape in her vision that spiraled and enlarged. It lasted about 20 minutes before gradually dissipating. Then about 30-60 minutes later, she developed a migraine headache with light and sound sensitivity.

Auras can also increase in frequency as people age and in those with longer histories of migraine.

When should I be concerned about my aura?

You should inform a medical provider when an aura occurs for the first time after age 40, when symptoms are exclusively negative (isolated vision loss, particularly in only one eye), when aura is prolonged (>60 minutes) or very short (<5 minutes) in duration, or when symptoms fail to resolve.

Are there other medical conditions I should be worried about?

In general, with migraineurs, we perform a detailed evaluation of your headache history, medical history and neurological exam to rule out any other conditions. We can also perform additional brain imaging to look for structural problems in the brain. In addition, we sometimes recommend following up with an ophthalmologist to make sure there are no eye issues that could be causing the vision changes. We almost always recommend this when the aura affects one eye only, which could represent a retinal detachment. However, if it is clear that the vision change is in a visual field (affecting both eyes), that part is unnecessary.

More specifically, when there are transient episodes of neurological deficits, we are first worried about transient ischemic attacks. Similarly, seizures can present with brief episodes with neurological impairments or alterations. Brain lesions such as tumors can present similarly. However, we would also expect to see other neurological deficits and not just auras, such as weakness in one limb or one side of the body.

Do I need to treat these auras?

Auras resolve on their own, frequently more rapidly than any medication would take effect. Most typical duration auras also do not tend to respond to acute migraine medication. Sometimes preventive measures may be helpful.

If the visual auras become more bothersome, are there medications I can take?

Yes, you can, but unfortunately there are no clinical trials evaluating treatment options for typical aura without headache. There are many case reports suggesting most people respond to the usual treatments for migraine with aura.

If you are having a prolonged aura and you want to abort it, case reports have suggested various medications such as isoproterenol inhalation, calcium channel blockers divalproex sodium, and lamotrigine. A prospective study examining bilateral greater occipital nerve blocks using bupivacaine 0.5% showed prolonged aura (>2 hours) improvement in 85% of people, usually within 30 minutes, and complete resolution in 60%. Basically, preventive migraine drugs need to be used to prevent auras. The acutely administered drugs tend not to improve or worsen aura.

Are there other headache conditions that present similarly?

There are several I can discuss with you. Retinal migraine, migraine with brainstem auras, and late onset migraine accompaniments come to mind.

Retinal migraine is an extremely rare condition that can present similarly with vision changes. ICHD-3 defines this as repeated attacks of fully reversible visual disturbances in one eye (monocular) associated with migraine headache. It can occur without a headache as well. 65% of people experience only negatives features, while 31% experience both negative and positive features, but only 4% have only positive features. Symptoms should resolve within 60 minutes.

Migraine with brainstem auras can also exist without headaches, previously known as "basilar migraine." There are typical aura symptoms in addition to the brainstem symptoms during most episodes. Brainstem aura can present with a variety of neurological manifestations. To meet criteria for migraine with brainstem aura, at least two of the following fully reversible brainstem symptoms need to be present and last 5 to 60 minutes: slurred speech (dysarthria), dizziness (vertigo), ear ringing (tinnitus), increased hearing sensitivity (hyperacusis), double vision (diplopia), impaired coordination or imbalance (ataxia) and decreased level of consciousness. You can also have one-sided eyelid drooping (unilateral ptosis) and hiccups.

As I already mentioned, late onset migraine accompaniments is a subcategory of typical aura without headache, normally seen after age 40. People begin to have migraine aura symptoms in mid or late life without headaches. Visual symptoms are the most common presentation in 92-100% of people, followed by sensory symptoms in 28-31%, speech changes in 18-33%, and motor symptoms in 2-6%.

Suggested Reading

Aiba S, Tatsumoto M, Saisu A, Iwanami H, Chiba K, et al. Prevalence of typical migraine aura without headache in Japanese ophthalmology clinics. *Cephalalgia* 2010;30:962–967.

Cuadrado ML, Aledo-Serrano Á, López-Ruiz P, Gutiérrez-Viedma Á, Fernández C, et al. Greater occipital nerve block for the acute treatment of prolonged or persistent migraine aura. *Cephalalgia* 2017;37:812–818.

Grosberg BM, Solomon S, Friedman DI, Lipton RB. Retinal migraine reappraised. *Cephalalgia* 2006;26:1275-1286.

He Y, Li Y, Nie Z. Typical aura without headache: a case report and review of the literature. *J Med Case Rep* 2015;9:40-44.

Headache Classification Committee of the International Headache Society (IHS). The International Classification of Headache Disorders, 3rd edition. *Cephalalgia* 2018;38(1):1–211.

Lai J, Dilli E. Migraine aura: updates in pathophysiology and management. *Curr Neurol Neurosci Rep* 2020;20:17-26.

Russell MB, Olesen J. A nosographic analysis of the migraine aura in a general population. *Brain* 1996;119:355-361.

Shah DR, Dilwali S, Friedman DI. Current aura without headache. *Curr Pain Headache Rep* 2018;22:77-84.

Vongvaivanich K, Lertakyamanee P, Silberstein SD, Dodick DW. Late-life migraine accompaniments: a narrative review. *Cephalalgia* 2015;35:894–911.

How Do Hormones Affect My Migraine?

Huma U Sheikh, MD

I have had migraines since I was 13 and they always tend to be worse around the time of my menstrual cycle.

Yes, that is not uncommon. Prior to puberty, migraine tends to be more common in boys but after puberty the prevalence increases in girls and then stays that way through the lifetime. For women, hormonal changes are a huge trigger for migraine attacks. This is most common during the monthly changes that occur with menstruation. However, hormonal changes during the time of pregnancy and menopause also influence a women's migraine frequency and severity.

Studies show that about 20% of women notice some relation of their migraine attacks during the time of their menstrual cycle and/or ovulation. It is most common with the subtype of migraine without aura. The most important component of the changes in hormones is the fluctuation in estrogen that occurs with the bleeding of menstruation as well as in ovulation. During this time, there is drop in estrogen which is thought to be the important component that is a trigger for a migraine attack. Estrogen plays a role in the development of pain in the brain, which is an essential part of migraine.

The ICHD-3 has two diagnoses related to migraine and menstrual cycle. The first is "pure menstrual migraine without aura". In this diagnosis a woman has migraine attacks exclusively on days of her menstrual cycle, but no attacks outside of that. The other more common diagnosis is menstrually-related migraine, in which women have migraine attacks during a women's menstrual cycle but will also have other attacks outside of that time. There are similar diagnoses for the subtype of migraine with aura.

How can I treat the migraine attacks that occur with my menstrual cycles?

There are several strategies that can be used to treat the migraine attacks that occur during menstruation or ovulation. There are no specific treatments made specifically for menstrual migraine but the other medications that are used can be tailored to help during this time. The main abortive medications used are triptans and ergots, medications that are made specifically for migraine, as well as other non-specific medications, like NSAID's. There have been studies looking at the use of different triptans for menstrual migraine. Sumatriptan, zolmitriptan, frovatriptan and rizatriptan have all been studied and found to be more effective than placebo for pain relief. These have all been studied as abortive therapy to take when the migraine attacks occur.

Triptans have also been studied extensively as prophylaxis for menstrual migraine. Several triptans including naratriptan and frovatriptan have been studied as "mini-prophylaxis." This means that a person will take it daily starting a few days below and during the menstrual cycle. Frovatriptan has the longest half-life and was shown to be helpful in the trials comparing this medication with no treatment. It is a possible option to be used for menstrually-related migraine. It is important to keep in mind that there is a risk of medication overuse headache as well as other side effects.

Naproxen has also been used as prophylaxis around the time of a woman's menstruation to help with the migraine attacks. This involves taking naproxen daily for the few days before and after onset of menses. It was found that this prophylaxis helped to decrease the number and duration of migraine attacks, although the number of patients in the study was small.

Since there is a hormonal component of menstrual migraine, one other strategy to help with menstrual migraine is to use hormonal therapies or contraceptives. This is based off of the fact that it is the drop in the estrogen that is a trigger for migraine and hormonal contraceptives will stabilize this. There have been a few studies looking at the use of hormones for prophylaxis of menstrual migraine. Hormonal therapies have been shown to be effective in generally lowering the number of headache days in menstrually-related migraine. However, they also show that headaches tend to increase on the days when the estrogen component is stopped. Extended or continuous combined hormonal contraceptive therapy may be effective, but it is important to take an individualized approach, as there may be other side effects. In women with migraine with aura, there are studies to show that hormonal contraceptive therapy may increase the risk of stroke, which is essential to keep in mind.

If a patient is also having headaches outside of their menstrual cycle, it can be a good option to start preventive medication. These could include the use of daily oral medications, or one of the newer injectable medications targeting a chemical in the migraine pathway known as CGRP. There are also now newer migraine specific drugs called “CGRP antagonists” or “gepants” which may play roles of either abortive or preventive medications. These may provide newer ways to help with migraine during the time of menstruation and ovulation.

How are hormonally related migraines different than regular migraine attacks?

In general, menstrually-related migraine is thought to have a similar pathophysiology as those with migraine unrelated to menstruation. However, for menstrual related migraine, the changes in hormone at the time of menstruation are a strong trigger for the onset of migraine attacks. Some studies have looked at the characteristics between migraine attacks related to menstruation versus those that are linked to other triggers. One study showed that those with menstrually-related migraine had more severe attacks, including more severe nausea, photophobia and phonophobia; and the headaches tended to last longer. Some studies have also shown that menstrually-related migraine tends to be more difficult to treat.

What will happen to my migraines if I decide to become pregnant?

During pregnancy, there are several changes that occur, including fluctuations in hormones. One of the changes include the rise in estrogen in the first trimester which becomes more stable during the second and third trimester. There are some studies to show the natural progression of migraine during pregnancy.

Studies show that most women will have improvement of their migraine attacks during pregnancy. There is a fluctuation in estrogen levels in the first trimester which may worsen migraine early on but typically they will improve in the second and third trimesters when the hormone levels are more stable. Although that is the typical pattern, some women may experience their first migraine attack during pregnancy.

The postpartum period is another time of huge fluctuation in hormone levels that therefore may again worsen headaches. Some women may notice a decrease in headaches with breastfeeding. About one third of women will notice that they have headaches soon after giving birth.

Although migraine attacks in pregnancy and after delivery are not uncommon, it is important to also be aware of headaches that may be a sign of another issue in the brain. Pregnancy can put women at high risk of clots in the brain as well as high spinal fluid pressure. It is important to keep these in mind if a woman has a headache that is not her usual migraine or is different in characteristic.

Treating migraine attacks during pregnancy and post-partum times can be difficult, since many of the medications may affect the growing fetus and young baby. There are some possible strategies, including lidocaine blocks and complementary methods like relaxation therapies and mindfulness that may be effective in treating migraine during this time. If these are not helpful, it is important to reach out to a healthcare provider for other treatment options, who balance the risks and benefits of treatment.

Will my migraine change when I go through menopause?

Menopause is again a time where there is a lot of fluctuation in hormone levels, typically month to month but also overall. This can influence a woman with a history of migraine but also sometimes can be the first time that a woman will experience migraine attacks.

Studies show that typically perimenopause, the time leading up to menopause can bring on more migraine attacks, which may be more severe and difficult to treat. However, after menopause occurs, most women will also notice that their migraine attacks are improved overall. About 60% of women will notice that their migraine symptoms improve during menopause. The two major hormones that play an important part in migraine patterns during this time are estrogen and progesterone. Women who had menstrually-related migraine are more likely to notice changes in their migraine during perimenopause and menopause.

What are lifestyle factors that can help my hormonal migraines?

Overall, there are several complementary treatments that can be used as primary treatment or adjuncts to help with migraine attacks. These can be helpful in migraine attacks that are hormonally triggered or triggered by other environmental factors. Biofeedback, cognitive behavioral therapy (CBT), mindfulness and yoga have both been shown to help with migraine attack and frequency. Some people also find that acupuncture can provide some relief but may require a few sessions to begin to notice a difference. In addition to medications, these are good options as add on therapy or in cases when medications are contraindicated or not tolerated due to side effects.

Suggested Readings

Abdullah M, Qaiser S, Malik A, Chaudhry M, Fatima T, Malik A, Iqbal N. Comparison Between Menstrual Migraine and Menstrual-Unrelated Migraine in Women Attending Gynecology Clinics. Cureus 2020 Oct 16;12(10):e10976

Ornello R, De Matteis E, Di Felice C, et al. Acute and Preventive Management of Migraine during Menstruation and Menopause. J Clin Med 2021; 10: 226

Sullivan E, Bushnell C. Management of menstrual migraine: A review of current abortive and prophylactic therapies. Curr Pain Headache Rep 2010;14: 376-384

Vetvik K, Macgregor E, Lundqvist C, Russell M. Prevalence of menstrual migraine: a population-based study. Cephalalgia 2014; 34:280-288.

My Headaches seem Worse with My Periods. Why is that?

Jan Lewis Brandes, MD, MS, FAAN, FAHS
Director and Founder, Nashville Neuroscience Group
Assistant Clinical Professor, Department of Neurology, Vanderbilt University School of Medicine
Nashville, Tennessee, United States of America

A common explanation is that your "headaches" are likely to be migraine. The so-called "hormonal headache" or menstrual headache around the menstrual cycle is much more likely to be migraine in origin. Migraine attacks are actually more common in boys than girls *until* the onset of menstruation in girls, after which, migraine attacks predominate in women and continue to do so throughout the rest of women's lives.

So, the first imperative here is to get an accurate diagnosis! If your headaches *are* migraine (see earlier discussion about criteria for migraine diagnosis), most researchers believe the explanation for the association with menses is estrogen withdrawal. However, it may be that it is the fluctuation in estrogen levels that are to blame for menstrual migraine. Before ovulation, a slight rise in estrogen occurs with a subsequent fall in estrogen. The rise in estrogen before menstruation begins is yet higher and the fall more precipitous, and that rate of fall or rate of change in estrogen may underlie attacks of menstrual migraine.

Is this why migraine is often viewed as being a woman's disease?

Absolutely. The role of estrogen is the determining factor in why migraine is found in a 3:1 ratio of women to men. And that difference is first apparent after the onset of menstruation, although it continues to plague women throughout all their hormonal milestones – menstruation, pregnancy, breastfeeding, perimenopause and for some women, even after menopause.

But I also get migraine attacks at other times of the month. Is that common?

Yes, in fact, only about 14% of women with migraine have attacks solely associated with their menstrual cycles. Termed "pure menstrual migraine" (PMM), the definition states that the migraine attack should occur 2 days before to three days after the onset of menstruation and at no other times of the month. Much more common is the pattern known as "menstrually related migraine" (MRM), or menstrually associated migraine. Approximately, 60-70% of women with migraine fall into this group – where some of their attacks are associated with menses but they have attacks at other times of the month.

In about 1/3 of women with migraine, menstrually related migraine begins at the time of menarche. Some studies reveal that women with non-menstrual migraine represent about 40% of women with migraine, but often those are self-reported and not based on careful diary records and recording of hormonal fluctuations.

Okay, so it definitely is menstrually related migraine. Can I use the same acute medications that I use for my nonmenstrual attacks?

Most definitely, all seven triptans have been studied in menstrual migraine and all showed benefit. All except eletriptan were studied in randomized, double-blind, placebo-controlled trials specifically for menstrual migraine. The fixed dose combination sumatriptan/naproxen was also found to be beneficial in RDBPC clinical trials for menstrual migraine.

For the newer gepants and lasmiditan, only retrospective data is available for menstruating women.

The most important question is not just which medication to use, but what does an individual medication do for an attack. After taking an acute medication, whether a nonsteroidal anti-inflammatory medication or a triptan, or a gepant or ditan, or even acetaminophen, the important question is, "am I headache free?" Because menstrual migraines are under hormonal influence which constitutes a more long-lasting trigger, a second critical question is, "if I get pain free or significant pain relief, does my headache come back in 24-48 hours?"

Those are the critical questions for treatment. If the answers are no and yes, then it may be that combinations of acute migraine medications or short-term prevention, or even hormonal strategies can be considered.

My menstrual migraines are always much worse. Is that common?

One important strategy is to see if these menstrual attacks are predictable. Keeping a simple headache and menstrual diary is the best method for starting to plot a treatment approach. Just noting days of headache and days of menses is really the first step!

Menstrual migraine is known by headache specialists as being particularly difficult to treat. These attacks are often longer lasting and more severe compared to migraine attacks not associated with menses. Women who have easily treatable menstrual migraine don't usually come to headache clinics, so there may be some bias there, but it in no way changes the severity or duration of severe menstrual migraine for a large proportion of women with migraine. It only presents more challenges for effective treatment. Greater understanding of hormonal influences on migraine is an area of active research and newer medication choices are also adding to treatment choices.

Is there anything I should do differently to treat them?

If migraine is occurring in a regular pattern around menses, then multiple studies have been conducted to see if starting an acute migraine treatment before the onset of a menstrual attack can *prevent* the menstrual migraine.

This approach is termed "short-term prevention" and the idea is to get a medication started before the drop in estrogen, and to try and prevent the subsequently triggered menstrual migraine.

The best evidence for a triptan medication in these studies of predictable migraines is frovatriptan. It was most effective when given twice a day, beginning two days before the anticipated migraine and continuing for three days afterward. A loading dose of 5 mg in the am and in pm was given and on subsequent days, two doses were studied. Results showed that the 2.5mg dose, given twice a day, on days -2 to +3 of menses was most effective. No evidence for triptan overuse (medication overuse) headache was seen in the patients who stayed on this short-term regimen for an entire year. Overall, in addition to the decrease in menstrually associated migraine days, other migraine days were reduced as well.

Naratriptan has also been studied in this short-term prevention regimen and also showed benefit, but some rebound effect was observed when naratriptan was stopped after a multi-day regimen. Sumatriptan has also been studied in this format.

Other medications, used for short term prevention for 5-7 days, to prevent menstrual migraine have included naproxen 500mg three times per day from -6 days to +7 days of menses, in addition to magnesium 360mg twice a day over two months.

Some retrospective data looking at gepants for menstrual migraine has shown benefit, but no prospective double-blind placebo-controlled trials have yet been conducted.

A short-term regimen obviously works best for women with predictable cycles, but variations of short-term prevention can be used based on an individual woman's pattern. For example, if the menstrual migraine typically starts near the end of menses, the short-term prevention could be started later rather than before menses. If the only attack is on a single day, the regimen could be shortened. And for a woman whose pattern begins with "menstrual migraine" before her actual menses begins, she could start the regimen by treating her as she would at onset of her migraine and then continuing the short-term prevention for the next 2-3 days.

So "short term prevention", while it means a specific course usually of a longer duration triptan or non-steroidal antiinflammatory drug use, may be extended or shortened or begun in a way that addresses a particular woman's pattern of hormonally influenced migraine.

My migraine attacks seem to be mostly during the placebo week of my oral contraceptives. Can I take my oral contraceptive pill (OCP)continuously?

Based on the hypothesis of estrogen withdrawal as trigger for menstrual migraine, yes. By eliminating the placebo week or placebo days from a fixed-dose oral contraceptive pill regimen of of active pill, followed by placebo days, the fall in estrogen should be reduced or even suppressed.

While the elimination of the placebo days may be helpful in preventing or reducing migraine for some women, there, as yet, appears to be no method for determining in advance who will benefit. So, there is some risk that a woman could have her migraine worsen, rather than have fewer attacks.

I keep reading about the association of migraine with stroke? Are oral contraceptives safe to use if I have migraine?

Studies of continuous oral contraceptive pill use have shown safety in large populations of women, but these have not been conducted specifically in women who have migraine. Undoubtedly, given the prevalence of migraine in women, many women with migraine were included, but they were not studied specifically. All studies in this have evaluated the lower dose ethinyl estradiol of 20-35ug.

The first randomized trial of combined continuous OCPs was published back in 1995, and this use of continuous OCPs was begun, off-label, by many gynecologists to treat dysmenorrhea, endometriosis, and the heavy bleeding, or "menorrhagia" that many women experience. So, for women struggling with difficult to treat menstrual migraine and the pain and discomfort of endometriosis or other painful menstrually associated conditions, a continuous OCP regimen may provide dual benefits.

For women who develop migraine aura, after starting an OCP, the usual recommendation is to stop oral contraceptives. But for many women who have migraine without aura, no identifiable risk factors for stroke, and who do not smoke, if their menstrually associated migraine is disabling and interfering with her ability to function at home or at work, then hormonal strategies certainly should be considered. Coordinating between your gynecologist and the clinician managing your migraine is ideal for managing the complexities of menstrual migraine and its hormonal influences.

But remember that hormonal options should not be pursued in a woman with migraine who continues to smoke, *ever*.

Other options for women whose migraine attacks appear related to estrogen withdrawal may be considered. EstroGel and estrogen patches have been studied in randomized clinical trials but tended to show a rebound headache effect when the estrogen was stopped or only if tightly dosed with menstruation. If these approaches seem appealing to try, they should only be done in the hands of experienced headache and gynecology specialists.

And remember that the migraine headache felt related to the withdrawal or drop in estrogen level is usually migraine without aura. But high-level estrogen states may trigger migraines with aura, so the use of added estrogen should best be avoided in women with aura. Continuous transvaginal estrogen ring dosing has been suggested as a benefit for menstrual migraine, but has only been observed in very small and non-controlled studies.

Do be aware that hormonal strategies can and will do exactly what they want to in migraine. What works for your friend, or for one patient, may have the exactly opposite effect in you! Or another person! That is why it is so important to keep a careful headache and hormonal diary, including all medications and noting any supplements when you discuss treatment choices. Be vigilant for changes in migraine when stopping or starting any hormonal manipulation, as very differential effects can occur.

Be wary of quick fixes, nutraceuticals, or even published reports of medications or supplements that are purported to work in menstrual migraine. Most involve extremely small numbers of patients, as few as six patients, in one well known trial, and often do not include a placebo group. Drug interactions can occur with supplements and cause unintended harm, so always discuss any novel addition with your clinical partner.

Are there any non-pharmacological treatments for menstrual migraine?

Probably the best evidence is for magnesium, dosed in a small group of women at 360mg daily. Another small trial showed benefit of 400 daily units of vitamin E. Most herbal products that are promoted for use in migraine have very limited data and safety information, and are not recommended.

A promising area for treatment of menstrual migraine in women who do not want to take medication, e.g., in someone who is trying to achieve pregnancy, is that of devices. One small trial has been conducted with transcranial stimulation with benefit in women with migraine, and there will certainly be others which should be studied specifically for menstrual migraine; these devices would potentially include non-invasive vagus nerve stimulation (nVNS), single pulse transcranial magnetic stimulation, and distal transcutaneous electrical stimulation (Nerivio).

What do the newer migraine preventive drugs, the calcitonin gene related peptide monoclonal antibodies, do for menstrual migraine?

Unfortunately, careful data collection from the large, successful trials of all four currently available CGRP monoclonal Abs approved for migraine prevention did not include formal recording of menstruation. But in "look back" or retrospective analysis of the data, a trend toward benefit is seen in erenumab, according to a recent study.

Since sex hormones affect CGRP, and some have suggested a stronger role in women for CGRP influence, these preventive medications will certainly be important to understand in menstrual migraine.

Why aren't there more clinical trials for menstrual migraine or studies that include subsets of menstrual migraine?

In part, because there has been a lack of recognition that clinical trials for a disease state should reflect the population most at risk, i.e., women. That was particularly the case with the large calcitonin gene related peptide monoclonal antibodies and the gepant trials. But that can change! It is not dramatically more expensive to include data on an electronic diary that shows days of menstrual flow in preventive or even acute trials. Advocacy helps influence the design of clinical trials and the questions they are designed to answer. So, work to be involved with groups who can influence those choices.

References

Brandes JL. The influence of estrogen on migraine: a systematic review. *JAMA*, **2006** Apr19: 295(15)1824-30. Doi: 10.1001/jama.295.15.1824.PMID: 16622144.

Lentsch SdV, Maassen VanDenBrink A. Changing levels of sex hormones and calcitonin gene-related peptide (CGRP) during a woman's life: Implications for the efficacy and safety of novel antimigraine medications. *Maturitas*, **2021**, *145*: 73-77.

Maasumi K, Tepper SJ, Kriegler JS. Menstrual Migraine and Treatment Options: Review. *J Head and Face Pain*, **2016** Dec 2. https://doi.org/10.111/head.12978.

MacGregor EA. Oestrogen and attacks of migraine with and without aura. *Lancet Neurol.* **2004**, *3*, 354-361.

Ornello R, De Matteis E, Di Felice C, Caponnetto V, Pistoia F, Sacco S. Acute and Preventive Management of Migraine during Menstruation and Menopause. *J Clin Med* **2021**, *10*: 2263.

Pavlovic JM, Stewart WF, Bruce CA, Gorman JA, Sun H, Buse DC, Lipton RB. Burden of migraine related to menses: results from the AMPP study. *J of Headache Pain*, **2015**; *16*:24. Doi: 10.1186/s10194-015-0503-y.

Vetvik KG, MacGregor EA. Menstrual migraine: A distinct disorder needing greater recognition. *Lancet Neurol.* **2021**, *20*:304-315.

Witteveen H, van den Berg P, Vermeulen G. Treatment of menstrual migraine; multidisciplinary or mono-disciplinary approach. *J of Headache and Pain*, **2017** *18*:45, DOI 10.1186/s10194-017-0752-z.

MIGRAINE IN PREGNANCY

SUSAN W. BRONER, MD

Do migraine headaches get better or worse in pregnancy?

While between 4 to 8% of women with migraine experience more attacks during pregnancy, many women improve. 60-87% of women see a significant reduction in their migraine frequency and severity, particularly during the second and third trimesters. Women with a history of menstrual migraine or migraine without aura are more likely to improve. Some women with migraine aura may worsen, and others experience migraine or migraine aura for the first time during a pregnancy.

Are there any effective treatment options in pregnancy?

While treatment options are more limited in pregnancy, there are still several acute treatment options for pregnant women with migraine headaches. Nonmedication approaches are the cornerstones of migraine prevention and first line approaches in pregnancy. Key components are tapering off caffeine, keeping hydrated, maintaining a regular sleep schedule, engaging in moderate exercise as tolerated, eating regularly and healthfully, and avoiding known triggers. The use of cold or heat packs and deep relaxation techniques may be used acutely. Acupuncture, biofeedback, meditation, and cognitive behavioral therapy can also be employed acutely and preventatively.

Where these are not enough, acetaminophen alone or with caffeine is considered a first line treatment and is generally considered safe. Although some studies have shown an association between maternal use of acetaminophen and an increased risk of childhood development disorders, such as attention deficit hyperactivity disorder and autism spectrum disorder, it is not yet understood if this association is causal or if some other underlying factor explains the association. Higher doses and longer use in pregnancy may increase this risk, so it is recommended to minimize its use.

The U.S. Food and Drug Administration has recommended the avoidance of non-steroidal anti-inflammatories (NSAIDs) after week 20 due to an increase of kidney malformation. Additionally, some studies show an association between NSAID use and miscarriage in early pregnancy or near conception. That being said, ibuprofen, naproxen, indomethacin, and ketorolac may be considered for use on a limited basis in the first 20 weeks of pregnancy. NSAIDS should not be used in the third trimester as they can cause premature patent ductus arteriosus closure in the heart, leading to potential fetal heart failure and death.

For those who have severe attacks that are not responsive to analgesic options, certain triptans are considered second-line treatments. Evidence supports their use over butalbital containing products. Several studies over the years suggest that triptans are not associated with major congenital malformations (MCMs), developmental issues, or prematurity. However, triptans may confer a slightly higher risk of spontaneous abortion. Given how disabling migraine may be, triptans can be considered for severe attacks. There is the greatest evidence for sumatriptan, naratriptan and rizatriptan. One needs to weigh both the risks of the medication with the risks of the condition. Remember, severe migraines may pose a risk to the pregnancy if they are associated with vomiting with subsequent metabolic disruption and hypotension.

Butalbital-containing products are not recommended for the treatment of migraine in general, and butalbital has been associated with the development of congenital heart defects in utero. The American College of Obstetricians and Gynecologists and the Centers for Disease Control have stated that opioids should only be used in pregnancy when other alternatives are not effective, and for only a limited duration.

Anti-emetics are often used in the treatment of the nausea that can accompany migraine, or for pain relief itself. Pyroxidine and doxylamine are considered safe to use for nausea and ginger may be a good non-medication alternative. Metoclopramide has not been associated with an increase in the risk of MCMs in pregnancy but may confer extrapyramidal side effects on the mother, with higher doses and longer duration of use increasing this risk. Data suggests that ondansetron is not associated with a high risk of MCMs, but there may be a small increase in the risk for congenital heart malformations and cleft lip with or without cleft palate. Diphenhydramine, dimenhydrinate and cyproheptadine appear to have little risk for the fetus, with no MCMs observed in studies.

Lidocaine is considered relatively safe in pregnancy, whether it is used topically, as a nasal spray or in a lidocaine-only occipital nerve block. Lidocaine nerve blocks can be beneficial for women with frequent migraine attacks or status migrainosus (migraines of duration greater than 72 hours). While there are no adequate controlled studies of lidocaine in pregnant women, animal studies have revealed no evidence of harm to the fetus. While cardiac side effects may occur with more invasive uses of lidocaine, low doses are less likely to cause this.

Am I considered "high risk" in pregnancy if I have migraine?

Most women with migraine headaches have normal pregnancies with healthy babies. Some studies, however, suggest that women with migraine have a small increased risk of low birth weight, preterm delivery, preeclampsia, need for cesarean section, and severe nausea and vomiting with pregnancy.

A more recent study looking at a large population of Danish women found that migraine was associated with an increased risk of pregnancy-associated hypertension disorders in mothers and increased low birth weight, pre-term birth, respiratory distress syndrome (but no deaths) and febrile seizures in their offspring. Therefore, women with migraine should share their diagnosis with their obstetrician and gynecologist.

What can I do to prevent migraines in pregnancy?

Nonmedication approaches are the cornerstone of migraine prevention in pregnancy. As outlined previously, lifestyle adjustments and other nonpharmacologic steps may be quite helpful in reducing migraine frequency.

Regarding supplements, there is limited data on coenzyme Q10 so this should probably be avoided. There is no evidence assessing potential risks of high doses of riboflavin, but physiologic doses are thought to be safe. Feverfew is contraindicated as it may result in spontaneous abortion. The data around magnesium is not clear. While once thought to be safe in pregnancy, fetal bone abnormalities have more recently been associated with prolonged (more than 5 days) IV magnesium sulfate treatment. There is no data on whether oral formulations for migraine prevention pose this risk and one meta-analysis suggests that the risk posed by oral magnesium supplementation in pregnancy for any reason is thought to be very low. Until further data is obtained, these risks should be reviewed with the patient and her partner.

A transcutaneous neurostimulator (TENS) unit called the Cefaly device has some evidence for migraine prevention and can also be used acutely.

If migraine attacks continue to be severe and frequent, or if there is significant frequent vomiting, the benefits of oral preventatives may outweigh the risks to the developing fetus. While most migraine preventatives are generally avoided in pregnancy, certain beta-blockers (labetalol, propranolol), SSRIs (sertraline) and, occasionally, the tricyclic antidepressant amitriptyline are employed. Prior to initiation, there should be a conversation between the prescribing provider, the obstetricians and the patient and her partner to weigh the risks and benefits of such oral medications.

In summary, most women with migraine experience a normal pregnancy, with a majority seeing a reduction in frequency and severity of attacks. Lifestyle approaches and trigger management are the cornerstone to minimizing migraine exacerbations. A variety of acute treatments are available and should be offered. Treatment options exist for those with more frequent or disabling attacks. A thorough discussion of benefits and risks should be undertaken involving the patient and her partner, the treating healthcare practitioner, and the obstetrician to provide relief for this disabling condition.

Suggested Reading

American College of Obstetricians and Gynecologists Committee on Obstetric Practice Society for Maternal-Fetal Medicine. Committee Opinion No. 573: Magnesium sulfate use in obstetrics. *Obstet Gynecol* 2013;122:727-728.

American College of Obstetricians and Gynecologists Statement on Opioid Use During Pregnancy. *Advocacy and Health Policy.* Mar 16, 2016.

Broner SW, Bobker S, Klebanoff L. Migraine in Women. *Semin Neurol* 2017;37:601-610.

Browne ML, Van Zutphen AR, Botto LD, et al. Maternal butalbital use and selected defects in the national birth defects prevention study. *Headache* 2014;54:54–66.

Burch R. Epidemiology and Treatment of Menstrual Migraine and Migraine During Pregnancy and Lactation: A Narrative Review. *Headache* 2020;60:200-216.

Calhoun, A.H. Migraine Treatment in Pregnancy and Lactation. *Curr Pain Headache Rep* 2017; 21, 46.

Ji Y, Azuine RE, Zhang Y, et al. Association of Cord Plasma Biomarkers of In Utero Acetaminophen Exposure with Risk of Attention-Deficit/Hyperactivity Disorder and Autism Spectrum Disorder in Childhood. *JAMA Psychiatry* 2020;77:180–189.

Li DK, Ferber JR, Odouli R, Quesenberry C. Use of nonsteroidal antiinflammatory drugs during pregnancy and the risk of miscarriage. *Am J Obstet Gynecol* 2018 Sep;219(3): 275.e1-275.e8.

Liew Z, Ritz B, Virk J, Olsen J. Maternal use of acetaminophen during pregnancy and risk of autism spectrum disorders in childhood: a Danish national birth cohort study. *Autism Res* 2016;9:951-958.

Makrides M, Crosby DD, Bain E, Crowther CA. Magnesium supplementation in pregnancy. *Cochrane Database Syst Rev* 2014 Apr 3;2014(4).

Negro A, Delaruelle Z, Ivanova TA, et al. Headache and pregnancy: a systematic review. *J Headache Pain* 2017;18(1):106.

Skajaa, N., Szépligeti, S.K., Xue, F., Sørensen, H.T., Ehrenstein, V., Eisele, O. and Adelborg, K. Pregnancy, Birth, Neonatal, and Postnatal Neurological Outcomes After Pregnancy with Migraine. *Headache* 2019;59: 869-879.

MIGRAINE AND BREASTFEEDING

JASMIN MARIE HARPE, MD, MPH

Should I avoid breastfeeding so I can treat my migraines after I deliver?

Although 80% to 90% of postpartum women in many countries initiate breastfeeding, as many as 80% of them need medications during breastfeeding. Breastfeeding is encouraged and is considered quintessential due to the tremendous health benefits of breast milk to the infant. These benefits include enhanced cognitive development, lower risks of infection, and enhanced immune system development. The World Health Organization (WHO) recommends exclusive breastfeeding for the first 6 months of life, followed by continued breastfeeding with appropriate complementary foods for up to 2 years or beyond. There are few studies on the safety of migraine medications during breastfeeding. Lactating women are often excluded from the drug development processes limiting data on drug levels in milk for risk assessment. Nonetheless, the available evidence suggests that there are safe options for the treatment of migraine attacks during lactation, even more so than during pregnancy.

What are my chances of getting migraines while breastfeeding?

About 30% to 40% of all women experience headaches during the postpartum period. Many are prior migraine or tension headache sufferers, while others may develop headaches for the first time. Though breastfeeding may confer weeks to months of potential benefits gained in pregnancy, many women experience migraine attacks during the first week after delivery. For the following six weeks, headaches tend to be more painful and last longer than usual. This is likely due to fluctuating hormones after birth. Later headaches improve as hormones return to previous levels.

Are there any medications I can take while breastfeeding if I have a migraine?

Women with migraine may be concerned about breastfeeding due to fears of exposing their newborn to medications. Treatment of migraine during lactation is typically less restrictive than during pregnancy. Many medications are believed to be safe during breastfeeding. Many over-the-counter remedies may be helpful, and acetaminophen and anti-inflammatory medications such as ibuprofen are considered first-line options. Aspirin, due to an association with Reye's syndrome in children, and naproxen typically are avoided. Diclofenac and ketorolac are considered reasonable prescription alternatives in the NSAID family. Sumatriptan, zolmitriptan and eletriptan are among acute medications with low levels in breast milk, but studies of triptans in nursing mothers are limited. Long half-life triptans such as naratriptan and frovatriptan should be avoided and pediatricians should be consulted about any need for "pumping and dumping" after taking acute medications. There are no data on the safety of the newer GGRP antagonists (ubrogepant, rimegepant) or 5HT-1F agonists (lasmiditan) in lactation. Sedation, dependency, or apnea are all concerns with opioid use so these drugs should be avoided. Any medications taken during pregnancy should be discussed with the infant's pediatrician.

Are there other options besides medication to treat a migraine headache while I am breastfeeding?

Non-invasive, holistic techniques to manage headaches during breastfeeding can be effective. Local application of heat or more commonly ice, resting in a quiet and dark environment, relaxation strategies such as employing cognitive behavioral therapy (CBT) techniques or napping all may provide relief.

Certain devices have not been adequately studied in breastfeeding women but are considered by many to be safe for use while nursing. Although several are commercially available, two are most widely used. The External Trigeminal Nerve Stimulation (e-TNS) device is one option for breastfeeding women. It may be used for acute or preventive management. Self-adhesive electrodes are positioned against the clean skin of the forehead. Precise micro-impulses are sent through the electrodes to the upper branch of the trigeminal nerve, where migraines begin. The neurostimulation can relieve headaches during an attack (Acute Setting) or prevents future attacks (Prevent Setting). Each session lasts about 20 minutes. The Remote Electrical Neuromodulation (REN) migraine device may be used for acute treatment of episodic or chronic migraine. This device is placed on the arm and activated by smartphone technology with the stimulation session lasting 45 minutes. It is felt to work through activation of natural internal neurological pain control circuits.

What if my migraine attacks get frequent while I'm breastfeeding?

For women who experience attacks that are frequent or difficult to control when the above strategies are not helping, preventative medications may be warranted. Although many medications are contraindicated certain classes of anti-depressants and blood pressure medications may be relatively safe and effective. The newer monthly or quarterly injections of monoclonal antibodies directed at the migraine target chemical known as CGRP have yet to be adequately studied. Although the use of botulinum toxin injections into the head and neck muscles for chronic migraine is appealing because of its relative lack of systemic side effects, safety of this drug in nursing is also not yet established. One safe alternative may be head and neck injections using solutions of local anesthetics, with or without steroids, in procedures known as occipital or pericranial nerve blocks. A discussion between the mother's neurologist or primary care provider and the infant's pediatrician is warranted to review the risk-benefit ratio of any medications to both mother and child and to inform what to watch out for in the infant should there be side effects.

Suggested Readings

American Academy of Pediatrics, Section on Breastfeeding. Policy statement. Breastfeeding and the use of human milk. *Pediatrics* 2012;129: e827-e841.

Burch R. Headache in pregnancy and the puerperium. *Neurologic Clinics* 2019;37(1):31–51. doi:10.1016/j.ncl.2018.09.004

Hutchinson S, Marmura MJ, Calhoun A, et al. Use of common migraine treatments in breast-feeding women: A summary of recommendations. *Headache* 2013; 53:614-627.

Ito S. Opioids in breast milk: Pharmacokinetic principles and clinical implications. *J Clin Pharmacol* 2018;58(10): S151-S163. doi:10.1002/jcph.1113

Negro A, Delaruelle Z, Ivanova TA, et al. Headache and pregnancy: a systematic review. *J Headache Pain* 2017;18(1):106.

Parikh SK. Unique populations with episodic migraine: Pregnant and lactating women. *Curr Pain Headache Rep* 2018; 22:80.

Stults EE, Stokes JL, Shaffer ML, Paul IM, Berlin CM. Extent of medication use in breastfeeding women. *Breastfeed Med* 2007; 2:145-151.

The World Health Organization. Guideline1: protecting, promoting, and supporting breastfeeding in facilities providing maternity and newborn services Geneva: World Health Organization; 2018. https://www.who.int/nutrition/publications/guidelines/breastfeeding-facilities-maternity-newborn-summary.pdf.

Uguz F. A new safety scoring system for the use of psychotropic drugs during lactation. *Am J Ther* 2021; 28:e118–e26.

I WANT TO HAVE A BABY, WHAT HAPPENS TO MY MIGRAINE MANAGEMENT?

MERLE DIAMOND, MD
PRESIDENT, MEDICAL DIRECTOR DIAMOND HEADACHE CLINIC & DIAMOND HEADACHE INPATIENT UNIT AT AMITA HEALTH SAINT JOSEPH HOSPITAL
CHICAGO, ILLINOIS

My companion and I are ready to start a family, what do I need to know about my current migraine regimen before trying to conceive?

Being diagnosed with chronic migraine and being concerned about your current migraine regimen and what that will mean for your migraine treatment is normal. This conversation is a frequent one for many headache patients who decide they want to attempt to conceive while on a medical treatment plan for their migraines. It is very important to give you as much information as possible as we start planning for a healthy pregnancy and safe outcomes for both you and your baby. Since migraines and headaches impact women for at least 3 decades of their lives, most in the reproductive years, it is very important to address all issues. First and foremost, it is important to share what we know about migraine epidemiology and pregnancy. A common but unproven old-wives tale, is that most patients go into remission with pregnancy. Often this is true, but there are certain indicators that can help us reassure patients. I understand that you are currently on a monthly CGRP monoclonal antibody, daily topiramate, as well as a triptan and gepant for acute attacks. We will likely need to stop these medications, and your headaches may worsen off them. With your current regimen, you stated you are having 6 migraine days per month lasting less than 24 hours. Currently, you are combining the gepant with the triptan to reduce headache recurrences. Prior to the monoclonal antibody and topiramate combination, you had 12 migraine days per month lasting 1-2 days. We will need to discuss suitable alternatives.

Will I still get migraines once I am pregnant?

Women have a nearly 60% chance of remission in the first trimester with another 20% remitting over the next two trimesters. In some, the migraine may first occur in pregnancy. Obviously, this is not the case for you. There are also certain factors that may help us to predict your frequency of migraine during pregnancy. Since you struggle with menstrually related migraine (getting your first migraine around the time you started your first menstrual cycle and having migraines with menses) you may do well during pregnancy. It also seems that those having migraine without aura are more likely to improved with pregnancy when compared to those with aura. Fortunately for you, these are all factors which put you in a group of patients who may indeed have few migraines during pregnancy. This is typically reassuring information that I like to share with any patient who is concerned with trying to conceive.

I am scared of when we actually conceive and the effects the medications I am currently taking will have. What do I need to know about this?

Great question, it is important to discuss with both you and your partner what your goals are. In some cases, some patients will only want to use medication as needed and not preventative medications. Some patients will want to be on some prevention as long as it is safe. Having an honest assessment about what can be done is important. This starts with a holistic approach to improving self-care with your diet and sleep hygiene and other non-pharmacologic approaches including biofeedback, physical therapy, cognitive behavioral therapy and perhaps the use of devices like neuromodulation. Maximizing these tools will often allow patients to be on less medication during a time where medication limitations can be difficult.

What medications do I need to stop prior to pregnancy?

Currently you are on a few medications which will need to be changed prior to pregnancy. Anti-CGRP medications in the form of monoclonal antibodies are not suggested during pregnancy. All the companies currently have pregnancy registries but do not have enough data to know about the safety of these drugs in pregnancy. These medications require a 6-month washout so that is important to recognize this. You are also on topiramate, which is an unsafe medication to use in pregnancy. This drug can be weaned within a month or two before becoming pregnant. The gepant also cannot be used during pregnancy as animal studies now show some teratogenesis, or negative impact on the fetus. As long as the triptan used is sumatriptan that drug is likely safe as an acute medication in pregnancy.

Can you give me more information on what I can use currently or do you think I will have to tough it out for nine months?

Migraine in pregnancy is anxiety producing. Patients need not only reassurance, but a tangible plan to utilize certain strategies, when necessary, while they are pregnant and when breastfeeding. It is important for you and your partner to think about what your comfort level is for medications versus more holistic treatments. Historically, there was a letter grading system for medications used in pregnancy. Medications were assessed based on retrospective datasets. Drugs were lettered ABCD or X based on the data that was available.
A – No risk
B – Thought to be safe
C – Not enough data yet
D – Not good
X – Bad

This rating system was updated in the past few years to get rid of the letter labeling. Historically, many clinicians as well as their patients have struggled to balance the effective treatment of mom's migraines with potential safety concerns for both mother and unborn child. So, how do we typically move forward in this setting? Let's start with acute therapy.

For the past several decades, many acute medications have been utilized to treat migraine in pregnancy. The best data shows that acetaminophen is safe, but it is often insufficient in treating the pain of migraine. Often women are given certain medications like codeine or hydrocodone combined with acetaminophen. Narcotics should be used judiciously to avoid addiction and medication overuse headache issues in the mom and the baby. Currently, sumatriptan which has had an active pregnancy registry, can be used safely for both mom and baby. Ergotamine products should be avoided as they can lead to a miscarriage. Other options that are available are metoclopramide and diphenhydramine. Occasionally IV magnesium can be used. Too much magnesium has triggered concern regarding the bone health of the baby.

Low dose prednisone can also be used to stop a prolonged headache cycle, but not long-term. It is also likely that neuromodulation and nerve blocks can be used successfully.

What can I use for prevention?

As we look at prevention, there are several options available. Riboflavin and magnesium can be utilized. The vast majority of beta-blockers can also be utilized for prevention. So, as you start to taper off topiramate, these could be added. Because you are on an anti-CGRP drug, the monoclonal antibody, you will need a washout of 5-6 months. Your topiramate is unsafe to utilize in pregnancy but can be weaned a month or two before you try to conceive. Other options for prevention during pregnancy might include memantine and some tricyclic antidepressants, including amitriptyline and nortriptyline. Cyclobenzaprine can be used as well. Some clinicians have advocated the use of onabotulinumtoxinA (Botox) in pregnancy although again, there is not a lot of data in the literature that shows how safe this drug is during pregnancy.

What now? What steps do I take or what plan should we follow?

Given what we've already discussed, I would highly suggest to discontinue your monoclonal antibody 6 months before attempting to conceive. This is a risk we do not want to take, as there is currently not enough pregnancy data on these medications which may cross the placenta as well as being secreted in breast milk. You would be able to start beta-blockers as they appear to be safe in pregnancy. Adding neuromodulation may be an important addition to your treatment plan. Lastly, there are options for acute medication that might be helpful, including combining acetaminophen with metoclopramide and/or diphenhydramine. We can also utilize sumatriptan for more severe attacks.

Suggested Reading

Bateman BT, et al. β-Blocker Use in Pregnancy and the Risk for Congenital Malformations: An International Cohort Study. *Ann Intern Med. 2018; 169:665–673. doi: 10.7326/M18-0338*

Brandes JL et al. *Migraine in Women. BC Decker Inc; 2004.*

FDA Pregnancy and Lactation Labeling (Drugs) Final Rule. U.S Food & Drug Administration, December 2014.

Marcus DA et al. Headache. *1999; 39: 625-632.*

Sances G. et al. Course of migraine during pregnancy and postpartum: a prospective study. *Cephalalgia. 2003; 23: 197-205.* Published by Blackwell Publishing Ltd.

Silberstein SD, Lipton RB, Goadsby PJ. Headache in Clinical Practice. 2nd Ed. New York, NY: Martin Dunitz; 2002: 257-267

Silberstein SD. Migraine and pregnancy. Neurologic Clinics. 1997; 15:209-31. 25.

I WANT TO TAKE BIRTH CONTROL PILLS. WILL THEY EFFECT MY HEADACHES?

VINCENT T. MARTIN, MD

I am thinking about starting a birth control pill. Will that help or hurt my migraines?

The effect of birth control pills on your headaches can depend on what type of migraine that you have- migraine with aura or migraine without aura. Those with migraine with aura have neurological symptoms that occur before or during headache. There are several types of auras. Most commonly auras visual events where you get flashing lights, zig zag lines or blind spots that start off small and gradually enlarge. Another type of aura is a sensory aura which is where you get numbness or tingling of the face, arm or leg. And finally, there is an aura called hemiplegic migraine where you get weakness or paralysis of your face, arm, or leg on one side.

Studies have shown that estrogen-containing combination birth control pills can trigger attacks of aura for the first time or can worsen the frequency of auras if you have had them previously. If auras are triggered by estrogen-containing birth control pills it would be recommended to stop the birth control pills because rarely strokes can occur in those patients. Some groups have recommended not using estrogen-containing birth control pills in those with migraine with aura because of a higher risk of stroke in those with auras. Certain "progestin-only" pills which do not include estrogen would be the preferred alternative.

Birth control pills are commonly used for contraception in women that have migraine without aura. We cannot usually predict what will happen with the frequency of migraine attacks when women start birth control pills. They can worsen headaches, have no effect, or improve the frequency of migraine. Sometimes headaches transiently worsen at the start of birth control pills, but if you stay with them the headache may decrease.

You had mentioned a "progestin only" pill. What are the different types of birth control pills?

There are two types of pills used for contraception - a combination birth control pill and a progestin only pill. Most combination birth control pills contain a synthetic estrogen called ethinyl estradiol as well as a progestin. Progestins are like a hormone in your body called progesterone. There are many different types of progestins. The progestin-only pill contains the progestin hormone, but no estrogen.

Does it matter what type of birth control pill is prescribed? There are so many….

There are no well conducted studies to guide us to choose one birth control pill over another in those with migraine. How someone does with a particular birth control pill largely depends on how their brain responds to the type of hormones in each birth control pill. For example, one pill could trigger attacks of migraine while another might prevent them or have no effect at all on migraine. So it becomes trial and error.

The dosage of estrogen in the pill can also affect the frequency of headaches. Higher dosages of estrogen in the birth control pills might sometimes worsen headache. This probably occurs because of greater estrogen falls during the placebo week of the pill. Therefore we generally recommend birth control pills with lower estrogen dosages, those containing 10-20 micrograms of ethinyl estradiol.

Progestin-only pills have been demonstrated in small clinical trials to decrease the frequency, severity, and duration of attacks of migraine. The progestin that has been best studied is desogestrel.

You mentioned before that birth control pills might be avoided in those with migraine with aura because they increase the risk for stroke. Is there an increased stroke risk with migraine?

Yes, there is an increased risk of stroke in those with migraine particularly in those that have migraine with aura. One study found that the risk of stroke in young women was 2.3 times higher in those with migraine with aura than those without migraine. Birth control pills are also a risk factor for stroke because of the estrogen in the pill. The risk is 7 times higher in a person with migraine with aura taking estrogen-containing birth control pills when compared to those having migraine with aura and not taking them. The risk goes from 5.9 stroke per 100,000 per year to 36.9 strokes per 100,000 persons per year when women that have migraine with aura take oral contraceptives. Given such a small stroke risk some physicians still prescribe oral contraceptives in those with aura. However, three large organizations have issued statements that estrogen-containing combination oral contraceptives are **contraindicated** in those that have migraine with aura. They include the World Health Organization (WHO), UK Faculty of Sexual and Reproductive Health, and the US Centers for Disease Control and Prevention.

Another factor that might influence stroke risk is the frequency of attacks of migraine with aura. Those with more than one attack per month had a significantly increased risk of stroke. So frequent attacks of migraine with aura might further dissuade one from prescribing an estrogen-containing birth control pill.

The higher the dosage of estrogen in the birth control pill the greater the risk for stroke. Pills with the highest dosage of estrogen (e.g., greater than 50 micrograms of ethinyl estradiol) have the highest risk. Moderate dosages (30-40 micrograms of ethinyl estradiol) confer a modest risk for stroke while low dosages (10-20 micrograms) have the lowest risk. For this reason, we generally prescribe birth control pills with the lowest dosage of estrogen.

Are there any other groups of women with migraine in which you would not use oral contraceptives?

Yes, the risk of stroke increases yet even more in those with other risk factors for heart disease. These risk factors include smoking, high blood pressure, diabetes, high cholesterol, and obesity. If a woman has multiple risk factors for heart disease or a past history of heart attack or stroke you might avoid estrogen-containing birth control pills altogether or use pills with the lowest estrogen dosage. Progestin only pills could be used as they do not increase the risk of stroke.

Birth control pills also increase the risk of clotting in the veins. This is a condition called deep venous thrombosis. Most physicians would avoid estrogen- containing birth control pills in patients with a history of deep venous thrombosis or pulmonary embolism, which is a blood clot that goes to the lungs.

I never knew that clotting was a risk with some birth control pills. I have heard that some people are predisposed to clotting in their families. Should I be checked for clotting disorders before starting birth control pills?

Yes, it is true that estrogen-containing birth control pills can increase the risk of clotting and even more so if a person has a genetic predisposition to clotting. The risk of inheriting a genetic disorder that predisposes to clotting is quite low. Since the risk is much less than 10% it is not practical to screen everyone wanting to start birth control pills for clotting disorders because these tests are quite expensive. The only situation where it might make sense to do so might be if you have one or more family members with a known genetic predisposition for clotting.

My headaches are the worst around my menstrual period. I have been told that I have menstrual migraine. Can birth control pills be used to help control my menstrual migraine?

Birth control pills can sometimes be used as a preventive treatment for attacks of menstrual migraine. Menstrual migraines are migraine attacks that consistently begin two days before to two days after the onset of menstrual bleeding with each menstrual cycle. They are thought to occur because of falling estrogen levels that occur just before the menstrual period. Birth control pills can be given to women to prevent these monthly falls in estrogen levels and thus reduce the frequency of menstrual migraine.

Typical estrogen-containing birth control pills contain 21 days of active hormones followed by placebo pills during the last week of the pack. The placebo pills are sugar pills and contain no hormones whatsoever. The fall in hormone levels will cause a menstrual period 3-4 days into the placebo week and often trigger a menstrual migraine. To prevent these falls in estrogen some health care providers will omit the placebo pills from three consecutive packs of birth control pills and only give a placebo week after the fourth pack of birth control pills. In effect, you would only have one menstrual period every three months. Some birth control pills called "extended duration" oral contraceptives give the placebo week every three months. Other pills have no placebo pills whatsoever. Doing this will reduce the number of menstrual periods per year and thus reduce your frequency of menstrual migraines.

I can see how reducing the frequency of menstrual periods will reduce the frequency of menstrual migraines. But I really don't want to any menstrual migraines-not even one every 3 months. They are just so severe and disabling. Anything that we can do to prevent them?

The headaches that occur during the placebo week of the birth control pill are predictable. They most commonly occur on the 3rd and 4th day of the placebo week. The fact that they occur predictably during that week gives us the opportunity to give targeted therapy just during that week to try to prevent these headaches. This is called "mini-prophylaxis". We could try giving certain medications called triptans beginning 1-2 days before the predicted onset of the menstrual migraine and continue it for 3-4 days taken twice per day. The triptans that are most used are naratrptan and frovatriptan.

An alternate approach would be to give supplemental estrogen during the placebo week of the birth control pill to prevent falls in estrogen that might trigger attacks of menstrual migraine. Often an estrogen patch can be placed during the placebo week to prevent these headaches.

I have also been told that I have chronic migraine. Hormones seem to be a big driver of my headaches!!!! Is there any evidence that controlling my menstrual migraines will help my chronic migraine?

Yes, one study found that 59% of persons with chronic migraine and menstrual migraine reverted to episodic migraine with hormonal therapies to control their menstrual migraines. But these results are preliminary and further studies need to be done to corroborate these findings.

Suggested Reading

Calhoun A, Ford S. Elimination of menstrual-related migraine beneficially impacts chronification and medication overuse. Headache 2008; 48: 1196-1193

Gialeraki A, Valsami S, Pittaras T, Panayiotakopoulos G, Politou M. Oral Contraceptives and HRT Risk of Thrombosis. Clin Appl Thromb Hemost 2018;24:217-225.

Martin V, Behbehani M. Ovarian Hormones and Migraine Headache: Understanding Mechanisms and Pathophysiology-Part 2. Headache 2006; 46: 1-22.

Merki-Feld G et al. Migraine start, course and features over the cycle of combined hormonal contraceptive users with menstrual migraine –

temporal relation to bleeding and hormone withdrawal: a prospective diary-based study. J Headache Pain 2020: 21:81.

Sacco, S, Merki-Feld G., Lehrmann E, Bitzer et al. Effect of exogenous estrogens and progestogens on the course of migraine during reproductive age: a consensus statement by the European Headache Federation (EHF) and the European Society of Contraception and Reproductive Health (ESCRH). J Headache Pain 2018: 19: 76.

Warhurst S et al. Effectiveness of the progestin-only pill for migraine treatment in women: A systematic review and meta-analysis. Cephalalgia 2018; 38: 754-764.

For Religious Reasons I Need to Fast. Will this Affect My Headaches and what Can I Do?

Rachel Colman, MD

Fasting can certainly affect headaches, especially migraine headaches. There are several reasons. The brain needs glucose to function at an optimal level. The brain always maintains careful control of the glucose level. When you do not eat your glucose level falls, and the brain sends out a signal that you are hungry, so you eat! If you do not eat in a timely fashion, your brain protects itself and you begin to break down stores of glycogen in the liver converting it to glucose for your brain to use. The brain in a sense "wants" to use the easier supply of glucose from food, so triggering hunger is seen as a negative signal. People with migraine can be triggered by this negative signaling pathway, and it can induce a migraine. This is quite a simplified version of what is happening on the chemical level, as there are many hormones and cascades that have been studied as the cause for hunger triggering a migraine, and it is likely a combination of many different factors at play in your brain chemistry.

The same is true for fluids and dehydration. Your body "likes" everything to be simple and when you do not provide your body with the fluids and the nutrition it needs, negative signaling occurs, which can lead to a migraine being triggered. It is well known that many foods can trigger the migraine attack for some as well. The biological and hormonal pathways that are linked in the brain to food, energy, nutrition, and fluids are closely related to migraine on many levels. There is another school of thought, that fasting does not lead to migraine in all cases, but rather that "hunger" is one of the common premonitory signs of an impending migraine. The premonitory phase of migraine includes the non-headache symptoms that occur prior to a migraine, which can include, fatigue, thirst, hunger, neck stiffness, frequent urination, light sensitivity, nausea, yawning, and mood changes. The premonitory symptom of hunger is often not recognized by the patient as a prodrome to migraine, and people assume that the hunger triggered the headache, hence try to avoid hunger, hoping they will then avoid the headache.

Another reason that fasting can trigger migraine is related to the intake of caffeine. Many people use caffeine daily. For many, not drinking their usual cup of coffee will trigger a headache. This headache is different from the one that is triggered from fasting alone. A person who does not have migraines can experience a caffeine withdrawal headache as well, and a person with migraine is liable to get a migraine type headache in this setting.

Caffeine is a stimulant that can be very useful in helping you stay alert. However, it is an addictive substance, and your body will develop a type of "dependence" to it. Within about 12-24 hours of not getting your usual dose of caffeine, your body will undergo withdrawal symptoms. Caffeine withdrawal leads to fatigue, restlessness, and headache, and your body "desires" the caffeine. This headache is often described as pounding and all over your head. If you are a person who has migraine, it can feel like your typical migraine, or may feel different. The headache is typically "cured" by taking more caffeine.

Often when fasting is planned, people will plan to slowly reduce their caffeine in the weeks prior to the fast, so they are no longer are dependent on it. I do recommend you trying to slowly reduce your intake if you use caffeine daily. Just a note of caution, some people try to wean off caffeine too quickly, i.e., in 2-3 days and stop the caffeine entirely the day before the fast. This may make you more prone to headache if you are not gradually physiologically weaned from the caffeine. You may feel fine the day you didn't have coffee (prior to the fast) but miserable during the fast, as this is 24 hours after your body "thought" it should have received a "dose" of caffeine. I recommend slowly reducing your caffeine intake starting 1-2 weeks prior to the fast, until you are having less than one small cup a day (6oz). For most people this will not lead to withdrawal when a dose is missed. However, there are some people who are more caffeine sensitive, and really need to slowly wean off the caffeine entirely to avoid a withdrawal headache.

I think it is also important to note that caffeine use itself can trigger migraine. Staying under two small cups per day is a good way to avoid more migraines on all days, not just fast days!

But Doctor. the fast is in two days? What should I do? I drink 3 cups of coffee a day.

Yikes! There is no time to gradually wean the caffeine at this point and reducing tomorrow may make the headache on the day of the fast even worse. While I never recommend this for any other reason besides fasting from caffeine (and only on rare occasions) there are over-the-counter caffeine tablets you can take on the day of the fast, if you are allowed to swallow pills. Caution is needed, as they often come in 200 mg tablets which is the equivalent to two strong cups of coffee. I have heard that a compounding pharmacist can even make caffeine suppositories for those who are unable to swallow pills on a fast day. A compounding pharmacist can also make a combination of acetaminophen or ibuprofen with the caffeine, in a suppository form, to help treat the headache as well as caffeine withdrawal. Over-the-counter tablets with this combination are also widely available. I recommend extreme caution with the use of "headache" or "migraine" combination medications. These tablets when taken frequently (more than 10 days per month) can trigger a new type of headache called "medication overuse headache." These caffeine-containing combination tablets are much more likely to trigger medication overuse headache as there are two agents of overuse: the caffeine and the pain reliever. Urgent need to treat a headache due to caffeine withdrawal while fasting is when I recommend using these medications.

Migraines, while not life threatening, can certainly be very disabling. I tell all my patients who need to fast for religious reasons to reach out to your religious advisor. I know in many cases people were told they do not need to fast, or were able to limit their fasting hours, due to the disabling nature of the migraine it would cause.

But Doctor, I already asked my religious advisor and they said I need to fast on this fast day. What can I do?

There are several tricks you can do to help prevent or minimize a headache from fasting.

1) Make sure you are well hydrated in the days leading up to the fast.

2) Carefully eat the day prior, with protein and complex carbohydrates at each meal. Avoid processed, salty, or sugary foods.

3) Be extra careful with your other triggers, avoid poor sleep, stressors, foods, sounds, and smells that are known to trigger you.

I do all that! I still get a headache later in the day. What can I do?

So sorry to hear that! Even with best efforts, migraine can hit in this scenario. If you are allowed to swallow pills during the fast, take your usual migraine medication, and try to nap. I know that some people are not able to swallow pills without water, or religiously cannot ingest anything during a fast. Luckily, there are other routes to get migraine medication to your brain! Given that migraine is known to cause nausea and vomiting, even non-fasting people sometimes cannot swallow their migraine medication. Migraine medications come in many different delivery routes. We can give you a nasal spray, an injection or even a suppository if needed. As I mentioned above, there are combination tablets with a pain reliever and caffeine that can be helpful in this scenario as well. Sleep can be a great help for migraine and is one of our best tools especially when fasting.

What about the month long fast of Ramadan? Is there anything I can do?

Fasting during the day for a whole month can be tough for people with migraine. In some the body gets adjusts to the new habit of only eating in the evening, and then the headaches may get a bit better after some time. For others the fasting will continually trigger a headache. I advise speaking with your religious advisor to see if you can have fluids, which will help, or any fasting modifications given the disabling migraines. I know some people try to switch to a more nocturnal work schedule. I had a colleague who requested working at nights during Ramadan, so they could continue to practice their faith and not have to worry about the terrible headaches, as then they were up overnight and able to eat and asleep during the day. Eating very complete and healthy meals when you do eat, trying to keep a balanced and nutritious diet with complex carbohydrates and protein, may help as well.

Is there any difference with a 25 hour fast, or just a 12 hour fast?

Great question! Since most people do not eat overnight, the headaches usually begin after the first or second skipped meal (breakfast or lunch time). When a fast starts at sunrise, I know many will choose to wake up early to eat a healthy breakfast and have some coffee, and that can help stave off a headache and hunger during the day. With a 24-hour fast getting in the last coffee and nutrients early in the morning is not possible, so people often notice migraines and headaches more frequently with this type of fast. All the recommendations I made for fasting apply to both types of fasts.

I have migraines, but my partner does not, and he always gets a bad headache on a fast day. Why?

Headaches triggered from fasting are likely tension-type headaches. These occur in many people in the setting of stress, poor sleep, skipped meals or dehydration. They often are bilateral, and possibly associated with light or sound sensitivity (but not both). They can be pounding and make you feel awful. As mentioned already, caffeine withdrawal headaches occur in people who use caffeine regularly, so that may be the culprit for your partner.

A tension-type headache responds well to over-the-counter medications like acetaminophen or ibuprofen. If you can swallow pills these medications can help. All my advice about pre-fast behavior and weaning caffeine slowly apply to everyone who is fasting, not just people with migraine. Feel free to share the information with your partner.

My cousin has cluster headaches. Will he be triggered by fasting?

Luckily, probably not. Cluster headache is a different type of primary headache disorder than migraine or tension-type headache. It occurs in episodes many times a day and cycles can last weeks to months. Each attack is shorter than a migraine. Cluster attacks are triggered by the brain (in an area called the hypothalamus) and are linked to your circadian rhythm (your bodies internal clock). Foods, fluids, and personal activity are not felt to be cluster attack triggers. Other similar primary headache disorders called "trigeminal autonomic cephalalgias" do not seem to have food triggers and are likely not triggered by fasting.

Do you think I could start an intermittent fasting type of diet?

Because fasting from food and water can trigger migraines, I recommend to all my patients with migraine to avoid fasting and dehydration. This includes fasting diets, skipping meals, and exercising in hot rooms. Having regular nutrition and fluids is one of the many things people who have migraine can do to help themselves live a lifestyle that prevents more migraines. If fasting does not trigger yours, then you should speak with your primary care MD regarding any new diet type.

Suggested Readings

Abu-Salameh I, Plakht Y, Ifergane G. Migraine exacerbation during Ramadan fasting. *J Headache Pain* 2010 Dec; 11(6):513-7.

Alstadhaug KB, Andreou AP. Caffeine and Primary (Migraine) Headaches-Friend or Foe? *Front Neurol.*2019 Dec 3; 10:1275.

Arca KN, Halker Singh RB. Dehydration and Headache. *Curr Pain Headache Rep* 2021 Jul 15;25(8):56.

Awada A, al Jumah M. The first-of-Ramadan headache. *Headache* 1999;39:490-493.

Dalkara T, Kiliç K. How does fasting trigger migraine? A hypothesis. *Curr Pain Headache Rep* 2013 Oct;17(10):368.

Goadsby PJ, Holland PR, Martins-Oliveira M, Hoffmann J, Schankin C, Akerman S. Pathophysiology of Migraine: A Disorder of Sensory Processing. *Physiol Rev* 2017;97:553-622.

Grewal P, Smith JH. When Headache Warns of Homeostatic Threat: The Metabolic Headaches. *Curr Neurol Neurosci Rep* 2017 Jan;17(1):1.

Kokavec A. Migraine: A disorder of metabolism? *Med Hypotheses* 2016; 97:117-130.

Lipton RB. Risk Factors for and Management of Medication-Overuse Headache. *Continuum* 2015;21:1118-1131

Martins-Oliveira M, Tavares I, Goadsby PJ. Was it something I ate? Understanding the bidirectional interaction of migraine and appetite neural circuits. *Brain Res* 2021 Aug 21:147629.

Conversations with Headache Patients: My Migraine Disease is Killing my Relationships! Is it Just Me?

Ashley Alex, MD

Assistant Professor of Neurology University at Buffalo Jacobs School of Medicine Buffalo, NY

Cynthia E. Armand, MD

Assistant Professor of Neurology Albert Einstein College of Medicine/Montefiore Medical Center Bronx, NY

My migraine attacks can be severe and prevent me from enjoying outings and company with family and friends. I feel a rift growing in my relationships. It can't just be me, right?

No, it is not just you! Like other chronic illnesses, migraine affects not only the person with the disease, but also the psychological well-being and interpersonal dynamics among all those in a relationship. Migraine is a neurologic disease that manifests not only as severe head pain, but also with symptoms including nausea, vomiting, sensitivity to lights, sounds, and scents, dizziness, an inability to concentrate, and mood changes. Due to such symptoms, persons with migraine often find it difficult to participate in activities with family and friends. This can cause internal guilt as well as strain on relationships. It is worth noting though that patients with migraine are often more critical about their inability to participate in activities than their loved ones.

The way you are feeling has been documented in research. The Chronic Migraine Epidemiology and Outcome (CaMEO) Study looked at the effect of migraine on daily living. About 20% of people indicated that migraine had caused significant problems in relationships or their termination. Those with chronic migraine were twice as likely to express a negative impact on their ability to establish and maintain a relationship, as compared to those with episodic migraine. In addition, about 3% chose not to have children, delayed having children, or chose to have fewer children because of migraine. So, yes, I want you to know that your feelings are valid and that you are not alone.

Why do my friends and family think that migraine is "just a headache?" Sometimes, I don't even bother telling anyone what I'm dealing with because I feel like they will think less of me!

Migraine is much more than just a headache, and your experience is a common one due the stigma associated with migraine. Stigma is the discrimination against someone based on the social perception of a characteristic or trait that they possess, with the trait in this case being migraine. Even though migraine is currently ranked the second leading cause of global disability, its stigma means that it is viewed as a minor personal problem by many who do not understand it. Migraine is an "invisible disease" without many prominent physical manifestations to show for the disability it causes. In addition, most people with migraine conceal their symptoms, which undermines their disability and contributes to feelings of isolation. This disrupts relationships, leading to poor quality of life. Internalizing these societal perceptions tends to compound the issue, causing those with migraine to avoid sharing their symptoms with others or even to avoid seeking medical care.

What can I do to make my loved ones understand what I'm going through?

I know it may be difficult to share what you are going through, let alone explain it, but it is important that you tackle your disease as a team with your loved ones. Living with migraine is best done with support. So, here are some tips:

1. Openly invite loved ones to your care appointments. This is an opportunity to chat with a healthcare provider to gain further understanding about migraine and debunk common misconceptions.

2. Follow-up these educational sessions with continued communication: talk about your disease and its personal impact.
   a. Tell your loved ones what is or isn't helpful during pain periods.

b. Do not downplay symptoms; this sends the message that what you are experiencing is not significant, when in fact the level of disability it causes is proof that it is.
c. Do not shy away from asking for help. Remember, support is paramount!
d. Do not feel guilty about making time for yourself to recover! Similar to flight attendants instructing one to put their own oxygen mask on before assisting others, you can only care and be present for your loved ones when you take care of yourself first.

3. The last tip is for your loved ones: take time to acknowledge your loved ones' efforts and thank them for their support. Continue to make plans with them to maximize quality bonding time whenever possible.

Being upfront and honest with those in your inner circle coupled with medical education during visits, will help to elucidate migraine's stigma. Even if precautions are taken, attacks may still occur. It is vital for both you and your loved ones to understand that migraine is no one's fault.

My children are often late to school or miss extracurricular activities because of my migraine attacks! Do others have this problem?

Yes, unfortunately the children of parents with migraine are often affected. This has been studied extensively from both the perspective of the parent as well as the child. Thirty-four percent of patients with chronic migraine have reported that their children have missed a day of school or had late arrival or pickup. One-fifth of patients noted cancelling a family vacation due to migraine. Patients with migraine often reported that they were easily annoyed by their children; more than half admitted they would have been better parents had it not been for their headaches.

When children of parents with migraine were interviewed, the greatest impact of migraine was on the parent-child relationship and overall well-being, i.e., sleep, physical and emotional health. With high frequency attacks, children reported a greater impact on their well-being and heightened uncertainty about their future and independence; however, with high intensity attacks, children reported greater emotional impact and burden of helping their parent daily. Single parents with migraine, as compared to partnered parents with migraine, reported that their children had to take over their responsibilities more often. About 50% of teens felt like they could not get help from a parent due to chronic migraine.

I don't want my children to resent me. How can I help my children understand?

Parenting with migraine is tough. Like with any relationship, it requires open communication, preparation, and support. One study showed that although three-quarters of children felt like they had enough information about migraine, more than half stated they would have liked help with managing the impact of migraine on their lives and less than half indicated that they would have liked training on how to care for a parent with migraine.

Here are a few tips you can use to help your children:

1. Educate your children about migraine. It's okay to speak to them about what helps during an attack and what can worsen your symptoms. This dialogue may calm any fears they have and inform them on how to help in times of need.

2. Acknowledge their feelings and provide emotional support. A child psychologist/therapist may be useful in teaching coping skills.

3. Reach out to other parents! Perhaps they can help with pick-ups and drop-offs which will allow your children to maintain participation in school events and extracurriculars, which can sustain routine in their lives and perhaps forge quality friendships.

I work in a highly technical field and my migraine disease is causing issues at work. What can I do about this?

Working with migraine is difficult and the added stigma can make this situation even more difficult to navigate. There is worry about work productivity as well as job and financial security. Within the workplace itself, there can also be stressful conditions, inflexible workplace conditions, and difficult bosses and colleagues. What can you do?

Have a discussion with your headache provider about your work obligations and environment so as to prepare you for any questions that employers may have. Discussion points should include details about specific work tasks, work hours (including any shift work), stress-inducing circumstances, and trigger-inducing activities. You should cover what work function you can and cannot perform during an episode of pain, and what parameters are necessary to recover from attacks.

If you find the work environment to be a contributor to worsened headache control, tell your employer, officially. The federal American with Disabilities Act (ADA) requires employers who have > 15 employees to accommodate the reasonable needs of employees which do not present an undue hardship to the employer. Therefore, collaborating with your employer can improve overall well-being, reduce disability and in-turn maintain or even boost productivity. It's a win-win for both of you!

Is there any way to protect my job?

There is indeed! The Family and Medical Leave Act (FMLA) protects eligible workers by providing up to 12 weeks of unpaid leave in a 12-month period while maintaining health insurance benefits. It is particularly beneficial for both episodic and chronic migraine patients since the 12 weeks of leave can be taken altogether or periodically as needed.

What if I do not want to take leave but need to explain potential work absences due to my migraine attacks?

FMLA documentation not only covers periods of leave, but also explains the impact of migraine disease as it relates to work function. Details about migraine attacks, work environment accommodations, potential late arrivals, early dismissals as well as time for scheduled doctor visits and treatments should all be documented. You may ask your employer about their FMLA forms, which will need to be completed and signed by your healthcare provider.

Suggested Reading

Buse, D.C., et al., *Life With Migraine: Effects on Relationships, Career, and Finances From the Chronic Migraine Epidemiology and Outcomes (CaMEO) Study.* Headache, 2019. 59(8): p. 1286-1299.

Buse, D.C., et al., *Adolescent Perspectives on the Burden of a Parent's Migraine: Results from the CaMEO Study.* Headache, 2018. 58(4): p. 512-524.

Buse, D.C., et al., *Impact of Migraine on the Family: Perspectives of People With Migraine and Their Spouse/Domestic Partner in the CaMEO Study.* Mayo Clin Proc, 2016.

Buse, D., D. Dodick, and A. Manack, *Perception of the Family Burden of Chronic Migraine: Results of the CaMEO (Chronic Migraine Epidemiology & Outcomes) Study (P5.039).* Neurology, 2015. 84(14 Supplement): p. P5.039.

Diseases, G.B.D. and C. Injuries, *Global burden of 369 diseases and injuries in 204 countries and territories, 1990-2019: a systematic analysis for the Global Burden of Disease Study 2019.* Lancet, 2020. 396(10258): p. 1204-1222.

Seng, E.K., et al., *When Mom Has Migraine: An Observational Study of the Impact of Parental Migraine on Adolescent Children.* Headache, 2019. 59(2): p. 224-234.

Shapiro, R.E., *What Will it Take to Move the Needle for Headache Disorders? An Advocacy Perspective.* Headache, 2020. 60(9): p. 2059-2077.

I'M DEPRESSED AND I HAVE HEADACHES. WHICH CAUSES WHICH?

JACOB M. APPEL, MD JD

My psychiatrist says that headaches can be related to depression. Is this true?

Yes, it is. A well-established bidirectional relationship exists between mood disorders, including depression, and headache disorders. This relationship has been established most strongly in patients suffering from migraines. Up to 57% of migraine patients report suffering from depression in population-based studies, while the overall prevalence of depression in the United States likely runs between 7% and 13%. In addition, both migraine and non-migraine headaches have been associated with increased long-term risks of attempting suicide. Baseline headache severity and presence of aura are key predictors of risk of self-harm. Since such a significant correlation exists between headaches and depression, neurologists treating patients with headache should be vigilant for mood symptoms. Diagnosing and treating depression early may reduce the risks of episodic headaches becoming chronic.

Are there specific types of headaches that are more likely to be associated with depression?

Several different types of headaches have been associated with increased rates of depression including migraine headaches and tension-type headaches. One large study. found that patients with migraine had 2.2 times the risk of depression when compared to individuals without migraines. Among patients with migraines, those patients with chronic migraines are approximately twice as likely to suffer from depression as patients with episodic migraines. Migraines with aura are more likely to be associated with depression than migraines without aura. Chronic morning headaches, which affect 1 in 13 individuals, are heavily associated with depression. One surprising finding is that while concussion and traumatic brain injury are associated with both headaches and depression, patients with non-traumatic headaches had higher rates of depression than those with a history of head injury.

Are there types of depression that are more frequently associated with headaches?

While the data is limited, this does seem to be the case. For example, one large study found that depressed patients with headaches were also more likely to display excessive sleep and other pain symptoms. Younger age in depressed patients was also significantly correlated with headaches.

Are any other psychiatric illnesses associated with headaches?

A large number of other psychiatric illnesses have also been associated with headaches. These include bipolar disorder, panic disorder, generalized anxiety disorder and post-traumatic stress disorder. Headaches are also associated with substance use disorders and with childhood trauma. Bipolar disorder (both type I and type II) and anxiety disorders, in particular, have been strongly correlated with migraines; some data suggests that rates of migraines are higher among patients with bipolar II disorder than bipolar I disorder. Conduct disorder has been linked to headaches in male children, but curiously, no similar finding has been found among girls. Certain personality traits, such as neuroticism, are also linked to headache disorders.

I have heard that stress can cause headaches. Is this true?

Absolutely. Stress, which induces the release of cortisol, a steroid hormone with widespread systemic effects, can trigger many different types of headaches. Major stressful life events have been tied to progression to chronic daily headaches. Stress-induced headaches have been tied to low feelings of self-efficacy in patients, so effective therapies may strive to augment a patient's sense of control.

So is it possible that my headaches are "all in my head"?

It is generally not that simple. While some headaches do present in a manner consistent with classic syndromes such as migraines and cluster headaches, others may prove harder to classify. Headaches may manifest in the context of conversion phenomenon—the presence of motor or sensory neurological symptoms in the absence of an apparent organic or physiologic cause.

Alternatively, if pain itself is the dominant symptom, they may be classified as belonging to a pain syndrome. In fact, headache is the most common presentation of pain syndromes. Some psychiatrists have posited that such headaches are the product of unconscious psychodynamic phenomena like unresolved interpersonal conflicts or the internalization of object-based relationships. Other theories attribute these headaches to the amplification of responses to otherwise benign stimuli while under psychological duress. Both conversion disorder and pain syndromes are "rule-out" diagnoses. Providers should exclude other neurological and psychiatric explanations for a patient's symptoms before rendering these "functional" diagnoses. Unfortunately, treatable organic pathologies at times may be misdiagnosed as conversion pain or somatization disorders.

Do we know why headaches and depression are related?

The relationship between headaches and psychiatric disorders is complex and much remains unknown. Coping with pain or illness has long been associated with mood symptoms, which makes sense even to non-clinicians. Most people recognize that physical suffering can have an impact on their psychological wellbeing. However, the high incidence of depression among individuals with headaches, as well as the order and chronology of onset, suggest that more is at play than merely a response to chronic illness. In the case of migraines and depression, the relationship is believed to be bidirectional: people with migraines are more likely to become depressed and people with depression are more likely to develop migraines. Whether genetic or environmental forces, or both, underlie this correlation is uncertain. Both migraines and depression have significant genetic diatheses, so it is perfectly plausible that underlying genetic linkages explain their concurrence. Several of the same neurotransmitters, including dopamine and serotonin, are implicated in both migraines and affective disorders. Allodynia (the experience of pain from stimuli that are not usually painful) is associated with both conditions. Reports indicate that migraineurs with depression have higher rates of cutaneous allodynia than those without depression, suggesting an underlying mechanism that involves centralized sensitization of neurons and a resulting decrease in a patient's pain threshold. More research is needed in this area.

Which comes first—headaches or depression?

More often than not, the affective symptoms precede the onset of headaches, but the two conditions may present in either order. Since either headache or depression can present first and the two are highly correlated, patients who present with one symptom should be screened and monitored over time for the other. It is worth noting that patients with migraines are five times more likely to develop new-onset depression than patients without a history of headaches, so a simple and short screening tool like the PHQ-2 or the PHQ-9, which can be self-administered, should be reviewed at the outset of neurology appointments at least annually. Patients who score positive for depression on screening tools should also be assessed for suicidality and a history of mania (indicative of bipolar disorder). Headache specialists may feel comfortable treating depression on their own or may choose to refer patients for psychiatric care. However, patients with bipolar disorder should generally be referred to a mental health professional. Needless to say, patients with acute thoughts of self-harm must be stabilized in an emergency setting. Pediatricians and pediatric neurologists should also screen for depression as depression in childhood is a significant risk factor for worsening of headaches among adolescents.

Are some people more likely to get both headaches and depression than others?

Gender predisposes individuals to certain types of headaches. For instance, women are roughly three times as likely to suffer from migraines as men. Women are also at greater risk of depression than men. Interestingly, women with migraines experience depression at higher rates than one would expect based on the incidence of depression among women in the general population. Both a long history of headaches and increased frequency of headaches are particular risk factors for depression among women suffering from migraines. A lifetime history of headaches is also associated with depression in older people.

Are headaches treated differently in depressed patients?

The general approach to treating headaches in the setting of depression or anxiety is to target the headaches themselves, but sometimes medications can be chosen that treat both the headaches and the comorbid psychiatric conditions. Tricyclic antidepressants (TCAs), such as amitriptyline, are often effective prophylaxis agents against migraines and tension headaches; they are also highly effective at treating patients with unipolar depression. It is important to remember that therapeutic doses of TCAs for the treatment of headaches generally run much lower than therapeutic doses for mood disorders. Fluoxetine, an SSRI (selective serotonin reuptake inhibitor) may provide some benefits with far fewer risks and side effects—especially in suicidal patients, who are at high risk of lethal overdose from TCAs. Mood stabilizers, notably carbamazepine and valproic acid, can perform double duty as treatments for bipolar depression and migraine headaches. Topamax is another anticonvulsant with proven efficacy in migraine prophylaxis but data on its use as a mood stabilizer is less persuasive. Cognitive side effects secondary to topiramate can occasionally be problematic. This concern with topiramate is particularly significant in patients with severe psychiatric illness, as they may not have the cognitive or functional reserve of healthier patients. Lithium can be used to treat mood instability and suicidality and is also an effective long-term treatment for cluster headaches. At the same time, certain headache treatments should be avoided in depressed patients. For example, beta blockers can be potent agents for preventing migraines, but have also long been thought to cause depression, although recent data is more equivocal. Levetiracetam, another anticonvulsant used in migraine prophylaxis, can cause a wide range of psychiatrist symptoms including anxiety, depression and even psychosis. Although often favored by neurologists for its ease of dosing and administration, it should be avoided or used cautiously in patients with a significant history of or predisposition to affective disorders. A careful choice of medications in patients with comorbid headache and depression can often prevent polypharmacy and increase adherence.

Can treatments for depression cause headaches?

Yes. Headache is a common side effect of SSRIs and SNRIs (serotonin norepinephrine reuptake inhibitors), and can also occur after initiating TCAs, monoamine oxidase inhibitors, mirtazapine and bupropion. Fortunately, in most patients, the headaches resolve in a period of days to weeks. Less frequently, headaches can result from discontinuation of SSRIs or SNRIs as part of a withdrawal syndrome. These symptoms are more common in medications with shorter half-lives such as paroxetine and venlafaxine, while less common with agents that remain in the bloodstream longer such as fluoxetine. It is highly unlikely that long term antidepressant use or its cessation will cause or exacerbate headaches.

Should I be worried that my headache medications interact with my psychiatric medications?

There is no need to worry, but headache medications and psychiatric medications can interact. Many of these interactions occur through the

CYP-450 system in the liver. For example, tricyclic antidepressants like amitriptyline can increase the serum levels of valproic acid, while valproic acid can increase levels of TCAs. Aspirin also increases valproic acid levels. NSAIDs can elevate lithium levels, risking toxicity, while lithium can also elevate NSAID levels. Often these interactions can be managed effectively with frequent monitoring and dose adjustments. MAOIs (monoamine oxidase inhibitors) are contraindicated with several headache medications including triptans, TCAs and carbamazepine. Providers should check for interactions carefully before prescribing medications to patients suffering from both headaches and psychiatric symptoms and when discontinuing their medications. Patients should be informed of the risks and interactions, especially as stopping one medication on their own can impact the levels of their other medications.

I am feeling discouraged. Having two major medical problems is challenging. Is there hope that I will recover.

Not only is there hope, but the prognosis is good. Hopelessness can be a symptom of depression. Most patients with depression make a full recovery with appropriate treatment. A wide range of medications and psychotherapies are available, and the two are not mutually exclusive. In fact, the combination of psychiatric medication and talk therapy has been consistently demonstrated to offer the quickest and most effective path to recovery. While there are no guarantees in medicine, there are many reasons for optimism. We will get through this together.

Suggested Reading

Amouroux, R., Rousseau-Salvador, C., Pillant, M., et al. Longitudinal study shows that depression in childhood is associated with a worse evolution of headaches in adolescence. *Acta Paediatrica* 2017:106, 1961-1965.

Breslau, N., Schultz, L., Lipton, R., Peterson, E. and Welch, K. Migraine Headaches and Suicide Attempt. *Headache* 2012;52:723-731

Colombo B, Annovazzi POL, Comi G. Therapy of primary headaches: the role of antidepressants. *Neurol Sci* 2004;25: S171–5

Dresler, T., Caratozzolo, S., Guldolf, K. et al. Understanding the nature of psychiatric comorbidity in migraine: a systematic review focused on interactions and treatment implications. *J Headache Pain* 20, 51 (2019).

Garvey, M. J., Schaffer, C. B., & Tuason, V. B. Relationship of headaches to depression. *The British Journal of Psychiatry* 1983;143:544-547.

McMurtray AM, Saito EK, Diaz N, Mehta B, Nakamoto B. Greater frequency of depression associated with chronic primary headaches than chronic post-traumatic headaches. *Int J Psychiatry Med* 2013;45:227-36

Mendonça MD, Caetano A, Viana-Baptista M; CHLO Headache Study Group. Association of depressive symptoms with allodynia in patients with migraine: A cross-sectional study. *Cephalalgia* 2016; 36:1077-1081.

Merinkangas KR, Angst J, Isler H. Migraine and psychopathology. Results of Zurich cohort study of young adults. *Arch Gen Psychiatry* 1990;47: 849–853

Mitsikostas D, Thomas A. Comorbidity of Headache and Depressive Disorders. *Cephalalgia* 1999;19:211-217.

Wang, S. J., Liu, H. C., Fuh, J. L et al. Comorbidity of headaches and depression in the elderly. *Pain* 1999; 82:239-243

I Get Excruciating Headaches Every Fall. What Can They Be?

Kate Mullin, MD

Associate Medical Director
New England Institute for Neurology and Headache
Stamford, Connecticut

Every autumn I get these headaches that wake me up from sleep and are so painful I have to pace around my bedroom. They last for weeks and then the vanish as fast as they came. My friends talk about their migraines, but I feel like what I have is different. What can this be?

It sounds to me like you may be experiencing cluster headaches. Can you tell me more about your headaches?

I am a 50-year-old man; they started when I was in my 20s. The headaches generally last around 40 minutes. They are right sided, one hundred percent of the time, and generally focused around my eye and temple. It feels like an ice pick piercing my eye at its worst. I experience anywhere from 2 to 6 attacks per day, for weeks at a time. But then, suddenly they will stop and sometimes I can go months even years between attacks.

This sounds very typical of cluster headaches, which is a primary headache disorder predominantly experienced by men. By definition, cluster headaches are severe, with unilateral, orbital, or temporal pain lasting anywhere from 15-180 minutes, if untreated. The attacks have a frequency from one every other day to up to 8 per day. Additionally, the headache should be accompanied by at least one of the following: ipsilateral eye redness or tearing, nasal congestion, eyelid edema, forehead, and facial sweating, miosis and/or ptosis and a sense of restlessness or agitation. Do you have any of those symptoms?

Yes! My right eye turns red and starts to tear. I think maybe my nose is running too. I always have to get up and pace around my room. My wife keeps telling me just to rest and lie down but I can't sit still until the pain stops. They're really awful, doc. Can they be treated?

Fortunately, there are a variety of treatments available to cluster headache patients. When a patient begins their cluster period, your neurologist or headache specialist will likely call you into the office in an effort to abort the cluster period in its entirety. This is often done with an occipital nerve block on the side of the headache. The nerve block contains numbing medication such as lidocaine as well as a low dose of a steroid. Your doctor may also put you on a brief course of oral steroids.

What if that doesn't work? What if I keep getting them? I'm losing sleep. Every morning like clockwork at 2am and then again around 5 am I get the headaches. I can't function with such disrupted sleep.

If the intervention at the beginning of the cluster period does not abort the headache cycle, then your doctor may put you on a preventative medication. The goal of preventative therapy is to produce a rapid suppression of attacks and to maintain that remission with minimal side effects until the bout is over. The first reported preventative shown to be effective was verapamil, a calcium channel blocker. Dosages can range from 240-960 mg daily. Verapamil can cause cardiac arrhythmias. Subsequently, periodic electrocardiograms should be obtained to monitor for PR prolongation. Constipation is the most common side effect and should also be monitored. If verapamil is contraindicated, many neurologists will add lithium carbonate for prevention at a dosage of 600-1200 mg daily. Lithium has a very narrow therapeutic window and potential for many side effects including tremor, dizziness, nausea or weakness. Renal and thyroid function tests should be performed prior to administration and lithium levels should be checked periodically.

A new monthly injectable medication called "Emgality" was recently FDA approved for cluster prevention. Emgality is a CGRP monoclonal antibody. The dosage is 300 mg monthly administered subcutaneously by three 100mg prefilled syringes during each month that the patient is actively in a cluster period. Emgality is well- tolerated and the only clinically significant adverse reaction in clinical trials was injection site reactions including redness, swelling, bruising etc.

While it is always our hope to stop the headaches from coming with a preventative treatment, you should also be given a medication to take at the onset of each attack to reduce the duration and severity of the individual attacks. Because cluster headaches are so severe and often brief, the preferred abortive medication is sumatriptan subcutaneous injection, as it is effective and fast acting. In a double-blind study, sumatriptan 6mg showed that in 74% of attacks, the severity of the headache at 15 minutes reduced compared to placebo at 26%. Often 20 r 3 mg for suffice to stop an attack. Some patients prefer zolmitriptan in nasal spray formulation if they are averse to needles. Zolmitriptan nasal spray is more effective than the oral formulation and also showed superiority to placebo in a small double-blind study. High flow oxygen is often effective in aborting a cluster attack, especially for patients having multiple attacks a day worried about overusing acute medications. The typical administration is 100% oxygen administered through a non-rebreather facial mask at a rate of 8-12 L per minute for 15 minutes or until the headache resolves.

Regarding your sleep disturbance, cluster headaches are often referred to as "alarm clock headaches" for just that reason. They tend to come like clockwork in the middle of the night. Many doctors will put their patients on melatonin prior to going to bed with the thought that your circadian rhythm and REM sleep cycles are involved in the timed attacks. Additionally, patients with cluster headaches are known to have reduced melatonin levels, particularly during a cluster bout. Cluster headaches often also begin around daylight savings in the spring and autumn when our sleep schedules became transiently disrupted.

Are there things that I can do to avoid getting attacks?

Alcohol, nitroglycerine, and histamine can trigger a cluster attack. Alcohol can induce an acute attack usually within an hour of intake. Exercise, elevated environmental temperature, and the smell of volatile substances such as varnishes and perfumes are also recognized as acute cluster triggers. It is best to avoid these substances while in the cluster period so as to not precipitate an attack. Unlike migraines, allergies, food sensitivities, hormones, and stress do not appear to play a significant role in precipitating attacks.

How do you know it's cluster headaches? What if you're wrong?

Cluster headaches are considered a Primary Headache. What that means is that they are not symptomatic from an alternative condition or diagnosis. In order to prove that a headache is primary, tests need to be done to rule out the secondary condition. For example, a thorough neurologic exam will be conducted. In between cluster attacks, the neurologic exam should essentially be perfectly normal- although some patients may have redness or slight dropping of the affected eye if they are actively cycling. Many doctors will order an MRI of the brain. Occasionally pituitary lesions can mimic cluster headaches, so it suggested to visualize the pituitary gland before giving the formal diagnosis.

Other primary headache types must also be considered when diagnosing cluster headaches. Sometimes migraines can look like cluster in that it's one sided and can have autonomic symptoms such as eye redness or tearing. Helpful features in differentiating cluster from migraine include the short duration of cluster attacks, circadian periodicity as well as the patterns of cluster cycles followed by periods of remission.

Hypnic headache is another primary headache condition that may be confused with cluster headaches. Hypnic headaches typically occur in an older population and predominately females, as opposed to the younger males of cluster. However, this headache type does awaken you from sleep in an alarm clock fashion similar to cluster attacks. Hypnic headaches are bilateral and do not have associated features such as eye tearing or nasal congestion.

Finally, there is a larger category of primary headache called Trigeminal Autonomic Cephalalgias (TACs) of which cluster is one of many. The other conditions, including paroxysmal hemicrania, hemicrania continua, SUNCT and SUNA are all classified by unilateral searing headaches accompanied by autonomic features such as eye tearing and nasal congestion. They are differentiated by the duration of each attack and the frequency of attacks. A thorough history regarding the duration of attack and number of attacks per day is key in differentiating cluster from the other TACs.

What if the headaches don't stop after a few weeks like they normally do?

There are two different classifications for cluster headache. Cluster Headache is classified according to the duration of the cycle and periods of remission. Episodic cluster is defined as at least two cluster periods lasting from 7 days to 1 year (when untreated) and separated by pain-free remission periods of ≥3 months. Episodic cluster is more prevalent, comprising approximately 80-90% of cluster patients. The remaining 10-20% of cluster patients are diagnosed with chronic cluster. Chronic cluster is defined by attacks that typically occur for one year or longer without remission, or with remission periods lasting less than three months. Owing to the severe pain and accompanying symptoms with long-lasting attacks without remission or short remission periods, individuals with chronic cluster headache experience a high degree of impairment.

I think my brother gets something similar to my headaches. Are cluster headaches genetic?

Studies have suggested that first-degree relatives, such as your brother, have a 5-8 times higher risk and second-degree relatives have a 1-3 times higher risk of cluster headache than the general population. A specific gene has not yet been located. It is thought that cluster headache is a complex genetic disorder with phenotypic and genetic heterogeneity which complicates attempts at gene identification. However, since cluster headaches are fairly rare, most do not have relatives with the problem.

Am I going to have these headaches forever?

Unfortunately, because cluster headache is such a rare diagnosis, we don't have a lot of data on the long- term prognosis. From what we know, it does seem like cluster headache is a lifelong diagnosis. However, the frequency and severity can fluctuate throughout your lifetime. A study was done that showed that about one-tenth of episodic cluster patients evolved into chronic cluster patients whereas one third of chronic patients transformed into episodic. This should provide hope that as you age your periods of remission become longer.

Suggested Reading

Francis GJ, Becker WJ, Pringsheim TM. Acute and preventive pharmacologic treatment of cluster headache. *Neurology*. 2010; 75(5):463–473

Headache Classification Committee of the Internal Headache Society (2018). Classification and diagnostic criteria for headache disorders, 3rd edition. Cephalalgia, Vol 38

Hoffmann J, May A. Diagnosis, pathophysiology, and management of cluster headache. Lancet Neurol. 2018 Jan;17(1):75-83.

Robbins MS, Starling AJ, Pringsheim TM, Becker WJ, Schwedt TJ. Treatment of Cluster Headache: The American Headache Society Evidence-Based Guidelines. Headache. 2016 Jul;56(7):1093-106.

Tepper DE. Cluster headache. Headache. 2015 May;55(5):757-8.

Tepper D. Oxygen for Cluster Headache. Headache. 2017 Oct;57(9):1493-1494.

Migraines are a Medical Condition...Why should I See a Psychologist?

Nomita Sonty, M.Phil, Ph.D

I have migraines why is my doctor referring me to a psychologist?

It is not uncommon for a person suffering with migraine headaches to be referred to a clinical psychologist by their doctor so that they may learn strategies to better manage head pain and everyday life. Migraines can interrupt your daily activities, increase unplanned absences from work and may even prevent you from fully engaging with your family and friends.

The more frequent your headaches and the longer their duration the more intrusive they are in your functioning. As these headaches become chronic you may also notice that you become terribly worried about having headaches. You may feel somewhat sad, anxious, frustrated and your sleep can become impaired. A clinical psychologist who specializes in pain management works with your medical team and is helpful in managing your pain, distress and sleep disturbance.

Additionally, it is not uncommon that some of you may prefer not to take medicines for your migraines or you may be planning a pregnancy during which you may not be able to take your current prescriptions. Under such circumstances you may choose to try a behavioral approach and are likely to be referred to a clinical psychologist.

Do all migraine sufferers need to see a clinical psychologist or am I crazy?

Not all migraine suffers are referred to a psychologist, but many are. Referral to the psychologist is not because a migraine sufferer is considered "crazy" but because it is recognized that many patients benefit from talking to a professional about their condition. Emphasis is placed on setting up realistic expectations and learning new skills to manage headache pain and migraine-related anxiety.

What will a clinical psychologist's evaluation look like?

Psychologists specializing in pain management have a basic understanding of the pathophysiology of migraines, its course and prognosis. They will conduct an evaluation during which they will ask questions on: 1) the history of your headaches, how they have progressed over time, and triggers such as stressors, life style, sleep patterns, food habits, and caffeine and alcohol consumption; 2) strategies you already use and how successful you are in managing your migraines; 3) your premorbid mental health history, medications you use and previous response to treatment; and 4) additional information about you including your education, employment, personal relationships, and social support. They will also want to know about your personality and how you cope with unpredictability in your life especially as related to your health. Some psychologists may use questionnaires to obtain this information.

Does stress cause or contribute to migraines?

Simply speaking, stress can be defined as any change in a person's ongoing pattern of life that forces them to accommodate. So, if we accept this definition then we can assume that any person who suffers from migraines is stressed. The degree to which they are stressed is variable and may depended on a number of factors. Migraines compound the stress of daily living with the cycle of pain, anxiety and sleep disturbance and the condition itself can become a major stressor. Scientific research has shown that psychological stress can contribute to migraine frequency and intensity but there is no clear evidence that stress causes migraines in a person who has never had them before.

Why do I get migraines on weekends and even when I am on vacation?

When a person is constantly experiencing stress and the stress is suddenly lifted they may develop a "let-down" migraine. Any change in the level of stress, which can happen at the end of a workday, on a weekend or on a vacation, can become a trigger for headaches. This is often confusing because you may expect that decreased stress should decrease your headaches. It is often recommended that the migraine sufferer transition gradually from one activity to another or from one schedule to another.

I don't want to make plans because I will have to cancel them once again.

Migraine headaches and related emotional and cognitive components create significant unpredictability in a person's life. Over the years you may have cancelled numerous plans with family and friends that you have now learned to avoid for fear that you may have to cancel them again. You are aware that migraines make you unreliable and this may make you feel embarrassed or ashamed. Often, my patients have lost relationships along the way because of this and they sometimes find it easier to isolate.

Also, when your migraines are uncontrolled, you may find yourself being able to do just the bare minimum so adding additional activity may feel burdensome. So, it is not uncommon to avoid plans that feels onerous or those that you feel may worsen your migraines.

Finally, if you have become depressed you may not have the energy or desire to make plans that involve people who do not have migraines or see migraines as just another headache which should respond to an over-the-counter medicine.

Somebody mentioned that my personality is causing my migraines...is that true?

There have been several attempts to study different personality types and migraines but research has concluded that there is no specific migraine personality. However, how you cope with symptoms varies from person to person and is determined by who you are and how you cope with illness or adversity. For example, those who need more control may find that the unpredictability caused by these headaches may cause anxiety. As another example, those who are inflexible may become frustrated when required to adapt to the changes that are often required while living with a chronic condition like migraines.

Is it normal to feel "foggy" even after my migraine has gone away?

Cognitive difficulties are often reported by patients after a migraine or sometime even between migraines. The term "postdrome" refers to lingering physical or cognitive complaints the day or two after a migraine – which patients often call their "headache hangover." Research shows that there may be difficulty with the speed of processing information, attention, concentration, and visual and verbal memory for many during and following migraine. Additionally, having depression and anxiety can make these cognitive issues worse.

What will a clinical psychologist do to relieve my migraines?

Once the evaluation is completed the psychologist will create a treatment plan that may consist of all or some of the following components:

1) Learning about headaches, monitoring them, and identifying the various triggers to better clarify underlying patterns.

2) Initiating relaxation exercises and biofeedback to increase awareness of how emotional responses can affect your body and your symptoms. Strategies used in conjunction with biofeedback may include progressive muscle relaxation, imagery, and mindfulness.

3) If you are starting to feel anxious about your headaches the psychologist may use Cognitive Behavior Therapy (CBT) to address beliefs as related to anticipatory anxiety and avoidant behavior. Some psychologists may use Acceptance Commitment therapy (ACT) in place of CBT.

4) Addressing lifestyle and habits to recommend strategies to improve hydration, physical activity, eating habits, alcohol use and socialization.

5) Adding techniques of stress management since stress may trigger an episode or exacerbate an existing headache.

6) Including sleep improvement techniques such as Cognitive Behavior Therapy for Insomnia (CBTi) if sleep is significantly disturbed.

7) Introducing apps for migraine monitoring such as Migraine Buddy or Migraine Tracker, apps for relaxation exercises such as Headspace or Calm, or apps for sleep improvement like CBT-i Coach.

8) Telehealth has become a newer resource for providing psychological services. Many patients find such services convenient and helpful. The efficacy of this approach for managing migraines and improving outcomes is yet unclear.

What is Cognitive Behavior Therapy (CBT) and how will it help my headaches?

CBT for migraines is a short-term, goal-oriented psychological approach that attempts to change unhelpful thoughts in order to change mood and behavior in the context of helping you manage your migraine headaches. In this form of therapy, it is assumed that your expectation and perception of your diagnosis, symptoms, and response to treatment will influence how you feel and adapt. These thoughts are often informed by both your internal and external environment. Thus, CBT uses a range of techniques to help decrease the frequency, intensity, and duration of your migraines, and to help you cope with the disruption your headaches may bring to your life. CBT with mindfulness-based therapies has also been shown to be effective.

I have heard about biofeedback for managing headaches...so what is it?

Among the many behavioral strategies used by psychologists, biofeedback is found to be effective in decreasing the frequency and intensity of migraines. In this technique you are connected by electrodes to receive signals from your body to help you learn to self-regulate certain biological activities. The most frequently used feedback formats for the treatment of headaches are skin temperature, galvanic skin response (GSR) and muscle tension. You can train in the psychologist's office, but there are also portable devices that you can use at home.

I'm afraid that my migraines are affecting my marriage... what can I do about that?

Chronic migraines frequently have an impact on the entire family. The burden of household responsibilities may fall on your partner or spouse and can affect the dynamic in your relationship. Your partner can feel helpless from an inability to help you feel better, or they may feel resentful that their plans are interrupted by your migraines. Poorly controlled migraines may have an impact on your sexuality or intimacy. Open communication with your spouse or partner is helpful. Sometimes, you may invite your partner into your session with the psychologist to address these issues or you may seek the help of a couple therapist.

What can I do help make my headaches better?

It is important to feel optimistic about managing your migraines. There are many options available to improve symptoms and your quality of life. When used in combination medications, psychotherapy, biofeedback, interventional blocks, and physical therapy have been shown to decrease migraines, anxiety, depression and to improve overall quality of life.

1. It will be important for you be engaged in your treatment by educating yourself about your migraines.

2. Have realistic expectations if diagnosed with chronic migraines

3. Adhere to the medication regimen prescribed by your provider

4. Follow the lifestyle recommendations suggested by your psychologist

5. Continue to exercise even if in a modified manner

6. Become aware of your triggers including stress. Look for cumulative stressors as they often cluster together to trigger headaches.

7. Develop a daily schedule of using techniques like progressive muscle relaxation, deep breathing, yoga, or mindfulness. Using these techniques during non-migraine periods is just as important.

8. Be flexible to make the necessary changes in your life to manage your migraines.

9. Be open to treating comorbid conditions like depression, anxiety, and sleep disorder.

Suggested Readings

Buse, DC, Rupnow, M & Lipton, R. Assessing and Managing All Aspects of Migraine: Migraine Attacks, Migraine-Related Functional Impairment, Common Comorbidities, and Quality of Life. *Mayo Clin Proc* 2009;84: 422–435.

Nicholson, R. Chronic headache: The role of the psychologist. *Curr Pain Headache Rep* 2010;14:47-54.

Perez-Munoz A, Buse, DC & Andrasik, F. Behavioral interventions for migraine. *Neurol Clin* 2019;37:789–813.

Probyn K, Bowers H, Mistry D, et al. CHESS team. Non-pharmacological self-management for people living with migraine or tension-type headache: a systematic review including analysis of intervention components. *BMJ Open* 2017 Aug 11;7(8):e016670.

DOES SLEEP AFFECT MY HEADACHES?

MARK BARBER, MD, MPH

ASSISTANT PROFESSOR OF NEUROLOGY
DIVISION OF HEADACHE MEDICINE ICAHN SCHOOL OF MEDICINE AT MOUNT SINAI NEW YORK CITY

Does sleep affect my headaches?

The short answer is: "yes." But that simple answer minimizes what is, in fact, an extraordinarily complex topic. There is an intricate, bidirectional relationship between headache and sleep that grows out of shared anatomical structures, pathways, and neurotransmitters. People with headaches consistently report worse sleep than those without headaches. While many identify lack of sleep as a headache trigger, some people's headaches start *during* sleep. For many, sleep can be therapeutic in aborting a headache.

Severe sleep disorders are five times more likely among people with migraine compared to those without. In one large study of patients with migraine, shorter sleep duration was associated with worse migraine burden. Migraine was triggered by sleep disturbance in 50% of participants, headaches had awakened or been present on awakening in 71% of participants, and 75% of participants had at some point been forced to sleep or relax because of a headache.

Your question about sleep and headache is an important one. Considering that headache is a disease state intrinsically tied to an individual's immutable neurobiology, the identification of a modifiable risk factor may confer a measure of control over one aspect of disease management. There is also some urgency to harnessing this control, since poor sleep has been identified as a risk factor for headache chronification. After they chronify, headaches become much harder to treat.

Why are sleep and headache so closely related?

The neurologic processes that give rise to both sleep and headache quite literally share the same real estate in the brain, so it is unsurprising that dysfunction of those regions could be implicated in the pathophysiology of both. The brainstem and diencephalon contain highly conserved neural networks that control sleep and arousal, and the trigeminal pain-signaling networks where headaches are thought to start converge at multiple levels within those neural networks. The suprachiasmatic nucleus of the hypothalamus, which receives projections from the retinal cells of the eyes that respond to environmental light, is considered fundamental to the regulation of sleep. It houses the body's "flip-flop switch," simultaneously promoting wakefulness while inhibiting sleep, and vice versa. Light helps synchronize a person's 'biological clock' with cues from the environment, and perhaps unsurprisingly, also acts as both a trigger and aggravator of headache attacks.

Evidence of the overlap between the shared pathophysiology of sleep and headache is abundant in the clinical presentation of numerous headache disorders. For example, yawning, thought to be driven by structures in the lower brainstem, is a telltale sign of migraine prodrome in many patients. Fatigue may span the prodrome, headache, and postdrome phases. Like sleep, migraines often occur with circadian variation. Some people report early morning migraines, corresponding to the part of the sleep cycle with the greatest portion of REM sleep. People with migraine are more easily aroused during REM sleep compared to people who do not get migraines. Disruptions to sleep routines can trigger headaches, like people who get headaches on the weekends. Cluster headaches and hypnic headaches demonstrate even stricter adherence to sleep cycles -- more on this later.

Does my bad sleep cause my headaches? Or do my headaches cause my bad sleep?

Yes.

Be serious.

This question quintessentially represents a chicken versus egg debate that has persisted as long as headaches have been studied. Is poor sleep a headache trigger, or a symptom of the early prodromal state of the headache itself? Patient-reported headache triggers are notoriously difficult to study because they vary widely and because introduction of a trigger does not consistently produce a headache attack in experimental studies. Further, patient-perceived migraine triggers (disrupted sleep, stress, acquiescence to food cravings, dehydration) may, in fact, be early premonitory symptoms of an attack to which the patient may later incorrectly attribute the cause of their headache. Still, in one meta-analysis, sleep was identified as the second most prevalent migraine trigger (after stress) among participants across included studies. Your doctor can clarify whether poor sleep and fatigue are the cause or effect of your headaches by taking a careful history, implementing deliberate behavioral modifications, and proposing stepwise treatment adjustments.

If poor sleep can trigger my headaches, how can I improve my sleep?

If you sleep poorly, it is important to rule out underlying medical comorbidities that may be contributing (more on this below). However, good old-fashioned sleep hygiene is always important. You are encouraged to go to sleep and wake up at a consistent time every day (including weekends and holidays), and you should aim to sleep for seven to eight hours nightly. Daytime naps are discouraged, and regular exercise is important, but not within three hours of bedtime. Caffeine and alcohol should be avoided, especially in close proximity to sleep. Screens and other sources of blue light should be avoided within an hour of sleep. The bedroom should be used exclusively for sleep and sexual activity, it should be adequately darkened during sleep hours, and external noise should be blocked out (consider using a noise machine or fan).

Caffeine merits special attention as it pertains to sleep and headache. Caffeine is a strong antagonist of receptors for the neurotransmitter adenosine, and clinically it acts as a stimulant to promote wakefulness. Its consumption or withdrawal may trigger or abort headaches, depending on the circumstances. For example, one of the most common over-the-counter headache remedies contains caffeine. However, chronic repetitive exposure to caffeine can lead to medication overuse headache, dependency, and chronic daily headache. Headache patients should limit caffeine consumption.

I've noticed that on days when I finally get the chance to sleep in, my headaches are more likely to occur. Why?

There is evidence that some people experience headaches reliably on weekends. A study in the late 1990s even hypothesized that this headache phenotype was its own entity, separate from the other primary headache disorders. With improved understanding of migraine pathophysiology acquired in the intervening decades, it seems more likely these headaches represent attacks of known primary headache disorders, like migraine, triggered by alterations in routine that occur on the weekend. The brain that is predisposed to headache prefers routine, so weekend changes in sleep schedule, caffeine timing, and perceived stress can trigger a headache. One study even found that *changes* in stress or sleep, as opposed to high stress or poor sleep themselves, were predictive of headaches on subsequent days.

I know that improved sleep will help my headaches, but even after trying all those sleep hygiene recommendations, I still can't sleep. What can I do?

Insomnia is challenging, but there are many approaches to dealing with this problem, and you are not alone. In fact, although only 23 percent of the general population in a large Korean study reported sleep difficulties, 45 percent of the people with migraine in that same study reported insufficient sleep. The good news is that addressing sleep improves migraine burden. Cognitive behavioral therapy for insomnia is especially effective. Smitherman et al recruited patients with chronic migraine and comorbid insomnia and randomized them to either a treatment group, which underwent cognitive behavioral therapy (CBT) for insomnia; or a sham control group, which underwent instruction in other lifestyle behavioral modifications. The authors found that there was a six day-per-month decrease in headache frequency among patients who underwent CBT treatment for insomnia, which was more than two headache days fewer than the control group. The effects persisted at follow-up.

In some cases, medication may be a helpful adjuvant to help with sleep. Many medications that are prescribed for migraine prophylaxis or treatment themselves cause drowsiness (including anticonvulsants, antidepressants, antihypertensives, and muscle relaxants), and physicians will sometimes recommend taking them before sleep in an effort to harness those sedating effects.

Melatonin, which is secreted by the pineal gland and whose production is regulated by the hypothalamus, helps control the body's circadian rhythm and has also been studied in relation to its effect on headache incidence and treatment. Dysregulation of melatonin secretion may lead to increased migraine susceptibility and even decreased inhibition of CGRP, a neuropeptide thought to be integral to pain generation in headache attacks. Melatonin is also sold as an over-the-counter sleep aid and its supplementation has been studied in migraine prophylaxis. Although it is generally thought to be helpful, results of dosing studies have been inconsistent, with most studies investigating low doses (1 to 3 mg nightly). High dose melatonin, on the order of 10 mg nightly, is effective in prophylaxis against cluster attacks in people with cluster headache.

Prescription sedatives like zolpidem and benzodiazepines are not routinely advised as sleep aids for headache patients, but the sleep medicine literature has published helpful guides to ensure such medications are prescribed safely and responsibly.

I've noticed as I've gotten older, I've started to wake up at the same every night with a headache. Why is this happening?

Aging affects headache and sleep in unique ways. Some people with a history of headaches that arise out of sleep, find that the headaches worsen as they get older. One study defines sleep-related migraine as being present when greater than 75 percent of migraines occur during sleep or with awakening. The incidence of sleep-related migraines increases dramatically as people age. Sixteen percent of patients with these headaches were between the ages of 20 and 30, while 58 percent were between the ages of 61 and 70.

You mentioned that your headaches occur at the same time every night, which raises the possibility of hypnic headache, first described by Raskin in 1988. It is a headache that occurs *only* during sleep and it awakens the patient, lasting from 15 minutes to four hours. It is distinguished from migraine because affected individuals tend to want to get up and perform tasks rather than stay in bed. Hypnic headaches are also distinct from cluster headaches because of the quality of the pain and the absence of autonomic symptoms, like eye tearing and nasal congestion. They typically start after age 50 and occur on more than fifteen days per month. Although the pathophysiology is not well understood, it is thought that age-related degeneration of the hypothalamus may play a role in the onset of these headaches. One study monitored patients with polysomnography and interestingly found that all attacks arose from REM sleep.

Could it be possible I have cluster headaches? I read about those occurring at night, like my headaches.

Cluster headaches typically affect younger people (who have their onset when younger, but may never resolve with aging) and have a male predominance, and while they often occur at the same time every night, they may also occur during the daytime. The intense pain of a cluster headache is among the most severe pains that people can experience. Like hypnic headaches, their pathophysiology may localize to the hypothalamus, linking them to the circadian patterns that are observed in so many different headache types. In fact, functional imaging has shown abnormal activity of the hypothalamus during cluster periods as compared to headache-free periods in the same patients. And as described above, high-dose melatonin may be helpful in preventing cluster attacks, probably because of its effect on hypothalamic regulation of melatonin in the pineal gland.

It's exhausting to deal with these chronic headaches and poor sleep. It's really starting to affect my mood.

Anxiety and depression have both been associated with trouble falling and staying asleep, and both are more prevalent among patients with headache disorders. One study sought to clarify whether poor sleep among patients with migraine was attributable to underlying anxiety or depression. The authors found that associations between migraine and sleep problems persisted even after controlling for anxiety and depression. Despite this, there is broad consensus that although mood symptoms may not themselves be responsible for the sleep disturbances observed among patients with migraines, treatment of mood disorders in patients with migraine improves migraine burden. Headache medicine providers often advise patients to seek mental health care as part of the treatment plan for their headaches, and certain selective serotonin reuptake inhibitors (SSRIs) are routinely prescribed for migraine.

I snore a lot, and my primary care doctor recently diagnosed me with sleep apnea. Could that be affecting my headaches?

It's possible. A study of patients who presented to a neurology clinic with headaches and were referred for polysomnography found that among those diagnosed with obstructive sleep apnea (OSA), those who underwent treatment with continuous positive airway pressure (CPAP) saw greater improvement in their headaches compared to those who did not use CPAP.

Although there is evidence that morning headaches have been directly linked to hypoxemia (low oxygen levels) or hypercapnia (elevated carbon dioxide levels) and resolve with its treatment, a comprehensive, population-based study from Norway found similar rates of OSA among those with chronic migraine as the general population. Vgontzas and colleagues propose numerous potential explanations for this unexpected finding, including the possibility that migraine patients have a lower threshold at which hypoxemia may trigger a migraine. Therefore, CPAP may still be warranted for migraine patients who report snorting, fatigue, or frequent nighttime awakenings.

I've noticed I grind my teeth at night; could that be causing my headaches?

Dental problems like temporomandibular joint (TMJ) dysfunction and bruxism can trigger migraines. There is a higher incidence of TMJ dysfunction among patients with headaches compared to those without. A systematic review from 2014 similarly found that sleep bruxism was associated with increased migraine incidence among adults. To explain the mechanism by which this might occur, the authors suggest that nociceptive afferent nerves from the muscles of mastication to the trigeminal nucleus caudalis cause an excitability threshold to be crossed and a headache attack to be triggered. Nighttime mouthguards or oral splints may help some patients avoid this trigger.

I find it hard to lay still when I'm trying to sleep, and my bed partner wonders if I have restless leg syndrome. Could this be affecting my headaches?

Restless leg syndrome (RLS) is a known risk factor for migraine. A systematic review of RLS from 2014 analyzed 24 studies and found that the prevalence of migraine among people with RLS ranges from 15 to 62 percent, which is significantly higher than the general population. The biochemical reason for this association is not well understood, but it has been observed that increased iron deposition in the brain has been associated with both migraine and RLS, and the accumulation of iron may be associated with frequency of attacks. RLS has been associated with not only migraine, but also other primary headache disorders, with the notable exception of cluster headache.

I've recently been diagnosed with narcolepsy, and I've always had migraines. Is there any association between the two conditions?

There may be. The incidence of migraine among narcolepsy patients in one study was 2 to 4 times higher than in the general population. In those patients with both narcolepsy and migraine, onset of narcolepsy symptoms occurred a full 12 years before migraines started. The biological explanation is not fully elucidated, but one hypothesis suggests there is dysfunction of areas of the brainstem that get activated during migraine attacks, including the dorsal raphe nucleus and the locus ceruleus, since those areas also play a critical role in REM sleep.

Citations

Brennan KC, Charles A. Sleep and headache. Semin Neurol. 2009 Sep;29(4):406-18. doi: 10.1055/s-0029-1237113. Epub 2009 Sep 9. PMID: 19742415; PMCID: PMC5605773.

Dahmen N, Kasten M, Wieczorek S, Gencik M, Epplen JT, Ullrich B. Increased frequency of migraine in narcoleptic patients: a confirmatory study. Cephalalgia. 2003 Feb;23(1):14-9. doi: 10.1046/j.1468-2982.2003.00343.x. PMID: 12534574.

De Luca Canto G, Singh V, Bigal ME, Major PW, Flores-Mir C. Association between tension-type headache and migraine with sleep bruxism: a systematic review. Headache. 2014 Oct;54(9):1460-9. doi: 10.1111/head.12446. Epub 2014 Sep 18. PMID: 25231339.

d'Onofrio F, Bussone G, Cologno D, Petretta V, Buzzi MG, Tedeschi G, Bonavita V, Cicarelli G. Restless legs syndrome and primary headaches: a clinical study. Neurol Sci. 2008 May;29 Suppl 1:S169-72. doi: 10.1007/s10072-008-0916-3. PMID: 18545926.

Gelfand AA, Goadsby PJ. The Role of Melatonin in the Treatment of Primary Headache Disorders. Headache. 2016 Sep;56(8):1257-66. doi: 10.1111/head.12862. Epub 2016 Jun 17. PMID: 27316772; PMCID: PMC5012937.

Glaros AG, Urban D, Locke J. Headache and temporomandibular disorders: evidence for diagnostic and behavioural overlap. Cephalalgia. 2007 Jun;27(6):542-9. doi: 10.1111/j.1468-2982.2007.01325.x. Epub 2007 Apr 18. PMID: 17441972.

Gori S, Lucchesi C, Morelli N, Maestri M, Bonanni E, Murri L. Sleep-related migraine occurrence increases with aging. Acta Neurol Belg. 2012 Jun;112(2):183-7. doi: 10.1007/s13760-012-0049-6. Epub 2012 Mar 24. PMID: 22450708.

Hale D, Marshall K. Sleep and Sleep Hygiene. Home Healthc Now. 2019 Jul/Aug;37(4):227. doi: 10.1097/NHH.0000000000000803. PMID: 31274586.

Holland PR. Headache and sleep: shared pathophysiological mechanisms. Cephalalgia. 2014 Sep;34(10):725-44. doi: 10.1177/0333102414541687. Epub 2014 Jul 22. PMID: 25053747.

Houle TT, Butschek RA, Turner DP, Smitherman TA, Rains JC, Penzien DB. Stress and sleep duration predict headache severity in chronic headache sufferers. Pain. 2012 Dec;153(12):2432-2440. doi: 10.1016/j.pain.2012.08.014. Epub 2012 Oct 13. PMID: 23073072; PMCID: PMC3626265.

Johnson KG, Ziemba AM, Garb JL. Improvement in headaches with continuous positive airway pressure for obstructive sleep apnea: a retrospective analysis. Headache. 2013 Feb;53(2):333-43. doi: 10.1111/j.1526-4610.2012.02251.x. Epub 2012 Sep 10. PMID: 22963547.

Karsan N, Bose P, Newman J, Goadsby PJ. Are some patient-perceived migraine triggers simply early manifestations of the attack? J Neurol. 2021 May;268(5):1885-1893. doi: 10.1007/s00415-020-10344-1. Epub 2021 Jan 5. PMID: 33399964; PMCID: PMC8068686.

Kelman L, Rains JC. Headache and sleep: examination of sleep patterns and complaints in a large clinical sample of migraineurs. Headache. 2005 Jul-Aug;45(7):904-10. doi: 10.1111/j.1526-4610.2005.05159.x. PMID: 15985108.

Kim J, Cho SJ, Kim WJ, Yang KI, Yun CH, Chu MK. Insufficient sleep is prevalent among migraineurs: a population-based study. J Headache Pain. 2017 Dec;18(1):50. doi: 10.1186/s10194-017-0756-8. Epub 2017 Apr 28. PMID: 28455722; PMCID: PMC5409905.

Klenofsky B, Pace A, Natbony LR, Sheikh HU. Episodic Migraine Comorbidities: Avoiding Pitfalls and Taking Therapeutic Opportunities. Curr Pain Headache Rep. 2019 Jan 12;23(1):1. doi: 10.1007/s11916-019-0742-8. PMID: 30637489.

Kristiansen HA, Kværner KJ, Akre H, Overland B, Russell MB. Migraine and sleep apnea in the general population. J Headache Pain. 2011 Feb;12(1):55-61. doi: 10.1007/s10194-010-0268-2. Epub 2010 Dec 17. PMID: 21165665; PMCID: PMC3056010.

Lanteri-Minet M. Hypnic headache. Headache. 2014 Oct;54(9):1556-9. doi: 10.1111/head.12447. Epub 2014 Sep 18. PMID: 25231430.

Lipton RB, Buse DC, Hall CB, Tennen H, Defreitas TA, Borkowski TM, Grosberg BM, Haut SR. Reduction in perceived stress as a migraine trigger: testing the "let-down headache" hypothesis. Neurology. 2014

Apr 22;82(16):1395-401. doi: 10.1212/WNL.0000000000000332. Epub 2014 Mar 26. PMID: 24670889; PMCID: PMC4001194.

Mitsikostas D, Thomas A. Comorbidity of Headache and Depressive Disorders. Cephalalgia. 1999;19(4):211-217

Morin LP. The circadian visual system. Brain Res Brain Res Rev. 1994 Jan;19(1):102-27. doi: 10.1016/0165-0173(94)90005-1. PMID: 7909471.

Nayak C, Sinha S, Nagappa M, Nagaraj K, Kulkarni GB, Thennarasu K, Taly AB. Study of sleep microstructure in patients of migraine without aura. Sleep Breath. 2016 Mar;20(1):263-9. doi: 10.1007/s11325-015-1207-x. Epub 2015 Jun 4. PMID: 26041648.

Ødegård SS, Engstrøm M, Sand T, Stovner LJ, Zwart JA, Hagen K. Associations between sleep disturbance and primary headaches: the third Nord-Trøndelag Health Study. J Headache Pain. 2010 Jun;11(3):197-206. doi: 10.1007/s10194-010-0201-8. Epub 2010 Mar 12. PMID: 20224943; PMCID: PMC3451918.

Pellegrino ABW, Davis-Martin RE, Houle TT, Turner DP, Smitherman TA. Perceived triggers of primary headache disorders: A meta-analysis. Cephalalgia. 2018 May;38(6):1188-1198. doi: 10.1177/0333102417727535. Epub 2017 Aug 20. PMID: 28825314.

Pinessi L, Rainero I, Cicolin A, Zibetti M, Gentile S, Mutani R. Hypnic headache syndrome: association of the attacks with REM sleep. Cephalalgia. 2003 Mar;23(2):150-4. doi: 10.1046/j.1468-2982.2003.00472.x. PMID: 12603373.

Rains JC. Sleep and Migraine: Assessment and Treatment of Comorbid Sleep Disorders. Headache. 2018 Jul;58(7):1074-1091. doi: 10.1111/head.13357. Epub 2018 Aug 10. PMID: 30095163.

Sateia MJ, Buysse DJ, Krystal AD, Neubauer DN, Heald JL. Clinical Practice Guideline for the Pharmacologic Treatment of Chronic Insomnia in Adults: An American Academy of Sleep Medicine Clinical Practice Guideline. J Clin Sleep Med. 2017 Feb 15;13(2):307-349. doi: 10.5664/jcsm.6470. PMID: 27998379; PMCID: PMC5263087.

Scher AI, Midgette LA, Lipton RB. Risk factors for headache chronification. Headache. 2008 Jan;48(1):16-25. doi: 10.1111/j.1526-4610.2007.00970.x. PMID: 18184281.

Schürks M, Winter A, Berger K, Kurth T. Migraine and restless legs syndrome: a systematic review. Cephalalgia. 2014 Sep;34(10):777-94. doi: 10.1177/0333102414537725. Epub 2014 Jun 20. PMID: 25142142.

Shapiro RE. Caffeine and headaches. Curr Pain Headache Rep. 2008 Aug;12(4):311-5. doi: 10.1007/s11916-008-0052-z. PMID: 18625110.

Smitherman TA, Kuka AJ, Calhoun AH, Walters ABP, Davis-Martin RE, Ambrose CE, Rains JC, Houle TT. Cognitive-Behavioral Therapy for Insomnia to Reduce Chronic Migraine: A Sequential Bayesian Analysis. Headache. 2018 Jul;58(7):1052-1059. doi: 10.1111/head.13313. Epub 2018 May 6. PMID: 29732536.

Smitherman TA, Walters AB, Davis RE, Ambrose CE, Roland M, Houle TT, Rains JC. Randomized Controlled Pilot Trial of Behavioral Insomnia Treatment for Chronic Migraine with Comorbid Insomnia. Headache. 2016 Feb;56(2):276-91. doi: 10.1111/head.12760. Epub 2016 Jan 27. PMID: 26813845.

Torelli P, Cologno D, Manzoni GC. Weekend headache: a retrospective study in migraine without aura and episodic tension-type headache. Headache. 1999 Jan;39(1):11-20.
doi: 10.1046/j.1526-4610.1999.3901011.x. PMID: 15613189

Vgontzas A, Cui L, Merikangas KR. Are sleep difficulties associated with migraine attributable to anxiety and depression? Headache. 2008 Nov-Dec;48(10):1451-9. doi: 10.1111/j.1526-4610.2008.01175.x. Epub 2008 Jul 1. PMID: 18624714; PMCID: PMC2692650.

Vgontzas A, Pavlović JM. Sleep Disorders and Migraine: Review of Literature and Potential Pathophysiology Mechanisms. Headache. 2018 Jul;58(7):1030-1039. doi: 10.1111/head.13358. Epub 2018 Aug 8. PMID: 30091160; PMCID: PMC6527324.

Vogler B, Rapoport AM, Tepper SJ, Sheftell F, Bigal ME. Role of melatonin in the pathophysiology of migraine: implications for treatment. CNS Drugs. 2006;20(5):343-50. doi: 10.2165/00023210-200620050-00001. PMID: 16696576.

STAFF CHILD NEUROLOGIST ATLANTIC MEDICAL GROUP I CAN'T SLEEP. HELP!

SHANNON BABINEAU, MD

CLINICAL ASSISTANT PROFESSOR OF NEUROLOGY AND PEDIATRICS SIDNEY KIMMEL MEDICAL COLLEGE OF THOMAS JEFFERSON UNIVERSITY

How does sleep effect migraine?

Sleep and migraine have a complicated relationship. Insufficient, irregular, and poor-quality sleep can trigger migraines as well as influence their severity and frequency. In addition, people with migraine are more likely to have disordered sleep. Migraine sufferers have a greater incidence of poor sleep quality and insufficient sleep. Poor sleep quality and sleep disorders put migraine sufferers at risk for progression of their disease to chronic migraine. Those with chronic migraine have a much higher rate of sleep disorders, with up to 80% identified as having insomnia. But it's not all bad, sleep can be one of the best treatments for a migraine when it happens, and many medications used to treat migraine are used because they induce sleep. Most importantly, good quality sleep and sleep habits can be protective against migraine and can even help protect against other triggers leading to migraine. Taking some time to think about your sleep and talking to your doctor about difficulties with sleep, can have a big impact on improving and controlling your migraines.

How can changes in sleep trigger a migraine attack?

Sleep related issues including lack of sleep, sleeping late or excess sleep, and tiredness, are some of the most common triggers of a migraine attack. However, it has been difficult to prove in scientific studies that an individual migraine attack is due to a poor night of sleep. In adults, studies have showed that frequent nighttime awakenings and poor sleep efficiency (the amount of time in bed spent sleeping) are more likely triggers for an individual attack than overall reduced sleep duration. However, in self-reported studies, adults and children note that lack of sleep, oversleeping, and poor-quality sleep are all likely triggers of a migraine attack. Duration and quality of sleep do seem to have an influence on migraine severity, frequency, and the progression to chronic migraine. Sufficient and good quality sleep seem to be protective allowing for overall lower frequency of migraine attacks. In addition, sufficient sleep can help protect against the negative effects of other triggers on migraine, particularly stress. While stress is known not only to trigger migraines but disturb sleep; getting adequate sleep seems to make stress a less powerful trigger for migraine. Oversleeping also may provoke migraines in some. This may explain why some patients experience additional migraines during weekends or holidays.

I wake up with migraines, is this normal?

It is not unusual for a migraine to start while someone is asleep. Migraines often start during REM (rapid eye movement) sleep, and REM sleep time increases in the early mornings. So, it is easy to see why migraine sufferers report early mornings awakenings as a common time for their migraine to begin. However, awakening with migraines can be a sign that there are other conditions at play. Headache upon awakening is the best well-evidenced sign of a sleep disorder. And there are several sleep disorders that are more common in people with migraine. Awakening with headache can also, rarely, be a sign of a more serious condition with increased pressure inside the head, so it is important to let your doctor know if you awaken with headaches.

What sleep disorders are more likely to happen to me if I'm a migraine sufferer? What should I be looking for?

Insomnia is difficulty falling or staying asleep leading to daytime symptoms, despite taking enough time for sleep. Typically, if it takes longer than 30 minutes to fall or return to sleep regularly, insomnia should be considered. Sometimes insomnia develops in the setting of a stressful life event, illness, medication, or shift work, and resolves when the issue is addressed. In some the insomnia does not resolve and there are certain factors that perpetuate the difficulty in sleeping, including maladaptive habits (irregular sleep times, daytime naps etc.), spending a lot of time in bed trying to sleep, anticipation of poor sleep, and fear of ill consequences from sleep loss. Insomnia is found more frequently in migraine sufferers than in the general population, particularly in those with chronic migraine. Improved management of insomnia improves migraine disability, and it is an often-overlooked condition in migraine patients. One of the best studied treatments for insomnia is a type of cognitive behavioral therapy (CBT). There are online programs as well as the option to use a practicing therapist to teach this skill. Migraine sufferers with insomnia found a reduction in migraine frequency when they learned CBT-I. (CBT for insomnia)

Sleep apnea is characterized by brief pauses in breathing while asleep. Symptoms include snoring, feeling tired during the day despite adequate sleep at night, awakening from sleep gasping/choking, and awakening with a headache. Those older than 50, with higher body mass index, or suffering from high blood pressure, are at greater risk for sleep apnea. It is not clear if sleep apnea is more common in adult migraine patients than in the general population, but migraine sufferers may be more sensitive to the body's changes from apnea, so they may be more symptomatic. Sleep apnea can cause more than headaches, it has been associated with high blood pressure, stroke, sudden death, and heart disease. Sleep apnea is not something you want to ignore, as it is important to have it treated. The most typical treatment is with continuous positive airway pressure (CPAP), but may also involve weight reduction and sometimes oral appliances.

Restless leg syndrome is an unpleasant or uncomfortable urge to move the legs during inactivity that is relieved briefly by movement. It occurs more frequently in those with migraine and the symptoms are more severe in those with migraine. Nighttime tooth grinding (bruxism) is also seen more commonly in those with chronic migraine and possibly more often in those with episodic migraine.

It is important to remember that mood disorders like depression, anxiety, and post-traumatic stress disorder (PTSD) are more common in migraine patients and in those with sleep disorders, compared to the general population. Also, sleep patterns can be affected by mood disorders. Those who are depressed may want to sleep more hours during the day, those with PTSD may have intrusive nightmares, and those with anxiety and depression frequently find it difficult to fall asleep. If migraine sufferers with mood disorders are left untreated, they will experience more disability from their migraines. It is important to discuss any mood symptoms you have or ask about screening for depression, anxiety, and PTSD at your next visit if you are struggling with both migraine and sleep difficulties.

What sleep disorders are more likely to happen to my child if he/she is a migraine sufferer?

In children, several medical studies have shown a higher rate of sleep walking, night terrors, and nighttime bed wetting in children that either have or will develop migraine later in life. Sleep apnea can also occur in children and is most common between those who are 2-6 years old. If your child wakes up with headaches or snores at night, and is also suffering with migraines, it is important to have them evaluated for sleep apnea. The anatomy of young children's mouth and throat make them susceptible to sleep apnea. At times surgery for tonsil/adenoid removal can alleviate symptoms of childhood sleep apnea and help the child's headaches. As children become older, obesity is also a risk factor for sleep apnea. Restless legs syndrome can also occur in children and is seen more commonly in children with migraine. Kids will describe restlessness of the legs, growing pains that are worse in bed, insomnia, and morning headaches. Iron supplementation has shown some promise in alleviating the symptoms of RLS in children.

I'm a teenager with migraine, I'm never going to get enough sleep, what should I do?

There are many factors that make it difficult to get a good night's sleep as a teenager. Teenagers still need 8-10 hours of sleep at night based on the recommendations of the American Academy of Sleep Medicine. In addition, teenagers naturally have delayed sleep onset. Teenagers' biological clocks are shifted so they are tired later in the evening compared to younger children and adults. School typically starts early in the morning, with most middle and high schools starting earlier than the American Academy of Pediatrics recommendation of 8:30 am. Many teenagers participate in after school activities and often face significant homework which can take up many of the afternoon and evening hours, leaving little time for proper rest. In addition, teenagers often have access to screens around bedtime. Screens are known to inhibit sleep and can worsen difficulties falling and staying asleep.

So, with all these things going against you, what should you do? It is important to move sleep up on the priority list. Of course, after school activities and socializing are important and schoolwork does need to get done. However, with limited hours in the day, it is important to map out what needs to happen each day and try to work with your family to balance activities through the week to maximize the ability to get to sleep on time.

nigraine. It may just be time, or it is possible that sleeping can interfere vith the irritation the brain is experiencing and/or release certain chemicals hat can combat migraine. If, you are suffering with a severe migraine and our treatments are not enough, an effective treatment strategy includes rying to get yourself to sleep and even asking for a medicine to help initiate leep. However, if migraines are frequent and sleep is frequently used to reat a migraine, particularly if this includes long sleep durations earlier in he day, it can disrupt nighttime sleep and lead to sleep disorders. It is mportant to explore with your doctor options for treatment of a migraine hat may be more effective at aborting the migraine, so that long sleep times re not required frequently.

:an my migraine medicines change my sleep?

'es, many migraine medications can help or hinder sleep. As mentioned bove, sometimes medications that can make you drowsy are helpful to have p your sleeve when you are suffering with a particularly severe migraine hat isn't going away. There are some migraine medicines that can help treat ymptoms of a migraine including pain and nausea as well as help you sleep, llowing for treating the migraine from different angles. There are also nigraine treatment medicines that can make it harder to sleep, most ommonly caffeine. Caffeine is a part of many over-the-counter migraine eatments and it is important to know that when you are taking these nedicines it may be harder to fall asleep. There are also preventive nedications used for migraine that may increase sleepiness. Sleep inducing nigraine prevention is given before bed to help improve sleep as well as revent migraines. However, these medications can sometimes cause aytime drowsiness and can affect the natural architecture of sleep (making nore or less REM sleep or slow wave sleep), so not everyone reacts well to nese medications. Lastly, there are some medications that can treat nigraine as well as sleep disorders such as restless leg syndrome. It is nportant to recognize that many of the lifestyle habits adopted to help with nigraine frequency, such as regular exercise, reduced caffeine, and regular leep schedules, can also help with nighttime sleep quality.

Learning and practicing good sleep hygiene is helpful as well. older, this can ensure you are a good sleeper even when no one remind you to get to bed on schedule. It's important to avoid da which sometimes can trigger a migraine, and certainly can make get a good night's rest. Caffeine should be avoided later in the completely. You should maintain a bedtime and a wake-up tim be consistent on the weekends. Make sure your bedroom is da and use your bed only to sleep (not for school or homework or c friends). Exercising regularly can also help and you should n screen in your room when you are trying to sleep (television, c phone).

What are some other techniques to help get good sleep?

There are several techniques that can be helpful if you are ha time sleeping. Cognitive behavioral therapy for insomnia mentioned, and is a great tool to use if you have difficulty fallin asleep. In addition, learning a bedtime relaxation technique like muscle relaxation, biofeedback, or meditation can be helpful. something called "stimulus control" which tries to break the between lying in bed and not sleeping. This focuses on going when you feel tired and if unable to fall asleep in 10–20 minu watching the clock, 10–20 minutes is equal to repositioning leaving the bedroom. Return only when you are sleepy again. time, you can do a non-screen related relaxing activity to h drowsy. It is important to maintain a bedtime and wakeup tim naps when you are trying to work on stimulus control. L restriction can help. This is used more typically for those with i the goal is to improve sleep efficiency. To be sleep efficient, (90%) of the time you are in bed is spent asleep. First, keep a s note the full amount of time in bed and time asleep. Then sta your time in bed to match actual sleep time, get your sleep effici of whatever amount of time you spend in bed. Then, try increase your time in bed so that it is closer to 7-8 hours at ni fixed wake up time regardless of actual sleep duration. It is i know that these sleep techniques can take time to master, unusual for migraines to worsen initially, but it's worth it in the

Sometimes I go to sleep when I have a migraine, why?

Many migraine sufferers find that they need to sleep in order t from their migraine. It's not well understood what about slee

Suggested Reading

Arruda, Marco A., et al. "Childhood periodic syndromes: a population-based study." *Pediatric neurology* 43.6 (2010): 420-424.

Gelfand, Amy A., and Samantha L. Irwin. "Lifestyle Advice for Pediatric Migraine: Blaming the Patient, or Evidence Based?" *Seminars in neurology*. Vol. 40. No. 03. Thieme Medical Publishers, 2020.

Pavkovic, Ivan M., and Sanjeev V. Kothare. "Migraine and sleep in children: a bidirectional relationship." *Pediatric neurology* 109 (2020): 20-27.

Rains, Jeanetta C. "Sleep and migraine: assessment and treatment of comorbid sleep disorders." *Headache: The Journal of Head and Face Pain* 58.7 (2018): 1074-1091.

Vgontzas, Angeliki, and Jelena M. Pavlović. "Sleep disorders and migraine: review of literature and potential pathophysiology mechanisms." *Headache: The Journal of Head and Face Pain* 58.7 (2018): 1030-1039.

YOGA AND MIGRAINES

DR ANAND KUMAR AND DR PRAVIN THOMAS

They say Yoga is good for migraines. What Yoga should I do?

The Yoga which has been scientifically studied in migraine is Hatha Yoga. There are many exercises and practices which are all referred to as Yoga, but only a few techniques have been studied in migraines.

Can Yoga help reduce my suffering from migraines?

Yes, it can. Yoga, an ancient Indian traditional system of knowledge based on the principles of mind–body medicine, has been observed to have a beneficial effect on various migraine measures, such as headache frequency, intensity, duration of attack, need for medications, and the nature of the pain in all age groups studied.

How can Yoga help me reducing my migraine-related pain?

A lot of research has validated the effectiveness of yoga in various diseases like headache, backache, epilepsy, and many other ailments. Yoga reduces migraine headaches by different mechanisms: 1. Yoga brings about a significant change in the involuntary functions of the nervous system, also known as the autonomic nervous system. It reduces the sympathetic activity of the autonomic nervous system which is often associated with pain. It reduces the sympathetic activity by increasing the activity of the vagus nerve (vagal tone). 2. It also increases the levels of nitric oxide (NO) which is an endothelium-derived relaxing factor–like substance which helps in reducing migraine attacks. 3. Regular practice of Yoga engenders a state of calm alertness and suppresses stress response systems. 4. It reduces muscle tension in the areas affected in migraine pains (head, neck and shoulders).

While doing Yoga, can I stop taking medications?

You should continue them until your clinician tells you that they can be reduced. The effect of Yoga will not begin immediately and so you have to continue both acute pain medications and preventive treatments as prescribed by your physician. You have to maintain a headache diary as well as a yoga log book. Gradually your acute pain medication requirement will decrease and slowly the preventive medications, if any, can be tapered and even stopped.

How frequently do I have to do Yoga for migraine prophylaxis?

Most of the studies showed a significant reduction in headache frequency, intensity and severity by doing yoga thrice a week for 30-60 minutes, over 10-12 weeks. However, if possible, you can practice yoga daily.

Are there any side effects of doing Yoga?

There are three essential elements of yoga**: Asanas (postures), Pranayama (breathing exercises), and Dhyana (meditation).** Until now there was no serious side effects reported in literature. But we have to keep in mind that one should be aware of the limits while performing Yoga, like any other physical activity. Incorrect postures and overdoing can theoretically cause sprain or ligament injury, especially if performed unsupervised.

Who can teach/help me performing yoga sessions?

Yoga is not only a science but also an art. You require a regimen of specific yoga exercises, supervised by a qualified yoga clinician for at least initial one month. After that you should be able to do them on your own, with the guidance of your yoga clinician. You can even ask for video consultations if it is feasible.

Can I stop yoga once migraine is relieved?

After early stopping of Yoga few patients reported recurrence of headache. Yoga is not just another therapy- this is also an art of living. When you start practicing Yoga you would most likely realize that not only is your migraine controlled but also your overall performance has increased, your quality of sleep has improved and there is overall increased sense of well-being. Now it's up to you, will you want to continue to have these all benefits by continuing yoga practice or not!

What precautions we have to take before performing yoga?

There are a few Dos and Don'ts for yoga sessions.

Do's

1. Yoga should be practised before meal or at least two hours after meals.
2. Preferably in the morning but can be done any time.
3. Should wear comfortable clothing.
4. Should be supervised, especially in the beginning stages until the techniques can be practised safely and independently.
5. Avoid distractions like television and phone calls.
6. Can be done in any comfortable position, on the bed, chair or the floor.
7. Take breaks between sessions- it is not essential to 'sweat it out'.

Don't's

1. Do not do it if you are feeling dizzy, uncomfortable or having a bad headache.
2. Do not force or overdo it.
3. Stop if breathing becomes a strain.
4. Do not perform complex exercises if you are alone at home.

Are there any contraindications for yoga?

No, any person can perform yoga, but it must be individualized by the yoga clinician according to the patient's baseline capacity and modified if there are any underlying disease conditions. For example, if any patient is suffering from chronic joint pains, he/she can perform **pranayama (breathing exercises), and Dhyana (meditation)** without any difficulty, but for **asanas (postures)** he/she will require some modifications.

Can children suffering from migraine also perform Yoga?

Yes, there are studies showing beneficial effect of yoga intervention in children aged 11–18 years with headaches. Yoga was effective, safe, acceptable and feasible in children and young adults.

What will be the cost of Yoga therapy? Is it cheaper than current medications of migraine?

Let me give you some figures about the current financial burden of this disease. In the United States alone, the direct cost of headache was about $3.2 billion including the costs of prescriptions and over the counter medications, whereas the indirect cost associated with migraine due to loss of productivity and reduced performance was estimated around $13 billion per year for migraine and $18 billion per year for any headache. Now if you calculate cost for yoga therapy, it includes only a one-time fee for a yoga therapist for one-month supervised yoga teaching sessions and one yoga mat.

Integration of yoga therapy as an adjuvant to conventional medical therapy is effective and safe in patients with migraine. Low cost, safe and effective treatments like yoga in the management of chronic disease conditions like migraine are always worthy of consideration.

Suggested Reading

Bhatia R, Dureja GP, Tripathi M, Bhattacharjee M, Bijlani RL, Mathur R. Role of temporalis muscle over activity in chronic tension type headache: effect of yoga based management. Indian J Physiol Pharmacol 2007; 51:333–344.

Boroujeni M, Marandi S, Esfarjani F, Sattar M, Shaygannejad V, Javanmard S. Yoga intervention on blood NO in female migraineurs. Adv Biomed Res 2015; 4:259.

Cramer H, Ward L, Steel A, Lauche R, Dobos G, Zhang Y. Prevalence, patterns, and predictors of yoga use: results of a U.S. Nationally representative survey. Am J Prev Med 2016; 50:230–235.

Hainsworth KR, Salamon KS, Khan KA, Mascarenhas B, Davies WH, Weisman SJ. A pilot study of yoga for chronic headaches in youth: promise amidst challenges. Pain Manag Nurs 2014; 15:490–498.

John PJ, Sharma N, Sharma CM, Kankane A. Effectiveness of yoga therapy in the treatment of migraine without aura: a randomized controlled trial. Headache 2007; 47:654–661.

Kim SD. Effects of yoga exercises for headaches: a systematic review of randomized controlled trials. J Phys Ther Sci 2015; 27:2377–2380.

Kisan R, Sujan M, Adoor M, et al. Effect of Yoga on migraine: A comprehensive study using clinical profile and cardiac autonomic functions. Int J Yoga 2014;7(2): 126–132.

Kumar A, Bhatia R, Sharma G, Dhanlika D, Vishnubhatla S, Singh RK, Dash D, Tripathi M, Srivastava MVP. Effect of yoga as add-on therapy in migraine (CONTAIN): A randomized clinical trial. Neurology. 2020 May 26;94(21): e2203-e2212.

Lipton RB, Bigal ME. Migraine: epidemiology, impact, and risk factors for progression. Headache 2005;45(suppl 1): S3–S13.

Sharma N, Singhal S, Singh A, Sharma C. Effectiveness of integrated yoga therapy in treatment of chronicmigraine: randomized controlled trial. JHeadache Pain 2013; 14:P116.

Wells RE, Burch R, Paulsen RH, Wayne PM, Houle TT, Loder E. Meditation for migraines: a pilot randomized controlled trial. Headache 2014; 54:1484–1495.

Can Cannabis (Marijuana) Help My Headaches?? Marijuana and Cannabis are used Interchangeably in this Article

Grace Forde, M.D.

Director of Neurological Services
North American Partners in Pain Management
Lake Success, New York

Doc, I have tried everything for my migraines, do you think that marijuana can help me?

Yes, I do. I have many patients using marijuana to treat their chronic, severe, intractable headaches with a significant decrease in the frequency and severity of their attacks. There is some evidence that suggest chronic, migraines might be related to an endocannabinoid deficiency syndrome. Patients with episodic migraines also use, and benefit from cannabis.

Decreased endogenous cannabinoids, that is cannabis produced by your body, can cause cortical spreading depression via increased glutamate signaling which can be a trigger for an aura and/or migraine attack. It can also cause unopposed action of CGRP (calcitonin gene related peptide) and NO (nitrous oxide), on dural vasodilation causing a trigeminal nociceptive response, which can lead to (neurogenic) inflammation.

Therefore, using cannabis prophylactically makes sense given the effect that the endogenous cannabinoids have on the pathogenesis of headaches.

Many more patients use it as needed to treat the acute episodic attacks either by smoking or vaping, more commonly, to rapidly abort or treat an attack. The tetrahydrocannabinol (THC) component of the plant is well known as a treatment for severe nausea and vomiting.

What dose and what kind of marijuana should I take?

We are unable to do the type of research that is needed in the United States, i.e., placebo controlled, randomized clinical trials because cannabis is considered a substance of abuse in the US by the federal government. Therefore, I am unable to give you any specific dosing instructions that will be the silver bullet for your migraine, however, I believe that there is a one-size-fits-all approach. Having, said that there are some common recommendations. Products that are high in cannabidiol (CBD) or those that contain a 1:1 preparation of THC: CBD are usually used as preventative treatment. These medications are more commonly used in oral formulations, because of the longer half-life and is usually given three times a day. For treatment of an acute attack, the 1:1 or high THC preparation is used, with the latter only used in patients who are not naïve to cannabis. The inhalation or sublingual preparations are more effective in acute therapy, especially inhalation, because of the rapid onset of action.

Can cannabis cause medication overuse headaches (MOH)?

Studies have been done using nabilone in patients using daily analgesics for their migraines. Nabilone (Cesamet) is FDA approved in the US for the treatment of chemotherapy induced nausea and vomiting. The studies show that nabilone was able to reduce daily analgesic intake, even in patients who were overusing multiple medications. These patients also had improvement in certain quality of life measures, such as the HIT-6. The headache impact test (HIT) is a tool used to measure the impact headaches have on your ability to function on the job, at school, at home and in social situations. There is also evidence to suggest that the THC component of the plant might cause MOH.

Do I have to smoke?

No, you do not have to smoke, in fact most of my patients use oral preparations. The tincture and/or sublingual can be used for acute attacks and the edibles or pills can be used prophylactically to reduce and/or prevent the frequency, severity, and duration of the attacks. Also, the edibles have a delayed onset of action, it typically takes about 90 mins to take effect. One of the biggest problems I see with the edibles is that people are impatient and would take a second and even a third dose shortly after taking the first dose, because they did not get an immediate effect, and this can lead to increase in side effects.

Do I have to take it every day or only when I have a headache?

If you are using it prophylactically you will need to take it daily, however, the number of times a day will vary from patient to patient, but on average, most patients take it three times a day with a typical range of 2-4 times a day. However, if the patient has low frequency headaches, they do not have to take the medication every day. It can be used on an as needed basis.

Do I have to stop my current meds?

Many patients can decrease their preventative medication when they start taking cannabis, however, cannabis can interact with certain medications, especially ones that are metabolized by the Cytochrome P450 system. Cytochrome P450 are a group of enzymes mainly found in the liver whose role is to metabolize many different types of drugs. The more common medications that are used to treat migraines, which can interact with cannabis because they are also metabolized by the cytochrome P450 system, includes, but is not limited to, desipramine, ergotamine, doxepin, imipramine, nortriptyline, eletriptan, and valproic acid. Caution should be used when combining these medications and one should seek expert consultation.

However, if you are well-versed in the mechanism of action of cannabis and the more traditional headache medicines you can use combination therapy with synergistic, (additive), results. The addition of cannabis can potentially decrease the dose or the number of medications you are currently taking prophylactically.

I don't want to get high!

The part of the plant that gets you "high" is tetrahydrocannabinol (THC). CBD is the antidote to THC. If you feel high from the THC, taking CBD will reverse that effect almost immediately [9]

Will I become addicted?

Addiction is a disease. Time and space would not allow me to go into details, but you can see ASAM definition of addiction. However, addiction refers to repeated use of a substance despite lack of benefit and obvious harm. In New York State one of the indications for medicinal cannabis is opiate addiction. There is evidence to show that the CBD part of the plant decreases reward, drug seeking behavior, anxiety, and sensitivity to other drugs of abuse,

What are the side effects?

Most of the side effects from cannabis comes from the THC component. They include, but is not limited to, "feeling high", somnolence, dizziness, dry mouth, anxiety, paranoia, and cyclical vomiting. The cyclical vomiting is treated by stopping the medication. Interestingly, chronic users who experience this side effect have learnt that very long, very hot showers, would alleviate this side effect. The cyclical vomiting is paradoxical, since the THC portion has been shown to be effective against chemotherapy induced nausea and vomiting.

Is it covered by insurance?

Cannabis is not covered by insurance companies in the United States, due to federal regulations, which put it on the same level as illicit drugs, such as heroin and cocaine. However, more people die from fentanyl-based products and other opioids. The number of deaths solely related to medicinal cannabis use is virtually zero worldwide.

Can I use it if I become pregnant?

There is insufficient evidence to state conclusively whether cannabis is harmful to the developing fetus and/or nursing infant, however, both the American College of Obstetricians and Gynecologists (ACOG) and the American Academy of Pediatrics (AAP) advise against it. There is evidence to suggest that cannabis use in pregnancy is associated with low birth weight, especially in heavy users, spontaneous preterm birth, stillbirth and a higher incidence of neonatal intensive care unit admissions.

What about breastfeeding?

Cannabis is expressed in breast milk, however, recommendations regarding breast feeding while using cannabis is mixed amongst lactation specialist, with those recommending it, citing their risk/benefit analysis. For the pro camp, the benefits of breastfeeding outweigh any potential risk. However, the Academy of Breastfeeding Medicine states that breastfeeding mothers should be counseled to reduce or eliminate their use of cannabis to avoid exposing their infants and advised of possible long-term neurobehavioral effects from continued use.

By 19 weeks' gestation in humans, the fetus has the complete array of cannabinoid receptors, however, the number of receptors is substantially higher in the fetal brain compared to adult brains. Additional insights regarding the impact of cannabis on the developing fetal human brain suggest critical interruptions in the endocannabinoid system are possible. For example, repeated delta-9-THC exposure disrupts endocannabinoid signaling, particularly with CB1 cannabinoid receptor, resulting in a "rewiring" of the fetal cortical circuitry.

Suggested Readings

1 The Use of cannabis for Headache Disorders: Bryson C. Lochte, Alexander Beletsky, Nebiyou K. Samuel and Igor Grant. Cannabis and Cannabinoid Research, Volume 2.1, 2017
2 The endocannabinoid system in migraine: from bench to pharmacy and back. Cristina Tassorelli, Rosaria Greco and Stephen D. Silberstein. Curr Opin Neurol 2019, 32:405-412.
3 Marijuana Use in Pregnancy and While Breastfeeding: Torri D Metz, MD, MS and Laura M Borgelt, PharmD. Obstet Gynecol. 2018 Nov: 132(5): 1198-1210.
4 Cannabis and Migraine: It's Complicated. Lassio L Mechtler, Fran M. Gengo & Vincent H. Bargnes. Current Pain and Headache Reports, 25, Article number 16 (2021)
5 Endocannabinoid System and migraine Pain: An Update. Rosario Greco, Chiara Demartini, Anna M Zanaboni, Daniele Piomelli and Christina Tassorelli. Front Neurosci. 2018:12: 172
6 Endocannabinoid system and pregnancy. Correra F, Wolfson ML, Valchi P, Aisemberg J, Franchi AM. Reproduction. 2016; 152:R191-R200.
7 Ontogenetic development of Cannabinoid receptor expression and signal transduction functionality in the human brain. Mato, S, Del Olmo E, Pazos A, Eur J Neurosci. 2003; 17:1747-54
8 Miswiring the brain: Delta9-tetrahydrocannabinol disrupts cortical development by inducing an SCG10/stathmin-2 degradation pathway. Tortoriello G, Morris CV, Alpar A, et al. EMBO J. 2014;33:668-85.
9 Acute effects of a single, oral dose of d9-tetrahydrocanabinol (THC) and cannabidiol (CBD) administration in healthy volunteers. Martin-Stanos

R, Crippa JA, Batalla A, Bhattacharyya S, Atakan Z, Borgwardt S, et al. Curr Pharm Des. 2012;18(32):4966-79.

10 Cannabinoids induce latent sensitization in a preclinical model of medication overuse headache. Caroline M Kopruszinski, Edita Navratilova, Barbora Vagnerova, Juliana Swiokla, Amol Patwardhan, David Dodick and Frank Porreca Cephalalgia 2020;40:68-78.

11 https://www.asam.org.

12 https://cannigma.com/onditions/addiction

13 https://sites.psu.edu/cannabinoid

OPIOIDS AND MIGRAINE

W. HOWELL JARRARD, MD

I hear different names for certain pain medications such as narcotics, opioids, pain pills, etc. Are these used to treat migraines? If not, how are these different from the medications that are used to treat migraines?

Our body naturally makes "anti-pain" substances that are called "endogenous opioid peptides". These endogenous opioid peptides work by activating receptors in our body's nervous system causing a multitude of effects, one of them being analgesia (or pain relief). Certain medications and illicit drugs mimic these endogenous opioid peptides and act as a temporary analgesic, but also cause a number of side effects. Chronic use can potentially result in the long-term consequences of dependency and possibly addiction. There are a number of these medications, some of which include oxycodone, hydrocodone, morphine, and codeine. In general, these types of medications are not used to treat migraine. Fortunately, there are a number of medications available both over the counter and by prescription to adequately treat migraine.

Common over the counter and prescription medications for migraine include the non-steroidal anti-inflammatory drugs or "NSAIDs". NSAIDs work primarily by inhibiting an enzyme that is involved in the production of peptides (or chemicals) that can cause inflammation throughout the body. When this inflammation is in the brain it can cause migraine attacks, thus when reduced, migraines can be alleviated. Common NSAIDs include ibuprofen, naproxen, aspirin, and diclofenac. Triptans are the most common group of prescription medications that are specifically used to treat migraine. Similar to NSAIDs, they work by decreasing inflammation. Specifically, they work to decrease "brain" inflammation by lowering the amount of certain peptides that are known to be involved in migraine attacks. The most commonly prescribed triptans are sumatriptan (Imitrex) and rizatriptan (Maxalt), but there are many more. Another recently developed group of migraine attack medications called "gepants" target a chemical in the migraine cascade known as CGRP (calcitonin gene-related peptide). These may also be very effective.

I have taken opioids for headaches and for other reasons and they did improve my pain. Why are they not a good option for migraines?

It is easiest to think of migraine as a chemical imbalance in the brain and nervous system that causes inflammation and hypersensitivity to pain during its attacks. Opioids can help temporarily "mask" the pain, but they do not address the underlying inflammation causing it. In addition, opioids can actually increase some peptides that cause inflammation, which may worsen pain in the long term. Thus, while opioids might improve pain initially during an attack, in the long run, with frequent use, they may actually worsen migraine. Other medications used to treat migraine target these peptides and inflammation, ultimately treating the underlying cause directly.

There are a limited number of reasons why doctors prescribe opioid medications. Common reasons are pain due to cancer, palliative care management and end of life care. Other than these uses, opioids are typically reserved for patients with significant pain that is expected to be temporary (i.e., post-operative pain). In regard to chronic pain, prior research studies have not shown any strong evidence that long term opioids provide significant pain relief or improve quality of life. When opioids were directly compared to medications such as NSAIDs and triptans in research studies, they did not work any better in treating migraine pain. In addition, there are numerous negative side effects of using opioids, most commonly being sedation, diminished concentration, severe constipation and changes in mood. Given these side effects and their lack of superiority in managing migraine attacks, opioid use is typically avoided in the treatment of migraines.

How might opioids make my migraines worse over time?

The short answer is that opioids increase central sensitization. To understand what this means we must think about how the brain perceives pain. Acute pain is caused by the brain receiving an irritative stimulus from somewhere in the body. Whether from a cut on the hand or from inflammation related to a migraine attack, our nervous system receives a signal that is sent to our brain, and we experience it as pain. Over time, pain that is repeated or persistent makes the brain more sensitive to any type of irritative signal. In other words, this can cause future pain to become more painful (termed hyperalgesia) and otherwise non-painful sensations to become painful (termed allodynia). This increased brain sensitivity is known as central sensitization and is the reason frequent migraine attacks inadequately treated can lead to overall worsening of migraine. Opioids temporarily mask pain and do not treat the underlying cause of migraine while also augmenting central sensitization. This augmentation can even occur with short courses of opioid medications. In other words, opioid use can make future pain and migraine attacks occur more frequently and more severely. In addition, their use can also change a normal stimulation, that is otherwise not painful, into an uncomfortable or painful sensation.

Can I use opioids as needed for severe pain when my usual migraine medications are not working?

When your migraine medications are not consistently treating attacks, it is important to speak with your doctor about potential reasons for ineffectiveness. Some of the more common reasons include inadequate dosing or route of medication intake, delay in medication administration, overuse of migraine medications or incorrect diagnosis. Once you have found a regimen that is more successful, your doctor might recommend a tiered approach to management with a backup medication. Generally, it is a great idea to have backup medications to treat your migraine attacks when your first medication is not working. Opioids are not good backup medications, even when used infrequently. They interfere with other medications we use to treat migraine and decrease their effectiveness. This interference can continue even when you are no longer using opioids. In other words, even if taken in the past, opioids can interfere with the effectiveness of your current and future migraine medications. There are many reasons why this occurs, but the simplest explanation is that opioids likely increase peptides involved in inflammation associated with migraine attacks.

If I need to stop my opioids now, then what will happen to my headaches?

If you have been on opioids for a short amount of time or are not taking them frequently (less than daily), then you can usually stop taking them immediately without significant side effects. If you have been taking opioids for a long time (months or years) or have been taking them daily, then it may be best to slowly wean off of them. This is usually done to minimize opioid withdrawal, which consists of a number of symptoms. Opioid withdrawal symptoms can occur within hours to days of the last dose and usually resolve within days to weeks. The time course is dependent on which opioid medication is used. If you are concerned about stopping your opioids, then talk with your doctor who may recommend a plan to wean on a case-by-case basis.

Whether stopping opioids suddenly or slowly weaning, it can be expected that your migraines may get worse before they get better. It is important to stay motivated and expect eventual improvement in the future. Improvement can be seen as soon as a few weeks after stopping the opioids but may take up to a few months. If your headaches worsen significantly during this time, there are medications that can be used temporarily to ease the transition off of opioids. Remember, while your pain may worsen at first, be confident that discontinuing opioids will improve your migraines in the long run.

Are there ever instances where opioids should be prescribed for migraine?

Generally, opioid use for migraine treatment is avoided due to side effects and potential long-term consequences, but there are a few special scenarios where they are considered. These special scenarios commonly include pregnant or elderly patients. In these patient populations, the typical migraine medications are either proven not safe to use or have not been scientifically studied for safety. For pregnant patients, there are fewer medications that are known to be both effective in treating migraine and safe to the mother and baby. When migraines are resistant to this smaller group of medications and headache symptoms are severe, then short-term treatment with opioids can be considered. Fortunately, the majority of women's migraines actually improve during pregnancy.

Elderly patients often have more medical conditions and take more medications that prevent the safe use of some migraine medications. When this occurs, opioids can be considered for infrequent use and with a low dose. It is important to remember that elderly patients tend to be more sensitive to the side effects of medications, especially opioids. New migraine medications with less safety concerns continue to be developed and are expanding treatment options for these special patient populations.

What should I do if I'm taking buprenorphine or methadone to treat a prior addiction?

Two of the most commonly prescribed medications for patients with prior opioid addiction are buprenorphine and methadone. When used correctly and monitored closely, these medications can assist in treating dependency and addiction to both illicit and prescription opioid drugs. Each medication works differently, but they both have some activity on opioid receptors. Because of this, it is likely that these medications have some long-term effects similar to opioids, the most concerning of which is interference with migraine medications. If you recently started these medications or your opioid addiction is difficult to manage without medication, then you should continue use and discuss migraine management with your doctor. If you feel comfortable stopping these medications, then discuss this with your doctor, as doing so may improve your migraines.

What if I'm prescribed opioids after a surgery?

There are times when a doctor may recommend a short course of opioids after surgery for post-operative pain management. It is important to ask your doctor about possible non-opioid pain medications that can be tried first (i.e., NSAIDs or acetaminophen). If your pain can be managed using non-opioid medications, then this is preferable. However, inadequately treated severe pain can lead to stress, which can trigger a migraine attack. Thus, consider opioid use for severe pain that is not alleviated with non-opioid medications. When used for a short period of time, opioids are less likely to have significant long-term effects on your migraines.

Suggested Reading

Ballantyne JC. The brain on opioids. *Pain* 2018; *159*: S24–S30.

Berna C, Kulich, R, Rathmell, JP. Tapering Long-term Opioid Therapy in Chronic Noncancer Pain. *Mayo Clinic Proceedings* 2018; *90*: 828–842.

Bigal M, Lipton R. Excessive opioid use and the development of chronic migraine. *Pain* 2009;*142*: 179–182.

Casucci G, Cevoli S. Controversies in migraine treatment: opioids should be avoided. *Neurological Sciences* 2013; *34*: 125–128.

Kelley N, Tepper D. Rescue Therapy for Acute Migraine, Part 3: Opioids, NSAIDs, Steroids, and Post-Discharge Medications. *Headache* 2012; *52*: 467–482.

Levin M. Opioids in Headache. *Headache* 2014; *54*: 12–21.

Lipton R, Buse D, Dodick D, et al.Burden of increasing opioid use in the treatment of migraine: Results from the Migraine in America Symptoms and Treatment Study. *Headache* 2020;*61*: 103–116.

Tepper S. Opioids Should Not Be Used in Migraine. *Headache* 2012*; 52*: 30–34.

"IS MY TMJ CAUSING MY HEADACHES?"

JENNIFER P. BASSIUR, DDS

ASSOCIATE PROFESSOR OF DENTAL MEDICINE
(ORAL SURGERY)
COLUMBIA UNIVERSITY MEDICAL CENTER
NEW YORK CITY

My jaw makes a clicking or popping sound when I open and close. Do I have TMJ? Is that the cause of my headaches?

TMD stands for "temporomandibular disorders" and refers to various musculoskeletal and neuromuscular conditions involving the temporomandibular joint, or TMJ, the masticatory muscles, and the associated structures. TMDs are a relatively common type of orofacial pain and sometimes TMDs can cause headache.

The clicking or popping sound that you are hearing likely due to a disc displacement. There is a small fibrocartilage disc inside your TMJ that may be slightly out of place. Disc displacements are a common TMJ finding. They may or may not be painful. The condition is sometimes called "internal derangement" and refers to a misalignment of the articular disc that interferes with the smooth motion of the TMJ, resulting in joint noises and sometimes sticking, catching or locking of the jaw. The popping sound that you are hearing is consistent with a disc displacement with reduction, meaning that the disc is recaptured or realigned when you open your mouth. When you open, the "pop" that you hear is that disc going back in place. Before your teeth come back together, that disc is again displaced.

Clicking and popping of the jaw is common and doesn't necessarily mean that there is joint degeneration or even a problem. Unless the sounds are associated with pain or a significantly reduced range of motion, most patients with pain-free clicking or popping do not require treatment. If it does become painful, the cause is usually inflammation of the retrodiscal or synovial tissues, joint capsule or ligaments, or pressure on the disc attachments.

Do I need an MRI? Can it be fixed? Am I going to need surgery?

Magnetic resonance imaging (MRI) is the best method to confirm disc position and movement in the open and closed-mouth positions. It can also be used to assess the presence or absence of joint effusion or bony changes. Given your current symptoms, advanced imaging may not be necessary and treatment is not dependent on imaging.

TMD isn't something that is "fixed," but your symptoms can be managed. For many patients, conservative, non-surgical modalities are highly effective. We may want to include therapies such as: heat and ice; medications, for example non-steroidal anti-inflammatories or muscle relaxants, or for more chronic TMDs, tricyclic antidepressants or antiepileptic drugs; and physical therapies like postural training, stretching and mobilization. Cognitive behavioral therapy and active relaxation exercises are also helpful. There are specific articular disorders for which surgical management may be effective, but generally, surgery or any irreversible treatment should only be considered when conservative therapy is ineffective. There are different features can help determine the most beneficial management strategies for you. For example, when your jaw pops, is the popping associated with any pain? Does your jaw ever get stuck closed or open? Is it worse when you wake up in the morning?

The popping doesn't hurt, but lower down, both sides of my jaw hurt, especially when I chew. My jaw has never gotten stuck and it gets worse as the day goes on. It is probably best in the morning. Do I need a nightguard?

What you are describing, and we can confirm on examination, is pain in the masseter area. It is more consistent with a myogenous, or muscular TMD, rather than pain from the temporomandibular joint, itself. A nightguard is often recommended for patients complaining of jaw pain. It is most beneficial for individuals whose symptoms are worse upon awakening. If you were grinding your teeth at night, what you may have heard described as, "sleep bruxism," and had painful TMD, you might be at greater risk for chronic migraine. But since you feel best first thing in the morning, and your symptoms worsen throughout the day, it is more important that we look at what might be exacerbating your symptoms while you are awake. If your teeth are touching much of the time, you might be clenching. It is not uncommon to be completely unaware of clenching. To get your teeth apart, say the letter, "N". In this position, your tongue should be up at the roof of your mouth, resting, but not bracing in that position. Your lips come together, but your teeth remain apart. In the beginning, it is necessary to check periodically that you are in this position. Other habits may also be contributing to your symptoms. Are you leaning on your hands? Are you constantly looking down at a phone or computer? Biting nails? Chewing gum? The masseters, along with the temporalis muscles, are your main chewing muscles. There is a lot of overlap between pain in these muscles and headache.

My teeth are touching a lot, but I don't think I do any of those other things. I do eat a lot of almonds. I get pain in my temples, too. But I thought that was a headache. Are you saying it is actually TMD?

We would have to look at some of the other symptoms that you experience during these episodes and also what makes your pain worse. For example, do you also experience sensitivity to light and sound? How about nausea or vomiting? Does chewing make the pain worse? Does exercise? Do you get headaches in other areas of your head or at other times? The pain in your temples could be due to a headache disorder, like migraine, or it could be a symptom of TMD, or more likely, it is a combination of the two. Both headaches and TMDs occur frequently and can share common symptoms, making it difficult to separate the two disorders. In addition, because they also share many of their multifactorial origins, they often coexist.

While you are having this pain, you should avoid hard and crunchy foods like the almonds. Chewing hard foods requires a lot of work and you want to minimize the work that you jaw is doing. Stick to a soft diet and foods that don't require a lot of chewing. One food that people don't think about as being difficult to chew is lettuce, but it also requires a lot of chewing and should be avoided until you are feeling better.

TMDs can trigger or perpetuate primary headache, but primary headache can also trigger or perpetuate TMD. Painful TMD has been also been shown to increase headache frequency. Headache does occur more frequently in patients with TMD symptoms, especially those with myogenous TMDs. At the same time, TMDs are more likely to occur in patients with migraine or tension-type headaches than in individuals that do not have headache. When headaches occur secondary to TMD, jaw movement or pressure on the TMJ or associated musculature often exacerbate the headache. We want to look at what may be causing and perpetuating both the headache and TMD. Even without a causative association, in order to most effectively reduce your symptoms, we would want to make sure we are addressing both the headache and TMD.

Suggested reading

De Leeuw R, Klasser GD, editors. Orofacial pain: guidelines for assessment, diagnosis and management. 6th edition. Hanover Park (IL): American Academy of Orofacial Pain. Quintessence Publishing; 2018

Conti PC, Costa YM, Gonçalves DA, Svensson P. Headaches and myofascial temporomandibular disorders: overlapping entities, separate managements? *J Oral Rehabil*. 2016 Sep; 43(9):702-15.

Graff-Radford SB, Abbott JJ. Temporomandibular Disorders and Headache. *Oral Maxillofac Surg Clin North Am*. 2016 Aug;28(3):335-49

Fernandes G, Franco AL, Gonçalves DA, Speciali JG, Bigal ME, Camparis CM. Temporomandibular disorders, sleep bruxism, and primary headaches are mutually associated. *J Orofac Pain*. 2013 Winter; 27(1):14-20

Graff-Radford SB, Bassiur, JB. Temporomandibular disorders and headaches. *Neurol Clin*. 2014; 32(2):525-37

Bellegaard V, Thede-Schmidt-Hansen P, Svensson P, et al. Are headache and temporomandibular disorders related? A blinded study. *Cephalalgia* 2008; 28:832-41

Glaros AG, Urban D, Locke J. Headache and temporomandibular disorders: evidence for diagnostic and behavioral overlap. *Cephalalgia* 2007; 27:542–9.

I Have Chronic Paroxysmal Hemicrania. Do I Have to Take Indomethacin Forever?

Murray Choueka, MD
Fellow in Headache Medicine
Department of Neurology
Icahn School of Medicine at Mt. Sinai
New York City
Alexander Mauskop, MD, FAAN
Professor of Clinical Neurology
SUNY Downstate Medical Center
Director, New York Headache Center
New York City

For the past 6 months, I have been experiencing severe pain on the left side of my head. The pain builds up quickly, lasts 25 minutes and then dissipates quickly. I noticed my eyelid droops and my eye gets teary during the episodes. These episodes happen between 5 and 15 times per day. What kind of headache is this?

You most likely have what is called "paroxysmal hemicrania." This type of headache disorder is characterized by attacks of severe, strictly unilateral pain which is orbital, supraorbital, temporal or in any combination of these sites. The attacks last 2-30 minutes and occur several times per day. The attacks are usually associated with ipsilateral conjunctival injection, lacrimation, nasal congestion, rhinorrhea, forehead and facial sweating, miosis, ptosis and/or eyelid edema. They respond absolutely to a drug called "indomethacin."

Do I need any brain imaging or lab tests?

Yes, you do need to have an MRI to be absolutely certain that you don't have a brain tumor or some other imitator of these headaches. Typically, it is a tumor, it is a benign tumor. There are three reports in the literature of patients who met diagnostic criteria for chronic paroxysmal hemicrania (CPH) who ended up having masses around the pituitary gland. For those above the age of 50, especially if they have fevers or visual changes, we may check inflammatory markers in the blood to rule out a disease called "giant cell arteritis."

When will my headache go away?

Approximately 20% of patients have an episodic version of paroxysmal hemicrania. These patients will have bouts of headaches lasting at least 7 days with subsequent periods of remission lasting many months. The other 80% of patients, like yourself, have the chronic form called "chronic paroxysmal hemicrania." The good news is that your headaches can be completely prevented with medications. You may have periods of weeks to months where your headaches go away even without taking medications.

I know someone who has cluster headaches. My headaches seem to be similar to his. How can I be sure my diagnosis of chronic paroxysmal hemicrania is correct?

In 1980, a group of neurologists, including the author of this book, Dr. Green, described the features of CPH and how they differ from cluster headache. Until then, it is very likely that most cases of CPH were misdiganosed as other headache disorders and subsequently treated insufficiently. The pain of cluster headaches can feel quite similar to that of CPH. Cluster headache attacks may last as short as 15 minutes and may occur up to 8 times per day. In addition, both CPH and cluster headache may be accompanied by autonomic features such as eyelid droop, tearing or nasal congestion on the side of the headache. Due to the overlap in frequency and duration of pain, there is a risk of diagnostic confusion. In your case, the fact that the attacks occur up to 15 times daily makes cluster headache an unlikely diagnosis. The best way to confirm the diagnosis of CPH is to try indomethacin. While CPH is exquisitely sensitive to indomethacin, cluster headache tends not to respond to it. On the other hand, cluster headache is very sensitive to subcutaneous sumatriptan or inhaled oxygen while CPH often does not respond to them.

I am interested in trying indomethacin. What is it and how should I take it?

Indomethacin is in a class of drugs called non-steroidal antinflammatory drugs (NSAIDs). This class of drugs includes aspirin, naproxen and ibuprofen, which you are probably familiar with. While there are some case reports of these NSAIDs being effective, they usually provide only partial relief. In the 1980s, indomethacin was proven to be the only medication that consistently provides complete pain relief in CPH. You will start by taking indomethacin 25 mg three times daily for a total daily dose of 75 mg. If headaches persist, you may increase the total daily dose by 25 mg every 2 days until your headaches are eliminated. While most patients respond to doses of 150 mg daily or less, some may need as much as 225 mg daily. Complete pain relief typically occurs within 24 hours of reaching the effective dose. The most common side effect is gastrointestinal discomfort. Some patients may go on to develop stomach ulcers or gastrointestinal bleeding. To minimize these adverse effects, you should take a daily acid reflux medication, such has famotidine or omeprazole. You should also take the medication with food and an antacid. Once your headaches dissipate, you can slowly lower the indomethacin to identify the lowest effective daily dose.

I am hesitant about taking indomethacin every day due to the side effects. Is there anything I can take when the headache starts to abort each headache?

Due to the brief duration of each headache, the headache will likely have dissipated by the time any drug you take reaches peak levels in your blood. Subcutaneous sumatriptan, which reaches peak levels in just 15 minutes, is usually ineffective in reducing the duration of paroxysmal hemicrania attacks. There is very limited evidence that oxygen can lower the intensity of the attack in some cases. The mainstay of treatment for CPH is therefore preventative medications.

I started taking indomethacin, titrated the dose up to 75 mg three times daily and my headaches have finally resolved. Now what?

To minimize the adverse effects, you should slowly reduce the dose of indomethacin. There is no perfect way to do this. You may reduce the dose by 25 mg per day every 2 weeks until you start to experience mild pain again. This time course is based on the fact that symptoms have been shown to reappear up to 14 days after discontinuation of indomethacin. When you reach the point where you experience pain again, you should increase the total daily dose again by 25 mg. If your pain again goes away, you know you are at the lowest effective dose although over time, this might be lowered even more.

Do I have to take indomethacin forever?

You will likely have to take indomethacin for a long time. Over years, you may find that you need less indomethacin to stay headache-free. It is possible that you may experience a period of years in which you will be headache-free while off of indomethacin. Occasionally, CPH can convert to episodic paroxysmal hemicrania (EPH) where patients have remission periods lasting years. Because the disease is so rare, there is very little long-term data to answer this question with certainty. Since EPH attack periods can last up to a year, it is often impossible to differentiate between EPH and CPH early on in the disease course. In these cases, you should attempt to wean off of indomethacin after a few months. If the headaches return, you should restart indomethacin and perhaps try weaning off again after one year.

I have been taking indomethacin for five years. I have attempted discontinuing it multiple times with a recurrence of attacks each time. Is there any hope that my disease will ever go into remission?

Yes. There have been case reports of long-standing remission in CPH, even after 10 years of continuously requiring indomethacin! In these reported cases, there were remission periods of 6 months to 1.5 years. We are hoping that some of the new antimigraine drugs will be effective for this headache.

Is there anything I did that caused me to develop CPH? Is it genetic?

There is no known genetic contribution. In fact, 80% of patients with CPH do not have a family history of a related headache disorder. To our knowledge, there is nothing you did that caused you to develop CPH.

Is there anything I should avoid that may trigger these headaches?

In some patients, the pain is triggered by certain sudden movements of the head or neck. Alcohol, stress, exercise and sneezing are also known to be triggers. If you know that you have one of these triggers, obviously you should avoid them as best you can.

Indomethacin has provided complete headache relief but the stomach pain is intolerable! Are there any other medications I can take?

Unfortunately, there are no other medications that have been proven to be completely effective for CPH. Celecoxib, aspirin, verapamil, gabapentin, lithium, carbamazepine and oxygen have all been reported to be ineffective. Some patients, however, may respond to one of these drugs. Aspirin may provide partial relief from pain. There are case reports of CPH responding to topiramate, sumatriptan and acetazolamide. One option would be to try indomethacin suppositories. Taking the drug by suppository may cause diarrhea and does not eliminate the risk of gastrointestinal side effects. However, due to the limited options for the prevention of CPH, it may be worth a try. There is some evidence that the natural supplement, Boswellia Serrata, can reduce or even eliminate pain in CPH, and cause fewer gastrointestinal side effects than indomethacin.

I have a friend who receives Botox for chronic migraine. Is this an option for me?

Yes, this is an option! OnabotulinumtoxinA (Botox) is very effective for chronic migraine. While the exact mechanism of action has not yet been fully elucidated, it is believed to work by desensitization of the peripheral nerve endings which in turn modulates areas in the hypothalamus and brainstem, including the dorsal pons. The dorsal pons is known to be activated in both CPH and chronic migraine. Thus, there is a theoretical reason to believe Botox might work for CPH. There are at least two case reports in which Botox was effective for CPH. Due to the excellent safety profile for Botox, there is little harm in trying Botox alone or as an adjunct to another medication.

What about nerve blocks or nerve simulators?

There have been some cases reported in the literature in which occipital nerve blocks or sphenopalatine ganglion (SPG) blocks reduced the intensity and frequency of attacks. There are other case reports where they were ineffective. Unfortunately, the evidence is very limited. There is at least one case reported in which bilateral occipital nerve stimulator implantation provided intermittent relief. Due to the risk of both short and long-term surgical complications, this should only be done as a last resort.

I have a friend who has CPH who did not completely respond to indomethacin. Does that mean they don't have CPH?

Not necessarily. The IHS diagnostic criteria state that patients must have a complete response to indomethacin for a diagnosis of CPH. In order for research to progress, it is important to have strict diagnostic criteria which prevent the accidental inclusion of patients with other headache disorders like cluster headache. However, in clinical practice, absolute adherence to diagnostic criteria is not necessary and may lead to incorrect or inadequate treatment. For example, those who have intolerable side effects to indomethacin prior to reaching a therapeutic dose do not meet strict diagnostic criteria for CPH. However, for clinical purposes, they should be treated as if they have CPH. The lack of complete response to indomethacin should prompt your friend's physician to consider an alternative diagnosis like cluster headache. They should also rule out secondary causes of headaches with magnetic resonance imaging of the brain and vessel imaging of the head and neck.

I plan to become pregnant next year. Is indomethacin safe to take during pregnancy?

The safety of indomethacin has not been thoroughly investigated. The FDA recommends avoiding indomethacin after 20 weeks of gestation due to the risk of oligohydramnios (too little amniotic fluid). Furthermore, there is a risk of premature closure of the ductus arteriosus with indomethacin use after 30 weeks of gestation. Even prior to 20 weeks, there is a possible risk of birth defects. After delivery, indomethacin can be restarted even if you are breastfeeding. Indomethacin levels in breastmilk are less than 1% of the maternal weight-adjusted dose. The good news for you is that your pain might disappear during pregnancy. In a study of 84 patients, 9 out of 10 patients who became pregnant had their headaches disappear during pregnancy.

Suggested Reading

1. Antonaci F, Pareja JA, Caminero AB, Sjaastad O. Chronic paroxysmal hemicrania and hemicrania continua: lack of efficacy of sumatriptan. *Headache*. 1998 Mar;38(3):197-200.

2. Antonaci F, Sjaastad O. Chronic paroxysmal hemicrania (CPH): A review of the clinical manifestations. *Headache*. 1989 Nov;29(10):648-56.
3. Baber N, Sibeon R, Laws E, Halliday L, Orme M, Littler T. Indomethacin in rheumatoid arthritis: comparison of oral and rectal dosing. *Br J Clin Pharmacol*. 1980;10(4):387-392.
4. Boes CJ, Dodick DW. Refining the clinical spectrum of chronic paroxysmal hemicrania: a review of 74 patients. *Headache*. 2002 Sep;42(8):699-708.
5. Cittadini E, Matharu MS, Goadsby PJ. Paroxysmal hemicrania: a prospective clinical study of 31 cases. *Brain*. 2008 Apr;131(Pt 4):1142-55.
6. Cohen AS, Goadsby PJ. Paroxysmal hemicrania responding to topiramate. *J Neurol Neurosurg Psychiatry*. 2007;78(1):96-97.
7. Eross E. A comparison of efficacy, tolerability and safety in subjects with hemicrania continua responding to indomethacin and specialized Boswellia serrata extract (5250). *Neurology*. 2020; 94(suppl 15).
8. Ertem DH. Are repetitive pericranial nerve blocks effective in the management of chronic paroxysmal hemicrania?: A case report. *Medicine*. 2019 Aug;98(31).
9. Evers S, Husstedt IW. Alternatives in drug treatment of chronic paroxysmal hemicrania. *Headache*. 1996 Jul-Aug;36(7):429-32.
10. Garza I, Cutrer FM. Pain relief and persistence of dysautonomic features in a patient with hemicrania continua responsive to botulinum toxin type A. *Cephalalgia*. 2010 Apr;30(4):500-3.
11. Gatzonis S, Mitsikostas DD, Ilias A, Zournas CH, Papageorgiou C. Two more secondary headaches mimicking chronic paroxysmal hemicrania. Is this the exception or the rule? *Headache*. 1996 Sep;36(8):511-3.
12. Grangeon L, Moscatelli L, Zanin A, Rouille A, Maltete D, Guegan-Massardier E. Indomethacin-Responsive Paroxysmal Hemicrania in an Elderly Man: An Unusual Presentation of Pituitary Apoplexy. *Headache*. 2017 Nov;57(10):1624-1626.
13. Headache Classification Committee of the International Headaches Society (IHS). The International Classification for Headache Disorders, 3rd edition. *Cephalalgia*. 2018;38:1-211.
14. Jensen NB, Joensen P, Jensen J. Chronic paroxysmal hemicrania: continued remission of symptoms after discontinuation of indomethacin. *Cephalalgia*. 1982 Sep;2(3):163-4.
15. Khalil M, Ahmed F (2013) Hemicrania continua responsive to botulinum toxin type a: a case report. *Headache*. 2013 Mar;53:831–833.

16. Kudrow DB, Kudrow L. Successful aspirin prophylaxis in a child with chronic paroxysmal hemicrania. *Headache*. 1989 May;29(5):280–1.
17. Lucas S. The Pharmacology of Indomethacin. *Headache*. 2016 Feb;56(2):436-46.
18. Matharu MS, Cohen AS, McGonigle DJ, Ward N, Frackowiak RS, Goadsby PJ. Posterior hypothalamic and brainstem activation in hemicrania continua. *Headache*. 2004 Sep;44(8):747-61.
19. Miller S, Lagrata S, Watkins L, Matharu M. Occipital Nerve Stimulation for Medically Refractory Chronic Paroxysmal Hemicrania. *Headache*. 2017 Nov;57(10):1610-1613.
20. Pareja J, Sjaastad O. Chronic paroxysmal hemicrania and hemicrania continua. Interval between indomethacin administration and response. *Headache*. 1996 Jan;36(1):20-3.
21. Pareja JA, Caminero AB, Franco E, Casado JL, Pascual J, Sánchez del Río M. Dose, efficacy and tolerability of long-term indomethacin treatment of chronic paroxysmal hemicrania and hemicrania continua. *Cephalalgia*. 2001 Nov;21(9):906-10.
22. Pascual J, Quijano J. A case of chronic paroxysmal hemicrania responding to subcutaneous sumatriptan. *J Neurol Neurosurg Psychiatry*. 1998 Sep;65(3):407.
23. Sjaastad O, Antonaci F. Chronic paroxysmal hemicrania: a case report. Long-lasting remission in the chronic stage. Cephalalgia. 1987 Sep;7(3):203-5.
24. Sjaastad O, Apfelbaum R, Caskey W, Christoffersen B, Diamond S, Graham J, Green M, Hørven I, Lund-Roland L, Medina J, Rogado S, Stein H. Chronic paroxysmal hemicrania (CPH). The clinical manifestations. A review. *Ups J Med Sci Suppl*. 1980;31:27-33.
25. Vijayan N. Symptomatic chronic paroxysmal hemicrania. *Cephalalgia*. 1992 Apr;12(2):111-3.
26. Villar-Martínez MD, Moreno-Ajona D, Chan C, Goadsby PJ. Indomethacin-responsive headaches-A narrative review. *Headache*. 2021 May;61(5):700-714.
27. Warner JS, Wamil AW, McLean MJ (1994) Acetazolamide for the treatment of chronic paroxysmal hemicrania. *Headache*. 19914 Nov;34:597–599.
28. Zidverc-Trajkovic J, Pavlovic AM, Mijajlovic M, Jovanovic Z, Sternic N, Kostic VS. Cluster headache and paroxysmal hemicrania: differential diagnosis. *Cephalalgia*. 2005 Apr;25(4):244-8.

Do I Need Surgery for Trigeminal Neuralgia?

Murray Choueka, MD
Fellow in Headache Medicine
Department of Neurology
Icahn School of Medicine at Mt. Sinai
New York City
Alexander Mauskop, MD, FAAN
Professor of Clinical Neurology
SUNY Downstate Medical Center
Director, New York Headache Center
New York City

I have been experiencing electric shocks on the left side of my face for the past few weeks. The shocks last only seconds, but they are so painful that I wince each time. The shocks are triggered by just about anything touching my face. Even the wind can trigger it! I also have pain when I eat or speak. My primary care doctor thinks I have trigeminal neuralgia and sent me to see you. Is this the right diagnosis?

It is very likely that the diagnosis is correct. Trigeminal neuralgia, also known as "*tic douloureux*", is characterized by sharp, often electric-like pains in one or more of the 3 divisions of the trigeminal nerve. This nerve provides sensation to the face. The pain episodes are very severe, last from a fraction of a second up to 2 minutes, and can occur many times per day. They often occur as a series of attacks lasting less than one hour. The triggers for pain are innocuous and include touching a specific part of the face, eating or chewing, brushing your teeth, or wind blowing across the face.

What is causing this pain?

Trigeminal neuralgia is often caused by compression of the trigeminal nerve as it exits the brainstem by an artery or vein. This compression causes abnormal excitation of the nerve, which is then perceived by your brain as severe pain. This type of trigeminal neuralgia is called "*classic trigeminal neuralgia*."

I have noticed that I sometimes feel a dull pain lasting minutes to hours between attacks. Should I be concerned about this?

It is common for patients with trigeminal neuralgia to experience this. There is another condition, called "trigeminal neuropathy", in which patients experience constant dull pain. However, it would be unusual for patients with trigeminal neuropathy to experience frequent lancinating pain. These patients, unlike you, also have a loss of sensation on part of their face even though they have pain. Trigeminal neuropathy is a potential side effect of some of the surgical treatment options for trigeminal neuralgia. In these patients, we sometimes see simultaneous evidence of both trigeminal neuralgia and trigeminal neuropathy.

What about the other causes of trigeminal neuralgia, are any of them dangerous?

Trigeminal neuralgia is usually disabling, but otherwise not dangerous. However, there are some dangerous causes that we need to watch out for. Some patients may have trigeminal neuralgia caused by a tumor or vascular malformation pressing against the trigeminal nerve. For some others, particularly young people, it may be the first manifestation of multiple sclerosis, a treatable autoimmune disease that affects the brain and spinal cord. There are some other less common dangerous causes as well. We can assess for all of these on the brain MRI you are scheduled for. For patients with evidence of trigeminal neuropathy, it is important to pay special attention to the entire length of the trigeminal nerve on the MRI to assess for a tumor pressing on the trigeminal nerve.

My attacks are often triggered by chewing on food. Should I see a dentist to assess for a tooth infection?

If your pain is mostly in the bottom part of your face and chewing or brushing teeth is the most common trigger, then I would recommend you visit a dentist to ensure you do not have a tooth abscess. At the same time, avoid unnecessary dental procedures. Some people are willing to have multiple teeth extracted in the hope of relieving this terrible pain. If dental X-rays or CT scan show no problems, it is best not to have your teeth removed.

I just read the report of my MRI and it states that I have "vascular compression of the trigeminal nerve by the superior cerebellar artery." I read on google about microvascular decompression surgery. I am very hesitant about doing surgery. Are there any medications I can take instead to relieve the pain?

Absolutely. There is no reason to rush into surgery. There are two anti-seizure medications, carbamazepine and oxcarbazepine, which are often very effective in reducing or even eliminating the pain. These drugs work by calming down the hyperexcitability of the trigeminal nerve. These drugs were initially developed to treat seizures. It was later discovered that they work well for various other conditions, such as trigeminal neuralgia. While most patients tolerate these drugs, around 25% of patients have to discontinue them due to side effects. Some of the more common side effects are dizziness, headache, rash, upset stomach and low blood sodium level. Let us try oxcarbazepine 300 mg twice per day and see how that works for you. If you tolerate it well and it provides some relief, we can go up on the dose further to provide even more relief.

I tried oxcarbazepine which provided moderate pain relief. However, I am so drowsy when I take it. I reduced the dose which helped with the drowsiness but now the medication provides only minimal relief. I also tried carbamazepine which also caused drowsiness. I am still hesitant about surgery. Are there any other medications I can try?

There are plenty of other medication options. However, they are generally less effective than carbamazepine and oxcarbazepine. You can try a muscle relaxant called baclofen, or other anti-seizure medications such as phenytoin, lamotrigine or topiramate. OnabotulinumtoxinA (Botox) injections in the face are often effective and are a very safe option to try in combination with another medication. In a Chinese double-blind, randomized controlled trial of 42 patients, 68% had significant pain relief compared to just 15% in the placebo group. Possible side effects include temporary facial weakness and facial asymmetry. The injections are given into the areas of pain which sometimes include the gums and even the side of the tongue. In a small study in 2019, 2 out of 8 patients had complete relief of pain after Botox injections into the sphenopalatine ganglion, a network of nerves located behind the nose.

You may have heard about a new class of medications called CGRP monoclonal antibodies that are being used for migraine. In a recent study of 9 patients taking erenumab, a CGRP monoclonal antibody, 8 of the 9 patients had significant pain relief. In another retrospective study, 6 out of 8 patients felt that erenumab was either probably or definitely effective for them. Erenumab is prescribed as a monthly subcutaneous injection which can easily be self-administered at home. Trigeminal neuralgia is more common among the elderly. Constipation and increased blood pressure, which are already prevalent among the elderly, are possible side effects of erenumab. Fremanezumab and galcanezumab, two other CGRP monoclonal antibodies, do not have these warnings on their labels. Although they have not yet been reported to help in the treatment of trigeminal neuralgia, they work in a similar manner to erenumab and may be worth a try. A few of our patients with trigeminal neuralgia have responded well to these two other monoclonal antibodies.

What should I do if the pain is so bad one day that I cannot function? Are there any abortive medications I can take?

Unfortunately, because the pain is so sudden and brief, the only treatment that can help is preventive. If the pain becomes unbearable, intravenous lidocaine, valproic acid, ketamine or phenytoin, usually administered in a hospital setting, may provide some short-term relief from attacks. These can be used as bridges to a more practical preventive medication or procedure.

I have tried everything and cannot bear the pain any longer. Can you tell me more about microvascular decompression surgery?

The purpose of the surgery is to separate the nerve from the blood vessel so that the nerve is no longer compressed. The surgery requires general anesthesia. The surgeon will first make an incision behind your ear and then make an opening in the skull to access the area of neurovascular compression. They will carefully place a small piece of synthetic material between the nerve and the blood vessel. Around 75% of patients will have marked pain relief from surgery which will persist for at least a year but usually much longer. Since the area of neurovascular compression is so close to the brainstem, there is a small risk of damaging the brainstem or nerves which can cause hearing loss, facial weakness or even a stroke. Due to the potential complications, the procedure should only be performed by a neurosurgeon with a lot of experience with this specific procedure.

That sounds scary! I am not ready for a hole to be drilled in my skull. I have heard of nerve ablation procedures for patients with back pain. Can this also be done for trigeminal neuralgia?

Yes. This procedure is called radiofrequency thermocoagulation. The anesthesiologist makes a small incision in the cheek, passes a cannula through an opening in the skull (called the foramen ovale), and destroys the trigeminal nerve using heat. The success rate is over 90%. There are generally fewer complications with this technique than there are with microvascular decompression. It is certainly reasonable to start with this procedure. If it does not work, the procedure can be repeated or you can opt to then have microvascular decompression surgery.

Another option is stereotactic radiosurgery. You may have heard radio commercials for cancer treatments using various stereotactic radiosurgery technologies like GammaKnife or CyberKnife. For trigeminal neuralgia, a narrow beam of radiation is carefully targeted at the trigeminal nerve root causing degeneration of the nerve. Around 85% of patients experience pain relief after radiation.

In a less popular procedure, called partial sensory rhizotomy, part of the sensory trigeminal nerve is cut surgically. While the success rate is high, the risk of adverse effects is higher than with the other options I presented to you.

While all these procedures are very effective at relieving pain, there are some worrisome side effects to know about. Some patients develop severe numbness in the face or weakness in the muscle that helps to chew food. Others develop a dry eye or damage to their cornea. A disabling possible side effect of these procedures is called *anesthesia dolorosa*. These patients have a severe, constant and unpleasant feeling in the part of the face that is supplied by the trigeminal nerve. Anesthesia dolorosa is incredibly hard to treat with medications and surgery.

Is the pain relief from these various procedures permanent?

The pain relief is indeed permanent for some patients. The procedure with the highest rate of long-term pain relief is microvascular decompression, where 70% of patients are free of pain without medications after 10 years. Stereotactic radiosurgery has the lowest rate of long-term pain relief with only 45% of patients maintaining complete pain relief without medication at 5 years. Radiofrequency thermocoagulation and partial sensory rhizotomy fall in the middle. Please keep in mind that both radiofrequency thermocoagulation and stereotactic radiosurgery can be repeated in the future should your pain recur.

A friend of mine has trigeminal neuralgia but does not have neurovascular compression on their MRI. What is causing them to have trigeminal neuralgia?

When the cause for trigeminal neuralgia is unclear even after an MRI, we call it "*idiopathic trigeminal neuralgia*." When the word idiopathic is used in medicine, it means that scientists have not yet identified the cause for the disease. In your friend's case, the MRI should be reviewed very carefully for evidence of a tumor or multiple sclerosis plaque. Often there is a vascular loop even though it is not appreciated on the MRI scan. Sometimes the loop seen on MRI is not actually touching the nerve if and when surgery is done. So, it is not perfect.

What is the long-term prognosis for me? Will the pain ever go away permanently without surgery?

Some patients have pain-free remission periods lasting from months to years. There are also periods in which the pain is more mild and other periods in which it is more severe. There is very little data on long term prognosis without surgery, likely due to the fact that the severity of pain often leads refractory patients to eventually undergo a procedure.

Suggested Reading

1. Barker FG 2nd, Jannetta PJ, Bissonette DJ, Larkins MV, Jho HD. The long-term outcome of microvascular decompression for trigeminal neuralgia. *N Engl J Med*. 1996 Apr;334(17):1077-83.
2. Burch R. Preventive Migraine Treatment. *Continuum*. 2021 Jun 1;27(3):613-632.

3. Crespi J, Bratbak D, Dodick DW, Matharu M, Jamtøy KA, Tronvik E. Pilot Study of Injection of OnabotulinumtoxinA Toward the Sphenopalatine Ganglion for the Treatment of Classical Trigeminal Neuralgia. *Headache*. 2019 Sep;59(8):1229-1239.
4. George N, Ahmed Z. The effect of Aimovig on trigeminal neuralgia: a retrospective case study. *Headache*. 2019 Jul;59(S1); P277LB.
5. Headache Classification Committee of the International Headaches Society (IHS). The International Classification for Headache Disorders, 3rd edition. *Cephalalgia*. 2018; 38:1-211.
6. Kanpolat Y, Savas A, Bekar A, Berk C. Percutaneous controlled radiofrequency trigeminal rhizotomy for the treatment of idiopathic trigeminal neuralgia: 25-year experience with 1,600 patients. N*eurosurgery*. 2001 Mar;48(3):524-32.
7. Ko AL, Ozpinar A, Lee A, Raslan AM, McCartney S, Burchiel KJ. Long-term efficacy and safety of internal neurolysis for trigeminal neuralgia without neurovascular compression. *J Neurosurg*. 2015 May;122(5):1048-57.
8. Maarbjerg S, Gozalov A, Olesen J, Bendtsen L. Trigeminal neuralgia--a prospective systematic study of clinical characteristics in 158 patients. *Headache*. 2014 Nov-Dec;54(10):1574-82.
9. Mogahed MM, Anwar GA, Mohamed RM. Comparative study between intravenous ketamine and lidocaine infusion in controlling of refractory trigeminal neuralgia. *J Anesth Clin Res*. 2017 Jul;8(8):1-4.
10. Nanda A, Javalkar V, Zhang S, Ahmed O. Long term efficacy and patient satisfaction of microvascular decompression and gamma knife radiosurgery for trigeminal neuralgia. *J Clin Neurosci*. 2015 May;22(5):818-22.
11. Parascandolo E, Levinson K, Rizzoli P, Sharon R. Efficacy of erenumab in the treatment of trigeminla neuralgia: a retrospective case series. *Neurol Clin Pract* 2021 Jun;11(3):227-231.
12. Robertson C. Cranial Neuralgias. *Continuum*. 2021 Jun;27(3):665-685.
13. Wu CJ, Lian YJ, Zheng YK, Zhang HF, Chen Y, Xie NC, Wang LJ. Botulinum toxin type A for the treatment of trigeminal neuralgia: results from a randomized, double-blind, placebo-controlled trial. *Cephalalgia*. 2012 Apr;32(6):443-50.

I Get Shooting Pain on My Face When I am Brushing My Teeth: What Can This Be?

Risako Shirane, MD MSc
Fellow in Headache Medicine
Department of Neurology
Yale School of Medicine
New Haven, Connecticut
Icahn School of Medicine at Mount Sinai
Mount Sinai Beth Israel/Mount Sinai West

For the past 2 years, I have been experiencing excruciating pain on my face when I brush my teeth, or when I apply make-up on my face. It feels like an electric shock is running through my cheek when this happens. Thankfully, the pain goes away once I stop these activities. What do you think is going on?

It sounds like you may have trigeminal neuralgia. Can you tell me more about the pain, including how often this happens and how long it lasts?

The first time I experienced this was about 2 years ago, when I was 60 years old. I experienced a severe, sharp, shooting pain on the right side of my face while brushing my teeth – it went away within a few seconds once I stopped brushing, so I didn't think much of it at first. Gradually I began to experience the same pain doing other things, like chewing or touching my cheek to put make-up on. I've noticed that during the wintertime, cold wind brushing against my cheek can sometimes trigger the pain. As I said, the pain lasts for a few seconds at a time, but they keep coming back for as long as I am engaged in these activities. Oddly enough, however, I have not been woken up by the pain at night even though my face touches the pillow.

That must be very bothersome. What you are describing to me sounds very typical of trigeminal neuralgia, a facial pain disorder that often affects older people with women more likely to be affected than men. Individuals with trigeminal neuralgia experience recurrent, severe, sharp electric shock-like pain that lasts from a fraction of a second to 2 minutes on one side of the face. The pain may rarely involve the forehead but most commonly is noted in the cheek and jaw. The pain is triggered by inoffensive stimuli such as light touch, brushing teeth, or cold breeze over the face, just like you described. Activation of facial muscles through chewing or talking can also elicit pain in some individuals. The pain may recur as a series of attacks for up to an hour if the stimulus is still present, however it typically subsides quickly once the trigger is removed. Some patients note a temporary respite in the pains after a series have been repeatedly triggered, a time known as a "refractory period." Trigeminal neuralgia pain does and should not travel beyond the face.

Although this is rare, the pain may become continuous or persist in the background as a lesser intense pain between severe attacks in a small subset of patients. These patients would then be diagnosed with trigeminal neuralgia "with concomitant continuous pain."

Lastly, about two-thirds of patients with trigeminal neuralgia experience rare to occasional nighttime awakenings related to pain, however this does not seem to occur as frequently as daytime pain attacks. This observation raises the possibility of protective effect of sleep on trigeminal neuralgia, though its mechanism remains unclear.

It does sound like I have trigeminal neuralgia. What causes this?

That's a good question. Typically, trigeminal neuralgia is caused by mechanical compression of the trigeminal nerve which relays sensory information from the face to the brain. The trigeminal nerve gives off three branches (ophthalmic, maxillary, and mandibular divisions) that innervate the forehead/around the eye, cheek, and jaw, respectively. The distribution of the pain depends on which branch is affected. The culprit causing nerve compression is usually an artery running near the root of the nerve. Over time, the compression of the nerve leads to the breakdown of its protective sheath called myelin, causing the nerve to be hyperexcitable and send excess signals to the brain that are ultimately felt as pain. However, there are likely other mechanisms that bring about trigeminal neuralgia in some patients because compression of the trigeminal nerve is not found in subset of patients with this disorder. Also, there may be some genetic component to this disorder, because up to 11% of patients have a family member affected by it. These patients may have onset of symptoms at an earlier age and experience other neuralgias or spasms of the face.

I see. How do I know if my symptoms are caused by compression of the trigeminal nerve?

We would have you undergo MRI and MRA studies of the brain to determine if there is indeed a compression of the trigeminal nerve. The MRI provides a detailed imaging of the brain and cranial nerves such as the trigeminal nerve, while the MRA gives anatomical information about the blood vessels. If vascular compression of the trigeminal nerve is present, it will most likely be visible on imaging. In approximately 15% of cases, an entirely different structural abnormality affecting the trigeminal nerve is seen. These include brain lesions caused by multiple sclerosis, benign tumors at the cerebellopontine angle (where the trigeminal nerve fibers enter the brainstem), and abnormalities of the skull base. Multiple sclerosis is an autoimmune disease that causes destruction of the protective nerve sheath within the brain, a process known as 'demyelination'. Multiple sclerosis is a concern particularly in female patients who present with trigeminal neuralgia at a young age in their second to third decades of life. In fact, trigeminal neuralgia may be the first symptom of multiple sclerosis in some individuals. It is also entirely possible for patients with multiple sclerosis to develop trigeminal neuralgia through both a demyelinating lesion in the brainstem where the trigeminal nerve fibers enter, as well as vascular compression of the nerve itself. This is called a 'double crush' mechanism.

Can trigeminal neuralgia be treated, or will I have to live with the pain for the rest of my life?

There are various treatment options available to treat trigeminal neuralgia. Once diagnosis is made, we can start medications such as carbamazepine or oxcarbazepine which are anti-seizure medications that can also treat certain types of nerve pain. They work by stabilizing the membrane of the nerves, thereby suppressing excess pain signals to the brain. Carbamazepine has the best evidence of effectiveness at treating trigeminal neuralgia; however, it does come with potential side effects that some patients are unable to tolerate. These include drowsiness, dizziness, rash, hyponatremia (lowering of blood sodium level), ataxia (difficulty with balance), and bone marrow suppression that may make individuals more prone to infections. While you are on this medication, your doctor will periodically monitor your blood electrolyte levels and cell counts. Another downside to carbamazepine is that it can interact with other medications. Oxcarbazepine is like carbamazepine in its mechanism of action, but tends to be better tolerated. However, the risk of hyponatremia is still present. Fear not, there are other anti-seizure medications that can be used in replacement of these medications, such as lamotrigine and gabapentin, though they may not be as effective. There is a new medication being actively studied for treatment of trigeminal neuralgia called "vixotrigine." If approved it will certainly help widen the pharmacotherapy options for many patients.

What would happen if the medication does not relieve the pain or if I am unable to continue the medication due to side effects?

Unfortunately, the medications discussed above may not be sufficient to treat the pain for some patients. In those cases, other adjunctive or alternative therapies need to be considered. If the brain imaging shows evidence of an artery compressing the trigeminal nerve, the best next step will be to consider a surgical treatment called "microvascular decompression" to relieve the compression of the trigeminal nerve.

Surgery sounds scary. Is this a big surgery?

The surgery is performed by a neurosurgeon and involves creating a small hole behind your ear where a very small probe and camera will be inserted into the skull. The procedure is done under general anesthesia. Data show that 68 to 88% of patients with trigeminal neuralgia due to vascular compression experience pain freedom at 1 to 2 years after the surgery. Another study has shown that 64% of patients have remained pain-free 10 years after surgery. Although more invasive than other procedures, it tends to be the most effective. If you are a good candidate for surgery this may be your best option to consider.

What if you cannot find evidence of an artery compressing the nerve? Is there anything else that can be done to treat it?

As mentioned earlier, vascular compression of the nerve is not found in a subset of patients with trigeminal neuralgia. For these patients, the next step after medication therapy would be to consider a neuro-ablative procedure. Stereotactic radiosurgery is a type of radiation therapy in which a beam of radiation is carefully delivered to a particular part of the trigeminal nerve. Most patients who undergo this treatment start to feel pain relief within 2 months, and one-third to a half of patients remain pain-free 5 years after surgery. Some patients may experience decreased sensation on the side of face treated with radiation, but this is rare. Other options include radiofrequency thermocoagulation, glycerol rhizotomy, or balloon compression. All these procedures aim to control pain by intentionally introducing injury to a part of the trigeminal nerve through heat, chemical or mechanical manipulation, respectively, so as to stop unwanted pain signals from travelling to the brain. These procedures may achieve satisfactory pain relief in the short term; however, the benefits may wear off in the long-term. Many patients will prefer this to microvascular decompression.

Can the disease start to affect the other parts of my face?

Trigeminal neuralgia commonly involves the unilateral maxillary (cheek) and mandibular (jaw) divisions more than the ophthalmic division (forehead and around the eye), though isolated involvement of the ophthalmic division can occur in a small number of patients. Trigeminal neuralgia can, in rare instances, involve both sides of the face. This bilateral involvement would, however, raise concern for underlying causes other than a simple vascular compression such as multiple sclerosis or tumor and prompt further investigation. Additionally, if patients have significant tearing, redness of the eye or facial sweating associated with the onset of the pain, other diagnoses such as trigeminal autonomic cephalalgia need to be considered. If local rash is noted, shingles is also a consideration.

Suggested Reading

Bendtsen L, Zakrzewska JM, Abbott J, et al. European Academy of Neurology guideline on trigeminal neuralgia. Eur J Neurol 2019; 26(6):831–849. doi:10.1111/ene.13950

Cruccu G, Finnerup NB, Jensen TS, et al. Trigeminal neuralgia: new classification and diagnostic grading for practice and research. Neurology 2016;87(2):220–228.

Di Stefano G, Truini A, Cruccu G. Current and innovative pharmacological options to treat typical and atypical trigeminal neuralgia. Drugs 2018;78(14):1433–1442.

Headache Classification Committee of the Internal Headache Society (2018). Classification and diagnostic criteria for headache disorders, 3rd edition. Cephalalgia, Vol 38

Maarbjerg S, Di Stefano G, Bendtsen L, Cruccu G. Trigeminal neuralgia—diagnosis and treatment. Cephalalgia 2017;37(7):648–657.

Maarbjerg S, Wolfram F, Gozalov A, et al. Significance of neurovascular contact in classical trigeminal neuralgia. Brain 2015;138(pt 2):311–319.

WHAT ABOUT MULTIPLE SCLEROSIS AND HEADACHE?

NEHA VIJAYVARGIYA SAFI, MD

MULTIPLE SCLEROSIS FELLOW
ICAHN SCHOOL OF MEDICINE AT MOUNT SINAI
NEW YORK CITY

STEPHEN KRIEGER, MD, FAAN

PROFESSOR OF NEUROLOGY
ICAHN SCHOOL OF MEDICINE AT MOUNT SINAI
NEW YORK CITY

I'm a 28yo woman with a history of TMD and depression who was recently diagnosed with Relapsing Remitting Multiple Sclerosis (RRMS). About one year ago, I developed painful vision loss in my right eye over the course of 3 days. I went to see an eye doctor who told me I had optic neuritis and sent me to a local hospital. I was admitted and had an MRI of the brain and was told by the neurologist that I had abnormal signal in my right optic nerve and one white matter lesion in my brain. I then had a spinal tap that was negative for oligoclonal bands. Thankfully, my vision improved after a course of IV steroids, and I've been following with my local neurologist ever since. Six months after my optic neuritis, I had a repeat MRI of the brain and was told I had several new lesions. My local neurologist diagnosed me with RRMS and started me on dimethyl fumarate. Looking back on my life through the lens of this new diagnosis, I've had migraines my whole life – have these been a symptom of my MS all along?

This is an excellent question! There have been several studies that have attempted to answer the question of whether headaches can be regarded as a symptom of MS. A majority of these studies have demonstrated that patients with RRMS have more than a 50% higher predisposition to headaches that the general population. They also show that the prevalence of migraine in people with MS varies anywhere from 35.5 to 61.8%. There are several theories as to why migraines may be more common in people with MS. One such theory has been demonstrated in animal studies suggesting that the breakdown of myelin in the cortex of the brain may increase cortical excitability and thereby accelerate cortical spreading depression, which is thought to be an important phenomenon underlying migraine. More studies are needed to confirm these hypotheses, but in general, we don't think of migraines as a classic presenting symptom in MS. Migraine is therefore not diagnostic for MS, and the treatment of migraine for someone with MS is not fundamentally different for someone without this diagnosis. But it's definitely treatable!

Given my MRI findings, could my MS lesions have been the cause for my headaches all along?

The overwhelming majority of headaches are not attributable to MS lesions themselves, as the brain doesn't feel pain directly and MS lesions don't generally cause pain individually. However, there is increasing evidence to suggest that lesions in certain locations in the brainstem may contribute to the pathophysiology of migraines. The periaqueductal gray matter, located in the midbrain, plays a major role in modulating pain by limiting the detection of painful stimuli by the high structures in the brain. In patients with MS, one study showed that those who had a demyelinating lesion within the midbrain close to the periaqueductal gray had a four-fold increase in migraine-like headaches, 2.5-fold increase in tension-like headaches, compared to those patients with MS who did not have a lesion in the same location. This suggests that by forming a lesion in close proximity to the periaqueductal gray, the brain loses its ability to modulate the incoming pain sensory information, and therefore, the individual is more likely to experience pain.

I'm already an anxious and depressed person at baseline, but this entire process of experiencing new neurologic symptoms and coming to a diagnosis of RRMS has been incredibly overwhelming. Ever since my diagnosis, I've had a new type of headache, where I feel a band-like pressure sensation around my forehead that feels like someone is squeezing my head in a vice. I've been noticing these more frequently and they seem to get worse when I'm running low on sleep.

These headaches sound like tension-type headaches. Tension-type headaches are reported at a similar prevalence in MS patients as they are in the general population, with the exception of a higher number of older men with MS reporting tension-type headaches in a single study. Regardless of this data, tension headaches are not typically thought of as a manifestation of MS. It's possible that stress combined with your underlying depression are contributing to these headaches. Although more studies are needed to determine if stress levels lead to tension-type headaches specifically in patients with MS, fundamental principles of treating tension-type headaches are likely to be effective.

While there are medications such as some antidepressants that can be used to manage tension-type headaches, there are lifestyle modifications that can also be quite helpful. Working to regulate sleep, eating regular meals, and limiting caffeine intake can help to improve these headaches. In addition, relaxation training, including progressive muscle relaxation and meditative relaxation can be used to improve tension-type headaches. Hopefully, some of these techniques can help you relieve this particular type of headache.

Now that I've been taking dimethyl fumarate for the last six months, is it possible that this medication could be making my headaches worse?

The good news is we don't believe your dimethyl fumarate is causing you to have headaches or worsening your pre-existing headaches. There are, however, other disease-modifying therapies (DMTs) that have been shown to have headache as a known side effect, which are worth keeping in mind should you ever need to change MS treatment.

Interferon-beta (IFN-β), an early injectable medication, is known to significantly worsen pre-existing headaches and headaches that occurred concurrently with the onset of MS in more than 50% of patients with headaches that preceded initiation of treatment with IFN-β. Not only did it exacerbate pre-existing headaches, but it also triggered new onset headaches in about 1/3 of patients in those who did not report a history of headaches.[8]

Fingolimod, an oral sphingosine-1-phosphate (S1P) receptor modulator, is another DMT used in the treatment of MS. Headache has been reported in up to 25% of patients on fingolimod in two clinical trials according to the package insert; however, headache was also reported in 24% of patients receiving placebo treatment in those same clinical trials. Hypertension has been reported as an adverse reaction in 8% of patients on fingolimod, and posterior reversible encephalopathy syndrome (PRES), has also rarely been reported in patients on fingolimod – both of which can result in secondary headaches. There has also been one case-series that highlighted 11 patients with MS who all reported new onset, bilateral, non-pulsatile, persistent headaches that began within the first week of starting treatment with fingolimod.

Natalizumab, an intravenous monoclonal antibody that targets the alpha-4 integrin adhesion-molecule, has also been shown to have headache as a documented side effect. Headache was reported in 32-38% of patients receiving natalizumab across three clinical trials. It was also a notable adverse effect included under the umbrella of infusion-related reactions during the administration of natalizumab.

The remaining DMTs have not proven to significantly increase the incidence of headache in patients with MS.

Oh, and one more thing – I think it might be related to my TMD, but in the last two weeks whenever I drink cold water or occasionally when I brush my teeth, I get a searing pain that shoots down along my right jaw line. In the beginning it only lasted a few seconds at a time and happened about 2 or 3 times a day, but now it's lasting up to 1-2 minutes at a time and happening up to 10 times a day. Is there any way this could be related to my MS?

Glad you mentioned this! The symptoms you're describing actually sound typical of trigeminal neuralgia, which unfortunately is more commonly seen in patients with MS, and we don't think this is a result of your TMJ problem. Data from the North America Research Committee on MS (NARCOMS) registry demonstrates that trigeminal neuralgia is present in 9.5% of patients during the duration of the MS disease course, and for up to 15% of patients, it can even precede a diagnosis of MS.

Seeing as your symptoms just started in the last two weeks, we would like to recommend a repeat MRI of the brain with and without contrast to see if there's a new MS lesion in the pons at the level of the trigeminal nucleus or the trigeminal root entry zone. Most of the time trigeminal neuralgia is not associated with new MS disease activity, but If we see a new lesion there, then we will consider treating you with a course of steroids to try and bring about a quicker recovery from these symptoms. In the meantime, there are treatments that we recommend for symptomatic relief of your trigeminal neuralgia. First line therapies include sodium channel blockers such as carbamazepine or oxcarbazepine. Other treatment adjuncts or second line treatment options include gabapentin, lamotrigine, pregabalin, or baclofen.

If these treatments fail, there are surgical options available such as microvascular decompression in the presence of an aberrant vascular loop or gamma knife radiosurgery to help alleviate the pain.

References and Suggested Reading

1. Beckmann Y, Türe S. Headache characteristics in multiple sclerosis. *Multiple Sclerosis and Related Disorders*. 2019; 27:112-116. doi:10.1016/j.msard.2018.09.022
2. Elmazny A, Hamdy SM, Abdel-Naseer M, et al. Interferon-Beta-Induced Headache in Patients with Multiple Sclerosis: Frequency and Characterization. *Journal of Pain Research.* 2020; 13:537-545. doi:10.2147/JPR.S230680
3. Fragoso YD, Adoni T, Gomes S, et al. Persistent Headache in Patients With Multiple Sclerosis Starting Treatment With Fingolimod. *Headache*. 2015;55(4):578-579. doi:10.1111/head.12526
4. Gee JR, Chang J, Dublin AB, Vijayan N. The Association of Brainstem Lesions with Migraine-Like Headache: An Imaging Study of Multiple Sclerosis. *Headache*. 2005;45(6):670-677. doi:10.1111/j.1526-4610.2005. 05136.x
5. Gilenya (fingolimod) [prescribing information]. East Hanover, NJ: Novartis Pharmaceuticals Corporation; December 2019.
6. Husain F, Pardo G, Rabadi M. Headache and Its Management in Patients with Multiple Sclerosis. *Curr Treat Options Neurol*. 2018;20(4):10. Published 2018 Mar 24. doi:10.1007/s11940-018-0495-4
7. Kister Ilya, Caminero Ana B, Herbert Joseph, Lipton Richard B. Tension-type Headache and Migraine in Multiple Sclerosis. *Current Pain and Headache Reports*. 2010;14(6):441-448. doi:10.1007/s11916-010-0143-5
8. Maarbjerg S, Di Stefano G, Bendtsen L, Cruccu G. Trigeminal neuralgia – diagnosis and treatment. *Cephalalgia.* 2017;37(7):648-657. doi:10.1177/0333102416687280
9. Merkler D, Klinker F, Jürgens T, et al. Propagation of spreading depression inversely correlates with cortical myelin content. *Annals of Neurology*. 2009;66(3):355-365. doi:10.1002/ana.21746
10. Penzien Donald B, Rains Jeanetta C, Lipchik Gay L, Creer Thomas L. Behavioral interventions for tension-type headache: Overview of current therapies and recommendation for a self-management model for chronic headache. *Current Pain and Headache Reports*. 2004;8(6):489-499. doi:10.1007/s11916-004-0072-2

11. Polman CH, O'Connor PW, Havrdova E, et al. A Randomized, Placebo-Controlled Trial of Natalizumab for Relapsing Multiple Sclerosis. *The New England Journal of Medicine*. 2006;354(9):899-910. doi:10.1056/NEJMoa044397
12. Przybylowski CJ. Radiosurgery for multiple sclerosis-related trigeminal neuralgia: retrospective review of long-term outcomes. *Journal of Neurosurgery*. Published online 2018:1-8. doi:10.3171/2018.5. JNS173194
13. Rains JC, Penzien DB, McCrory DC, Gray RN. Behavioral Headache Treatment: History, Review of the Empirical Literature, and Methodological Critique. *Headache*. 2005;45(s2): S92-S109. doi:10.1111/j.1526-4610.2005. 4502003.x
14. Tysabri (natalizumab) [prescribing information]. Cambridge, MA: Biogen Inc; June 2020.
15. Villani V, De Giglio L, Sette G, Pozzilli C, Salvetti M, Prosperini L. Determinants of the severity of comorbid migraine in multiple sclerosis. *Neurological Sciences*. 2012;33(6):1345-1353. doi:10.1007/s10072-012-1119-5

THE DIAGNOSIS IN THE BACK OF YOUR HEAD: OCCIPITAL NEURALGIA AND OTHER PAINFUL CRANIAL NEURALGIAS

PAUL G. MATHEW, MD, DNBPAS, FAAN, FAHS

ASSISTANT PROFESSOR OF NEUROLOGY
HARVARD MEDICAL SCHOOL
MASSACHUSETTS GENERAL BRIGHAM HEALTH CARE/HARVARD VANGUARD MEDICAL ASSOCIATES
BOSTON, MASSACHUSETTS

I have a long history of migraine. Is it possible to develop another type of headache in addition to migraine?

Many people experience changes in their migraines over their lifetime. These include changes in migraine frequency, intensity, and associated features, such as nausea. These changes can fluctuate based on exposure to trigger factors including stress, changes in sleep, hormonal fluctuations, weather fluctuations particularly around the change of seasons, career changes, and family events such divorce or childbirth. Having a diagnosis of migraine does not mean that a patient cannot develop another headache disorder. For example, someone with migraine can acquire an infection of the brain, for example, meningitis, which almost always causes headaches.

My migraines started to get worse in my 40s, and I now have two types of headaches. One of my headaches involves a quick stabbing pain that tends to occur when I turn my head while driving or when I lay down on my back. What is that?

Occipital neuralgia is a painful disorder that occurs when the nerves that exit from the upper neck, which is referred to as "the cervical spine" are either compressed or irritated. This results in the patient experiencing jolts of pain lasting seconds at a time along the scalp in the back of the head where these nerves travel. Occipital neuralgia can develop after a traumatic neck injury like a car accident, from occupational or lifestyle choices that involve chronic poor posture over years/decades, or at times without a clear initiating event. As noted in the question, certain neck movements and contact to the skin overlying the affected nerve can trigger an attack. When the nerve compression or irritation is persistent, the patient can eventually develop a steady achy pain with superimposed stabs of pain. Occipital neuralgia can affect one or both sides of the head, and will typically also involve some degree of neck pain. Nerve compression/irritation of the nerves of the lower cervical spine can cause similar symptoms that involve the arm on the same side, which is referred to as cervical radiculopathy. Cervical radiculopathy can occur with occipital neuralgia and contribute to overall worsening of pain and disability.

How common is occipital neuralgia and how come none of my other doctors made this diagnosis?

Occipital neuralgia a common diagnosis that can occur in patients with other headache disorders including migraine. In one study, approximately 25% of patients who presented to a headache clinic complaining of headache had a diagnosis of occipital neuralgia often in addition to another headache disorder. The most common headache disorder to occur with occipital neuralgia is chronic migraine, which is a term used when migraines occur 15 or more days per month. When evaluating a patient with headaches that include features such as throbbing quality, light sensitivity, sound sensitivity, nausea, and vomiting, it is only logical that a physician would most often make the diagnosis of migraine. Once this diagnosis has been made, the physician may not ask additional questions about other forms of head pain. In addition, patients will often assume that all of their pain is due to migraine, and will not mention the other head pain that they may be experiencing. As such, if the diagnosis is never made, then occipital neuralgia specific treatments are not recommended.

Why did my migraines get worse after I developed occipital neuralgia?

I often tell my patients that headache can be a good thing, because like a car alarm, it can warn you if something is wrong like the presence of a brain tumor or an infection. Unfortunately, in the case of migraine, that car alarm is also setting off the headlights (light sensitivity), the radio (sound sensitivity), and the car is going in reverse (nausea and vomiting). When someone with migraine develops occipital neuralgia, it is as if someone is now periodically kicking the tires of a car with an already sensitive alarm system, and setting it off more frequently. Likewise, when a patient develops frequent attacks of occipital neuralgia, it can serve to interrupt sleep, increase stress, and ultimately increase migraine frequency.

The medications that I have been prescribed have been somewhat helpful, but nothing seems to really improve my pain significantly. Why is that?

Although occipital neuralgia can be responsive to medications used to treat migraines and nerve pain, including amitriptyline and gabapentin, migraine specific medications like sumatriptan tend to be far less effective for the treatment of occipital neuralgia. For example, patients with migraine and occipital neuralgia may note that sumatriptan improved their throbbing headache pain around their temples as well as their light and sound sensitivity, but did little to improve the disabling stabbing pain in the back of their head and associated neck pain. In order to confirm the diagnosis of occipital neuralgia, a patient's pain must improve with occipital nerve blocks. An occipital nerve block is an injection that is performed on one or both sides of the back of the head depending on where the pain is located. The injection consists of a local anesthetic, which is a medication that causes temporary numbness in the area of the injection. Some of the more commonly utilized anesthetics include lidocaine and bupivacaine. Depending on the diagnosis and the physician's experience, steroids like methylprednisolone, dexamethasone, or triamcinolone may also be included along with an anesthetic medication.

Nerve blocks did not work in the past and were very painful. My headache specialist recommended that we proceed with additional nerve blocks. Is this a reasonable approach?

In the case of occipital neuralgia, a nerve block can provide pain relief by the numbing effect of the anesthetic. Occipital nerve blocks can vary tremendously in terms of technique and medications used for the procedure. In addition, one of the most critical factors for predicting nerve block success can be the volume of injection, which can range from 0.5cc to >6cc per side. This is because occipital neuralgia may be due to compression of the occipital nerves by surrounding muscle and connective tissue, and the injection may actually be exerting hydrodynamic pressure to decompress the nerve. In one study that evaluated the effectiveness of 6cc occipital nerve blocks, patients experienced a complete remission of their stabbing occipital neuralgia pain for an average of 206.95 days with some patients experiencing a remission for over 840 days. In my practice it is not uncommon for patients to receive occipital nerve blocks for the treatment of occipital neuralgia, and they deny any further attacks for months if not years. If the pain returns, nerve blocks can be repeated often with a similar, if not longer duration of benefit.

I recall performing nerve blocks on both sides of the head for one of my patients, and afterwards she commented, “Dr. Mathew, my entire head feels numb”. I then commented to her husband, who was in the room, “this is the one time in your marriage that you can refer to your wife as a numbskull and get away with it.” They appreciated the humor, and he fortunately did not attempt to call her this affectionate name after the numbness resolved.

After receiving nerve blocks, my doctor recommended revisiting medications that did not work that well in the past. Is this a reasonable approach?

Occipital neuralgia can serve as a significant trigger of migraine in patients who have both disorders. As such, if the occipital neuralgia is under control, medications that were inconsistently effective in the setting of poorly controlled occipital neuralgia may be surprisingly effective for the treatment of migraine. In my clinical practice, I have found that adequate treatment of occipital neuralgia tends to result in a decrease of the frequency and intensity of migraines. In some cases, headache preventative treatments can be slowly withdrawn once the occipital neuralgia is well managed.

Can neuralgias occur in other areas besides the back of the head?

The term neuralgia refers to pain, numbness, tingling, and/or other unpleasant sensations caused by a damaged or irritated nerve. One of the best-known neuralgias is trigeminal neuralgia. The trigeminal nerve is the nerve that provides sensation to the face and scalp in the front of the head. Like occipital neuralgia, trigeminal neuralgia involves very intense stabbing pain, but unlike occipital neuralgia, trigeminal neuralgia almost always involves either side of the face. In cases involving both sides of the face, MRI imaging with contrast and other studies should be considered for further evaluation to look for pathological causes of the pain. The trigeminal nerve has three branches. Sensory information about the forehead is transmitted by the first branch (V1), sensory information about the cheeks is transmitted by the second branch (V2), and sensory information about the jaw is transmitted by the third branch (V3).

The nervous system is arranged like the structure of a tree. If something happens to the trunk, all of the branches above that point of the tree will be affected. Likewise, if there is nerve compression closer to where the trigeminal nerve exits the brain, all three branches (V1, V2, and V3) might be affected. On the other hand, if there is compression of the nerve after it exits the skull, only a single peripheral branch might be affected. Similar to occipital neuralgia, neuralgia pain involving these peripheral branches of the trigeminal nerve can be responsive to nerve blocks. Supraorbital and supratrochlear nerve blocks can address neuralgia pain involving the area around the eyes and forehead. Auriculotemporal nerve blocks can address neuralgia pain around the temples. Like with occipital nerve blocks, trigeminal nerve blocks can have a volume dependent duration of benefit lasting months and at times years.

One of my patients was a 68-year-old Naval Officer who at the age of 25 fell from a 20-foot tower in Vietnam after an explosion. After this head trauma, he began to experience constant daily post-traumatic headache with migraine features, but he was also experiencing stabbing pains in the right temple that occurred independently of the intensity of his migrainous headache pain. He subsequently received a 3cc auriculotemporal nerve block, which was composed of bupivacaine. Two years after this procedure, he denies any attacks of auriculotemporal neuralgia, and he experiences less than 5 headache days per month.

Is physical therapy useful for the treatment of occipital neuralgia?

Physical therapy is one of the most important modalities for the treatment of occipital neuralgia. It is often through joint and tissue mobilization that neck tension and associated occipital neuralgia pain be fully addressed. I remind patients that they may feel somewhat better with attending physical therapy sessions, but the true benefit is often only appreciated after weeks or months of continuing the stretching and strengthening routines that are recommended by the therapist after the formal therapy sessions have concluded. I often use the analogy of the personal trainer. Seeing a personal trainer for 5 sessions will not lead to a 30 lb. weight loss, but rather continuing the recommended exercises over months may lead to achievement of this goal. When patients feel better after receiving nerve blocks, I advise them that the pain relief they are experiencing is an opportunity to incorporate the recommended physical therapy routines into their daily schedule, and such routines when performed daily may prevent occipital neuralgia flares from recurring.

If medication, nerve blocks, and physical therapy fail to adequately control occipital neuralgia, are there any other options?

If none of these options are providing adequate relief, injections under x-ray guidance where the nerves exit the spine in the neck could be considered. If the injection under x-ray guidance provides temporary relief, a procedure called radiofrequency ablation (RFA) could be considered. RFA involves the delivery of electrical currents to modulate pain signals and at times create thermal lesions of the occipital nerves. If all of these modalities fail to control refractory occipital neuralgia, nerve decompression surgery could be considered. Occipital nerve decompression surgery involves making an incision in the back of the head and neck, followed by separation and at times excision of some of the structures that are causing compression of the nerve. Unfortunately, there are no imaging studies that can accurately confirm nerve compression, which can at times only be appreciated while in the operating room with the nerves exposed. This surgery should only be considered in patients who have found inadequate relief with maximum medical therapy with medications, injectable therapies like nerve blocks, and physical therapy.

Suggested reading

1. Burstein R, Blake P, Schain A, Perry C. Extracranial origin of headache. Curr Opin Neurol. 2017 Jun;30(3):263-271.
2. De Simone R, Ranieri A, Bilo L, Fiorillo C, Bonavita V. Cranial neuralgias: from physiopathology to pharmacological treatment. Neurol Sci. 2008 May;29 Suppl 1: S69-78.
3. Gfrerer L, Hansdorfer MA, Ortiz R, Chartier C, Nealon KP, Austen WG Jr. Muscle Fascia Changes in Patients with Occipital Neuralgia, Headache, or Migraine. Plast Reconstr Surg. 2021 Jan 1;147(1):176-180.
4. Jose A, Nagori SA, Chattopadhyay PK, Roychoudhury A. Greater Occipital Nerve Decompression for Occipital Neuralgia. J Craniofac Surg. 2018 Jul;29(5): e518-e521.
5. Krel R, Mathew PG. Procedural treatments for headache disorders. Practical Neurology (US).2019;18(4):76-79.

6. Mathew PG, Cooper W. The Diagnosis and Management of Posttraumatic Headache with Associated Painful Cranial Neuralgias: a Review and Case Series. Curr Pain Headache Rep. 2021 Jun 23;25(8):54.
7. Mathew PG, Najib U, Khaled S, Krel R. One and Done: A Case Series of Large Volume Occipital Nerve Blocks for the Treatment of Occipital Neuralgia. American Academy of Neurology Annual Meeting, Philadelphia, PA, May 2019, American Headache Society Annual Scientific Meeting, Philadelphia, PA, July 2019.
8. Mathew PG, Najib U, Khaled S, Krel R. Prevalence of occipital neuralgia at a community hospital-based headache clinic. Neurol Clin Pract. Dec 2019, 10.1212/CPJ.0000000000000789.
9. Williams KA, Lawson RM, Perurena OH, Coppin JD. Management of Chronic Migraine and Occipital Neuralgia in Post 9/11 Combat Veterans. Mil Med. 2019 Jul 1; 184(7-8): e207-e211. doi: 10.1093/milmed/usy405.

Why Do I Still have a Headache after My COVID Infection?

Allison Navis, MD
Assistant Professor
Division Neuro-Infectious Diseases
Icahn School of Medicine at Mount Sinai
New York City

I had COVID 8 months ago. I was never hospitalized, but felt quite sick with fevers and shortness of breath for 2 weeks. I also had a really bad headache at the time that went away, but 1 month later it returned and now I have a headache all the time. I never had headaches before. What is going on?

Headaches are a frequent symptom with COVID infection, and one of the most common reasons for which people with persisting symptoms after COVID infection (what we will call 'long-COVID') come to see me. For people that have a history of headaches or migraines that were well-controlled, we commonly hear that these have worsened after having COVID. However, many people coming in never suffered from headaches prior to their COVID infection.

One of the most common descriptions that I hear from people is that they always have some pressure or pain, but it's mild at baseline. The pain commonly worsens (flares) and this can be in the setting of certain triggers, or without a clear cause. It can worsen multiple times a day, or week. Often people can remember the week, or day, that the headache started. These are all common symptoms for what we call "new persistent daily headache."

While new persistent daily headache is one of the more common headaches that I hear about, it's not the only one. Some people develop migraine headaches, while others get episodic tension-type headaches. For a very small percentage of patients, other headache types may occur such as idiopathic intracranial hypertension also known as "pseudotumor cerebri.".

As a result, it becomes very important to get a good headache history and make sure we aren't missing any other headache types.

Why did the headache come back? I thought I was getting better?

It's not uncommon to hear of people feeling much better after having COVID and then symptoms returning after some period of time; whereas others describe their COVID symptoms never resolving. While we are still working to clearly define long-COVID, we commonly think of it as the persistence or development of new symptoms at least 4 weeks after COVID infection has resolved. So, having symptoms return after feeling better would still be considered part of long-COVID.

I notice that when my headache worsened, my brain fog and fatigue get pretty bad.

Most people coming in with long-COVID have multiple symptoms and commonly describe them fluctuating together. So, for example, mental strain might exacerbate physical fatigue which may then cause worsening of other symptoms like headaches.

What is causing the headache? Did COVID damage my brain?

We don't know what is causing any of these persistent symptoms and the diagnostic workup is typically normal in long-COVID- not just for headaches but for many of the other symptoms.

We still don't understand the neurological effects of COVID during active infection. So far, the data we have from active COVID, points away from primary damage in the brain from infection, and looks more like secondary damage from inflammation, the vasculature or metabolic derangements. However, I would not extrapolate what we know from active COVID infection to long-COVID, as most of the studies assess the most critically ill patients- those who were hospitalized patients or died. So, I wouldn't jump to assume something similar is occurring in long-COVID, especially since many people had "mild COVID", that is they weren't hospitalized or had complications.

While long-COVID may be a unique entity, it could be part of a post-infectious process and may not even be specific to COVID. We have seen similar symptoms in people who have had other infections. There is also a lot of clinical overlap with other syndromes like myalgic encephalomyelitis (MECFS) and postural orthostatic tachycardia syndrome (POTS). Unfortunately, we don't fully understand what causes post-infectious syndromes, MECFS or POTS. Current hypotheses range from immune dysregulation/inflammation playing a role, or metabolic and hormonal changes. The role that the blood vessels play is also still unclear. We know that COVID can affect the vasculature, but we are not seeing strokes or extensive microvasculature ischemic changes on imaging for most people, which is also reassuring.

Do I need an MRI or other tests?

For most primary headache disorders, brain imaging appears normal. Neuroimaging in long-COVID has not shown any major changes for most people that would explain symptoms so I have not been immediately ordering imaging on everyone. While there are no established criteria for workup at this time, my general approach has been similar to any headache workup- assessing for any red flag symptoms or concern for a secondary headache disorder.

I typically order imaging in anyone who had severe COVID infection with or without complications, who have concerning comorbidities such as immunosuppression, new onset headache after 50 years of age, or any focal neurological deficits. If there is concern for raised intracranial pressure, imaging including venogram and lumbar puncture would be warranted.

However, if there aren't any concerning, red-flag symptoms, I think it is safe to go ahead and try to treat the headaches first.

What can be done to help?

We have many options for treating headaches and the approach to treating headaches associated with long-COVID is no different than treating any other headaches. Since you are having daily headaches, I would recommend starting a daily medication. These medications can take several weeks to start working, but when they do, you should notice an improvement in the frequency and severity of the headaches.

These medications were often developed to treat other things, but can also be beneficial for headaches. They mostly fall in the category of anti-epileptic drugs, anti-depressants or anti-hypertensives. If insomnia is a major issue, medications that can be sedating like tricyclic antidepressants may be a good first choice. However, for people with cognitive issues symptoms or fatigue, those medications may worsen symptoms. In the setting of fatigue, I often try the serotonin norepinephrine reuptake inhibitors (SNRIs) first, as they can be more activating and may offer slight benefit to the fatigue. Alternative options for headaches that meet migraine criteria are the new CGRP antagonists, or botulinum toxin injections for chronic migraine.

In cases of new persistent daily headache, or status migrainosus, a short course of steroids may be helpful while daily preventatives are initiated. However, steroids should be used with caution in those with contraindications such as poorly controlled diabetes and never be used long-term.

I don't like to take medicines, is there anything else that I can do to help alleviate the headaches?

Like with any headache, there are always factors that can exacerbate. Dehydration, caffeine intake and sleep disruption are among the most common factors.

In general, maintaining good hydration is essential. Avoiding caffeine can also help for some. Many people with long-COVID also experience sleep disruptions, or insomnia, and that may be playing a role for some. It's also important to assess for sleep apnea. In that case, a sleep study can be beneficial in making a diagnosis and initiating treatment.

In addition, frequent use of over-the-counter analgesics can cause worsening of headaches (something we call "medication overuse headache"), so if you are taking one of those medications more than 2 times per week, we would recommend stopping use and that could improve symptoms.

If you are getting episodic headaches, keeping a headache log can be helpful to determine triggers, as they can be different for everyone. For long-COVID patients, many experience severe fatigue which can worsen after exertion- something referred to as" post-exertional malaise." Headaches may also be exacerbated in this setting so we often recommend avoiding any exertion that worsens fatigue, taking a gradual approach to increasing exertional tolerance, and only increasing duration or level of exertion in small increments. For others, mental strain can exacerbate symptoms. In those situations, we recommend limiting the amount of time spent working and taking frequent breaks.

However, these adjustments may not be sufficient to completely alleviate headaches. In some situations, headaches may even be the trigger for worsening of other symptoms like fatigue and brain fog. In those cases, medications to alleviate the headache can be very beneficial in overall improvement.

How long will this last? It's been 7 months and I still feel terrible.

There aren't any studies to date that focus on long-term outcomes so unfortunately, I can't say. We don't even have a good idea at this time of how many people go on to develop long-COVID. In my experience, many people do improve, but it can take a while. It's best to not compare how you are feeling today with one week ago as improvement is often gradual and not noticeable in short timeframes. But many people will notice their symptoms are getting better when they compare how they feel today to several months prior. It is also common to hear that some symptoms might improve while others do not. Or that things can ebb and flow, with periods of improvement followed by flares.

Since it's been 7 months and there hasn't been any improvement, I would recommend trying to treat with one of the above medications. If we are able to get the headache under control with medications, we can try to taper them down and see how you feel.

While I wish I could provide more concrete data on outcomes and optimal treatment, we are only at the beginning of learning about, and understanding long-COVID. However, many people do feel better and there are options for headache treatment, so I remain optimistic that we can get your headaches under control and with time things will improve.

References

1. Kayaaslan B, Eser F, Kalem AK, Kaya G, Kaplan B, Kacar D, Hasanoglu I, Coskun B, Guner R. Post-COVID syndrome: A single-center questionnaire study on 1007 participants recovered from COVID-19. J Med Virol. 2021 Jul 13. doi: 10.1002/jmv.27198. Epub ahead of print. PMID: 34255355.

2. Graham EL, Clark JR, Orban ZS, Lim PH, Szymanski AL, Taylor C, DiBiase RM, Jia DT, Balabanov R, Ho SU, Batra A, Liotta EM, Koralnik IJ. Persistent neurologic symptoms and cognitive dysfunction in non-hospitalized Covid-19 "long haulers". Ann Clin Transl Neurol. 2021 May; 8(5):1073-1085. doi: 10.1002/acn3.51350. Epub 2021 Mar 30. PMID: 33755344; PMCID: PMC8108421.
3. Fernández-de-Las-Peñas C, Navarro-Santana M, Gómez-Mayordomo V, Cuadrado ML, García-Azorín D, Arendt-Nielsen L, Plaza-Manzano G. Headache as an acute and post COVID-19 Symptom in COVID-19 Survivors: A Meta-analysis of the Current Literature. Eur J Neurol. 2021 Jul 30. doi: 10.1111/ene.15040. Epub ahead of print. PMID: 34327787.
4. Vanichkachorn G, Newcomb R, Cowl CT, Murad MH, Breeher L, Miller S, Trenary M, Neveau D, Higgins S. Post-COVID-19 Syndrome (Long Haul Syndrome): Description of a Multidisciplinary Clinic at Mayo Clinic and Characteristics of the Initial Patient Cohort. Mayo Clin Proc. 2021 Jul;96(7):1782-1791. doi: 10.1016/j.mayocp.2021.04.024. Epub 2021 May 11. PMID: 34218857; PMCID: PMC8112396.
5. Salmon-Ceron D, Slama D, De Broucker T, Karmochkine M, Pavie J, Sorbets E, Etienne N, Batisse D, Spiridon G, Baut VL, Meritet JF, Pichard E, Canouï-Poitrine F; APHP COVID-19 research collaboration. Clinical, virological and imaging profile in patients with prolonged forms of COVID-19: A cross-sectional study. J Infect. 2021 Feb;82(2):e1-e4. doi: 10.1016/j.jinf.2020.12.002. Epub 2020 Dec 4. PMID: 33285216; PMCID: PMC7833274.
6. Mao L, Jin H, Wang M, Hu Y, Chen S, He Q, Chang J, Hong C, Zhou Y, Wang D, Miao X, Li Y, Hu B. Neurologic Manifestations of Hospitalized Patients with Coronavirus Disease 2019 in Wuhan, China. JAMA Neurol. 2020 Jun 1;77(6):683-690.
doi: 10.1001/jamaneurol.2020.1127.
PMID: 32275288; PMCID: PMC7149362.
7. Romero-Sánchez CM, Díaz-Maroto I, Fernández-Díaz E, Sánchez-Larsen Á, Layos-Romero A, García-García J, González E, Redondo-Peñas I, Perona-Moratalla AB, Del Valle-Pérez JA, Gracia-Gil J, Rojas-Bartolomé L, Feria-Vilar I, Monteagudo M, Palao M, Palazón-García E, Alcahut-Rodríguez C, Sopelana-Garay D, Moreno Y, Ahmad J, Segura T. Neurologic manifestations in hospitalized patients with COVID-19: The ALBACOVID registry. Neurology. 2020 Aug 25;95(8):e1060-e1070. doi: 10.1212/WNL.0000000000009937. Epub 2020 Jun 1. PMID: 32482845; PMCID: PMC7668545.

"WHY DOES MY HEART BEAT FUNNY AND MY HANDS FEEL COLD?

WADE M. COOPER, DO

Ever since childhood, my hands and feet get cold easily. Is this related to migraine?

Yes, it certainly is. Part of our nervous system includes the autonomic nervous system, which regulates many of our body functions even without having to think about it. For example, if you are sitting in a chair and stand up, your body must adjust to this change in posture by raising blood pressure to maintain blood flow to your head and brain. This includes an increase in heart rate and contractility, squeezing down of blood vessels in your extremities, and expanding blood vessels in your neck and skull. This type of regulation is maintained by the autonomic nervous system, which includes a sympathetic component and a parasympathetic component. The activating sympathetic nervous system is responsible for things you experience when you are stressed, such as an increase in heart rate, sweating, pupil enlargement, and cold hands and feet. The parasympathetic nervous system generates body effects related to relaxing, such as a slower heart rate, an increase in body temperature, and muscle relaxation. These two components are generally in good balance for day-to-day functioning of the nervous system. However, in people with migraine this system can be a bit out of balance, where they have an elevated sympathetic level at baseline, with an irregular parasympathetic response. Not only can this be seen in blood tests that demonstrate this autonomic dysfunction imbalance, but also in our patients who describe the symptoms of autonomic dysfunction including palpitations, near fainting episodes, gut dysfunction such as irritable bowel syndrome, temperature intolerance, and – you guessed it – cold hands and feet.

I've been told I have funny heart beats, but they are nothing to worry about. Are you saying cardiac problems can be part of migraine?

Yes. We know people with migraine are more likely to have palpitations, lightheadedness, and fainting episodes called syncope. These arise from problems regulating blood pressure with position changes seen in some with a history of migraine. For example, autonomic cardiovascular reflex studies which examine the peripheral blood vessel responses to various stimuli demonstrate patients with migraine have a more active sympathetic nervous system during the acute phase of migraine. This overactive sympathetic activity causes release of chemicals that both signal constriction of blood vessels around the brain and stimulate the heart to beat faster, leading to a higher resting heart rate, differences in heart rate variability, and at times palpitations. When cardiologists evaluate patients for symptoms of skipped beats and palpitations, they are searching for structural problems within the heart muscle, valves, or a problem with the nerve conduction through the heart itself. When this all comes back as normal, the cardiologist may conclude the symptoms are not related to a problem within the heart, but rather a problem with the autonomic nervous system.

I hate when my heart skips a beat. It makes me feel anxious. Do you think the anxious part is related to autonomic dysfunction too?

We know that anxiety is more common in people with migraine than in those without. There are several reasons for this, but one of which is a difference in the autonomic nervous system. People with a higher baseline of sympathetic activity coupled with differences in parasympathetic activity seen with migraine are more likely to experience anxiety. Studies have demonstrated that those with migraine have lower resting norepinephrine levels between migraine attacks compared to those without migraine. Because of this, some authors believe people with migraine develop an "upregulation" of sympathetic receptors. When the body activates the sympathetic nervous system, those with upregulated receptors will have a larger, more intense response to a burst of norepinephrine, causing symptoms of anxiety or a panic attack. Curiously, the migraine brain has super-sensitive alpha-adrenergic receptors, which are implicated in anxiety and post-traumatic stress disorder as well as migraine. Furthermore, these same patients have a reduced parasympathetic capacity, meaning they have a hard time turning off the anxiety response once it is stimulated.

I get how the autonomic nervous system can affect other aspects of my body, but what about my head?

Autonomic dysfunction helps drive many different symptoms in migraine. For example, some migraine pain appears to arise from dilation of blood vessels inside the head partly resulting from a reduction in sympathetic tone and an increase in parasympathetic tone. Facial flushing and nasal stuffiness involve the same dilation effect of blood vessels in the face in nose. Lowered parasympathetic activity and vagal tone results in gastroparesis (slowed stomach function) and may increase the chance for vomiting. Excessive skin sensitivity where normal things like brushing hair or wearing a hat causes pain, known as allodynia, are associated with increased parasympathetic nerve activity. In fact, 4 out of 5 patients with chronic migraine experience at least one symptom related to autonomic dysfunction during the migraine attack, including eyelid droop, ear fullness, tearing, or nasal drainage.

I see how autonomic dysfunction can lead to feeling anxious and wound up. Is this why I find it hard to sleep sometimes?

There are many factors that impact sleep, but the autonomic nervous system plays a big role in this. We know that before we sleep our sympathetic activity begins to slow down, and our parasympathetic activity picks up. This results in peripheral dilation and a reduced body temperature that helps us sleep. People with an overactive sympathetic nervous system have a hard time initiating sleep, with features of racing thoughts and a sense of restlessness. Unfortunately, this can lead to the inability to get to deep stages of sleep where our body typically experiences pain recovery and brain restoration. Some people think this is why people with chronic migraine and centralized pain syndromes such as fibromyalgia almost always have poor sleep.

Is there a way to shut down the overactive autonomic nervous system for someone with migraine?

As we have discussed, the autonomic nervous system is present throughout the body and has many different roles. One location of particular interest is called the sphenopalatine ganglion (SPG). This structure is about 1cm in size and is connected to the trigeminal nerve that carries pain into the sinus cavities and face. This ganglion has pain sensitive nerves that extend into areas related to headache, including the optic nerve, the soft tissue behind the eye, and into most of the face. It even shares pain nerves in the lining of the brain and in the front and sides of the skull. In addition to these pain nerves, the sphenopalatine ganglion is a relay point for the parasympathetic nerves affecting blood vessel constriction or dilation. There is a way to place numbing medication near this nerve bundle by either going through the nostril with a flexible tube (no needles) or by using a long needle that is placed under the cheek bone. When the numbing medication is in contact with this nerve bundle, it can reduce the body's ability to start or continue a migraine attack. Recent evidence has shown that performing this procedure, called a SPG block, can cause temperature change in the skull confirming effects on the autonomic system. Even though this is commonly done for chronic headache or facial pain, this procedure has also been shown to decrease heart palpitations and even reduce blood pressure for 4 weeks after a single treatment.

Are there treatments that can be effective for helping someone with an overactive autonomic nervous system?

There are several medications that are commonly used for migraine prevention that provide some benefit to those with autonomic hypersensitivity. Those include beta blocker medications such as propranolol and atenolol, and tricyclic medications such as amitriptyline and nortriptyline. There are several medications that are less commonly prescribed for routine migraine that may be of special benefit in cases of dysautonomia. The first is clonidine, which is a selective Alpha-2 adrenergic agonist medication. Because this medication is quite effective in treating hypertension, you have to be careful when using this in people with variable or low blood pressure. This same mechanism of reducing sympathetic effects on blood vessels also reduces the triggering effects of migraine. For patients who may not be able to tolerate clonidine, there is guanfacine which operates in a similar manner but less potent. Curiously this medication is FDA approved for adjunctive treatment of attention deficit hyperactivity disorder in children and adolescents. Prazosin is an Alpha-1 receptor agonist that is rarely used in treating hypertension, which is what it was first marketed for, but more commonly utilized in patients with posttraumatic stress disorder (PTSD). It also may be helpful in Raynaud syndrome, where the extremities experience inappropriate vasoconstriction. In addition to the above medication options, patients with autonomic dysfunction should remain well hydrated, and do their best to manage situations that can trigger sympathetic activation such as stress, hot temperatures, sleep deprivation, and overuse of stimulants such as caffeine.

Finally, there are some non-pharmacologic therapies that can normalize an overactive autonomic nervous system such as biofeedback and progressive relaxation. These can be learned by working directly with a mental health professional or more recently by using various applications for hand-held devices. These behavioral approaches may be quite effective in patients with autonomic dysfunction, and once learned they can be applied in various settings such as before sleep or before someone starts their workday.

Suggested Reading

Avnon Y, Nitzan M, Sprecher E, et al. Autonomic asymmetry in migraine: augmented parasympathetic activation in left unilateral migraineurs. *Brain* 2004; 127:2099–2108.

Gazerani P, Cairns BE. Dysautonomia in the pathogenesis of migraine. *Expert Rev Neurother* 2018; 18:153-165.

Jafari B. Sleep architecture and blood pressure. *Sleep Med Clin* 2017; 12:161–166.

Jansen-Olesen I, Baun M, Amrutkar DV, et al. PACAP-38 but not VIP induces release of CGRP from trigeminal nucleus caudalis via areceptor distinct from the PAC1 receptor. *Neuropeptides* 2014; 48:53–64.

Katsaras DN, Arvaniti CK, Flevari PG, et al. Sphenopalatine ganglion block: an external gate to modulate cardiac autonomic tone and suppress premature ventricular beats? *Ann Transl Med* 2018; 23:457.

Miglis MG. Migraine and Autonomic Dysfunction: Which Is the Horse and Which Is the Jockey? *Curr Pain Headache Rep* 2018; 22:19.

Robbins MS, Robertson CE, Kaplan E, et al. The Sphenopalatine Ganglion: Anatomy, Pathophysiology, and Therapeutic Targeting in Headache. *Headache* 2016; 56:240-258

Triantafyllidi H, Arvaniti C, Schoinas A, et al. Bilateral sphenopalatine ganglion block reduces blood pressure in never treated patients with essential hypertension. A randomized controlled single-blinded study. *Int J Cardiol* 2018; 250:233-239.

Zhang Y, Ren R, Sanford LD, et al. The effects of prazosin on sleep disturbances in post-traumatic stress disorder: a systematic review and meta-analysis. *Sleep Med* 2020; 67:225-231.

The Migraine Patient with Orthostatic Intolerance: Postural Orthostatic Tachycardia Syndrome, Orthostatic Hypotension with and without Syncope

Mark Stillman, MD

Ever since I started getting periods, I have had 'sick' headaches and a feeling of fogginess and light-headedness. It is especially bad in the summer, and I have to lie down to prevent myself from blacking out. Is this common?

Before I can answer that, I need to ask a few more questions. Are these headaches one-sided or both sides? Do they throb? How severe are they and how long do they last if unsuccessfully treated? I understand you are nauseated and may even vomit, but does light or sound make them worse. And do they come before, during or after the onset of menstrual flow?

After you answer that, tell me whether your light-headedness and dizziness are related to sitting or standing upright and get better when lying down? Tell me whether any of the following sound familiar

- A sensation of your heart beating out of your chest?
- Shortness of breath?
- Weakness in your legs or skin color changes in feet or hands?

The answer is yes to all those questions at one time or another. The headaches are either right sided or left sided, throbbing and sometimes severe enough that I must stay in bed. They can last for a few days and begin 2 days before I start my period. They are severe enough to interfere with my ability to function and the nausea and sensitivity to light and sound prevent me from working in customer service, even if I am not vomiting. I am missing a lot of work as a result. But when I am not on my

period, I can still get light-headed and foggy, particularly if I must stand for long periods of time. My heart feels like it is in my throat, and I will have to lie down. I cannot workout anymore in the summer if it is hot outside!

It is apparent you have two separate conditions, both of which are common. Recurrent, benign, debilitating headaches in a woman of child-bearing age, lasting up to 72-hours and followed by a return to normal are invariably migraine headaches. Almost a fifth of the women world-wide get these during their lifetime. Complicating the situation is a condition called orthostatic intolerance, one that is often overlooked and mistaken as something else. Busy or unaware clinicians may dismiss a patient complaining of orthostatic intolerance – frequently a young female in her teens or 20's – as being as being anxious to the point of panic, "dehydrated", or even feigning illness!

Orthostatic intolerance refers to the following situation: the development of any combination of the following symptoms when a patient assumes an upright posture (i.e. sitting or standing upright from a lying position), and remit with assuming a supine posture: palpitations (a sensation that the heart is beating) and rapid heartbeat, chest discomfort, shortness of breath (air hunger; the inability to catch one's breath), fatigability, exercise intolerance, lightheadedness or dizziness, fainting and near-fainting, confusion and disorientation, anxiety, visual fading or visual dimming, duskiness of fingertips and toes, and lower extremity weakness. In adults aged 19 or older, postural tachycardia syndrome (POTS), a common form of orthostatic intolerance, refers to the development of dizziness, with or without syncope (fainting and loss of consciousness), accompanied by a sustained increase in heart rate from baseline of greater than 30 beats per minutes (or a sustained heart rate of >120 beats per minutes), when assuming an upright posture.

Why me? Why do I have to suffer from this?

We do not rightly know but if you look at the phenomenon from the viewpoint of evolution, there may be some clues. When land animals moved from the horizontal position (being 4-legged) to the upright position (swinging in the trees or standing upright), the body had to account for the pull of gravity on the blood and serum in the veins and arteries.) In humans, standing upright from the lying position results in the displacement by gravity of up to 750 mL of blood volume from the chest and abdomen. This deprives the right side of the heart its normal volume of blood flow and limits that volume of cardiac output to the brain and body. In normal conditions, to maintain blood pressure, the volume receptors in the heart and aorta sense this deficiency and signal the arteries and veins in the body to constrict. This reflex system is tuned to carefully maintain the blood pressure and flow of blood to the most essential organs of the body (brain and kidneys) even at the expense of other organs and structures, such as the and the feet and hands.

There are various reasons why such a system may malfunction. A person who is losing fluids from whatever cause (rapid blood loss, intractable diarrhea or vomiting, or use of diuretics) may lose enough volume to provoke difficulty standing upright so severe that is leads to syncope (loss of consciousness) due to lack of cerebral blood flow. Some medications in common use today may lead to inability to maintain blood pressure and perfusion of vital organs such as the brain; these medications may belong to classes of drugs used to treat hypertension or psychiatric disorders, for example. A carefully taken history will determine this. Finally, there are cardiovascular and hematological causes of instability, some better understood than others, that lead to orthostatic intolerance.

For reasons unknown, some people have a defective cardiovascular control (also known as autonomic) system - one that is not as robust as that of 'normal' individuals. This may explain your situation, and there is suggestive evidence that migraine sufferers are frequently seen in this group of patients. It is incumbent on your physicians to determine if there is an obvious, explainable illness responsible for your malfunctioning autonomic system, such as adrenal disease, valvular heart disease, neurological disorder, or renal disease.

How can you be sure this is what I have?

As with most things in medicine, the history tells us a lot, but history should be confirmed by examination and sometimes, even more rigorous testing. A useful starting point for the general physician is the 3-minute Active Standing Test using a hand-held sphygmomanometer or a portable automatic blood pressure arm cuff. The pulse rate, or beats per minute (bpm), and systolic and diastolic blood pressures should be measured first in the supine position (after a period of 5-10 minutes of supine rest) and then repeated while continuously standing every 30-seconds for a full 3 minutes. This test can detect orthostatic hypotension (sustained decrease from baseline supine blood pressure of ≥20 mmHg in systolic readings or a ≥10 mmHg decrease in diastolic readings) or POTS (postural orthostatic tachycardia syndrome; sustained tachycardia >30 bpm over baseline after standing, or sustained tachycardia >120 bpm) in the absence of concurrent orthostatic hypotension. "Sustained" is defined as occurring at all time points between 60 and 180 seconds after standing up.

An important caveat concerning the bedside Active Standing Test is its lack of sensitivity in detecting manifestations of orthostatic intolerance. A negative test is not particularly helpful as this test is better – that is, more specific - in diagnosing the conditions POTS and orthostatic hypotension when it is positive. No further formal testing is needed before initiating therapy if the Active Standing Test is positive.

However, in real life, a diagnosis of orthostatic intolerance frequently requires greater stress on the cardiovascular system, such as standing in line or gardening for hours on a hot summer day. Accordingly, the clinical recognition of orthostatic intolerance in controlled laboratory situations often requires greater persistence so that the laboratory setting can simulate real life events. This attempt at simulating real-life events is known as the principle of ecological validity, and it has only been *partially* addressed by the American Academy of Neurology in its guideline on the use of head-up tilt table testing.

The head-up tilt table is a flat table to which a patient is comfortably bound in the supine position. Under controlled circumstances, the table is gradually inclined over a period of minutes to a 60-degree head-upright position. The patient remains passive; in other words, the study patient makes no active attempt to stand during the tilt. During the maneuver, heart rate and blood pressure are continuously monitored by EKG and a non-invasive blood pressure monitor. Study endpoints include the development of orthostatic hypotension (systolic or diastolic) and/or tachycardia that persists longer than 3 minutes, and either of these can be punctuated by loss of consciousness (syncope) from a vasovagal response (syncope associated with rapid development of bradycardia and hypotension.)

Currently, the standard test in autonomic neurology laboratories is limited to only 10 minutes of 60-degree tilt. This 10-minute limit follows the recommendations of the American Autonomic Society, the European Federation of Autonomic Societies, the Autonomic Research Group of the World Federation of Neurology, and the Autonomic Disorders Section of the American Academy of Neurology as provided in a consensus statement on the definition of POTS. Recent evidence suggests extending the duration of maximal tilt beyond 10-minutes, as 10-minutes may not stress the cardiovascular system enough to invoke the desired abnormality in a patient with suspected orthostatic intolerance. This appears to be true among migraineurs with and without auras, and even more surprising is the finding that migraine sufferers *without* a history of orthostatic intolerance may exhibit abnormal tilt table responses if tilt is extended for as long as 45-minutes.

Virtually all migraineurs without or without auras who also complain of the orthostatic intolerance between headaches demonstrate an abnormal 45-minute head-up tilt. And nearly 70% of those migraineurs who have never had postural dizziness, or other such symptoms will also have an abnormal head-up tilt table test. The migraine sufferers without a history of orthostatic intolerance tend to develop an abnormal tilt in the later parts of the tilt while the migraineurs with the postural history will more likely develop test abnormalities in the first 10-minutes.

So what does that mean for me?

With your history, if your Active Standing Test is positive, we have confirmed a diagnosis of either orthostatic hypotension or POTS and can stop there, unless we feel your condition requires further characterization in the laboratory. As mentioned, even if you have a <u>normal</u> Active Standing Test, we may need to do a formal tilt table test and one that is prolonged past the usual 10-minutes. For the general clinician or neurologist, as long as there is no glaring abnormality (a drug effect, active diarrhea or blood loss, or a nerve disorder, for example), the work-up can stop with a positive test; the treatment will be empirical for the great majority of patients.

What do you mean by further characterization?

Orthostatic intolerance has many causes. The normal cardiovascular response to the effects of gravity on blood requires an integrated response from the brain, spinal cord and peripheral nerves that innervate blood vessels. Important components include an intact endocrine system as well. The specialty tests will interrogate the central nervous system's autonomic components (reflexes), the peripheral nervous system (sensory and motor function), the endocrine system (hormonal levels), and the structure and capacity of the body's blood vessels, blood components (cells and serum). All this requires expertise from an academic autonomic laboratory.

Will I have to live this way for the rest of my life? How do you treat my condition?

Appropriate questions. Irrespective of migraines, there are otherwise healthy adults who develop or acquire symptoms of orthostatic intolerance following a brief illness, usually a viral illness. The syndrome occurs because of the development of damage to the nerves that function in the reflex pathways controlling minute-to-minute blood pressure. The nerve disease is called pandysautonomia and many times it remits on its own. For the migraine sufferer who exhibits a tendency to get dizzy and faint - like you - the condition may remit with time. But with intercurrent illnesses, such as the flu, it may return for a period and require aggressive management temporarily.

The treatment of this condition can be multifaceted, and it may require periodic adjustment along with the treatment of your migraines. We will discuss this more in a few moments. There are general principles for management of orthostatic intolerance – either POTS or orthostatic hypotension with or without syncope. These include:

- Sitting a few minutes before standing up after a period of prolonged duration of lying flat

- Placing the head of your bedframe on bricks to elevate the head of the bed by approximately 6 inches. This will enable your body to adjust better to the upright position each morning

- Avoiding prolonged exposure to heat without adequate access to fluids, especially in locations where there is nowhere to sit or squat down. If symptomatic you may have to squat on your haunches for several minutes if you are unable to lie flat

- Remaining well hydrated. This usually requires drinking more than two or three liters or quarts of balanced electrolyte solutions a day (brands such as Gatorade, Powerade, or Pedialyte, for example). Water is an acceptable replacement

- The use - during the day when upright - of fitted support stockings that provide 20-30 mmHg, concentric pressure to the calves and thighs. These require a prescription but are often covered by insurance. Unfortunately, the times when they are especially necessary are when it is hot and humid and you are sweaty and flushed (vasodilation of the skin to release body heat); the stockings can be uncomfortable and hot in the summer, and they are not attractive when worn with shorts. While a fair number of patients need to don mid-thigh support stockings to be able to function normally, many patients can make do with knee-high stockings

- Using salt liberally. This means three to five grams sodium a day for some people but using salt for cooking and at the dinner table, as well as the ingestion of salty foods such as chips, may be necessary

- Avoid all prescriptions and over-the-counter agents that may stimulate the cardiovascular system or act as diuretics. This includes caffeine in all forms, including the ever-popular energy drinks as well as alerting agents (for late night studying), anti-cholinergic nasal decongestants and adrenergic nasal sprays (such as Afrin, Neo-synephrine, and generic equivalents), over-the-counter headache remedies containing caffeine, and pseudoephedrine-containing decongestants (such as Sudafed, Alka-Seltzer Plus, Allegra-D, Zyrtec-D, or generic equivalents). The "-D" indicates pseudoephedrine or a derivative and can not only drive the heart rate so high that it induces dizziness and/or syncope but also induce abnormalities in the brain's blood vessels that might lead to catastrophic headaches!

You should also keep in mind that some medications normally used to prevent headaches and other conditions, such as depression, can make orthostatic intolerance more difficult to manage, or even worse. These medications include the old migraine preventive drugs called tricyclic antidepressants (for example, amitriptyline or nortriptyline) and newer and, particularly, older antipsychotic agents used for nausea or to abort migraine headaches. Some examples include chlorpromazine and prochlorperazine. These two classes of drugs can speed the heart rate up to levels that may induce dizziness, and they also can cause orthostatic hypotension as a side effect. Another important class of medication to be wary of is the anticonvulsant class of medication that behave like acetazolamide (Diamox), a diuretic. Included in this grouping are topiramate (Topamax) and zonisamide (Zonegran).

For patients with documented orthostatic intolerance with or without a migraine problem, I always start with the above recommendations. Many patients may stabilize with this alone. Cardiologists will start with the recommendation of cardiac rehabilitation exercises, that over a period of weeks start in the supine positions (supine exercise bicycles) and gradually advance to isotonic exercises standing upright. This type of physical therapy requires trained therapists and a prescription. A "poor man's" replacement for this is going to the pool and for the first few weeks walking in the shallow section of the pool for half an hour three times a week. Over a period of weeks gentle swimming can be added to the routine. This type of isotonic exercise improves blood flow from the lower extremities to the heart and less the tendency to have POTS.

Unless I feel there is a need to pursue certain diagnostics testing, there is an additional routine regimen I generally utilize for migraine sufferers. As most patients exhibit tachycardia or rapid heart rate, I treat them with a beta-blocker such as nadolol, metoprolol, or propranolol. These agents have the added benefit of being excellent migraine preventives as well to slow the rapid heart rate, dizziness symptom complex. I start low and push the daily dose high enough to drive the heart rate at rest to about 60 beats a minute. If the above beta blockers cause fatigue or depression, I may attempt a trial of another beta blocker that does not penetrate the brain as avidly, such as atenolol (and thus abandon using it for migraine prevention). My next empirical choice, either as an add-on agent or as a replacement, is a volume expander such as fludrocortisone. If a trial of this steroid is ineffective or poorly tolerated, I move to an alpha-agonist such as midodrine. Another option for patients who may also suffer from orthostatic hypotension is pyridostigmine, a medication that blocks the degradation of the neurotransmitter acetylcholine and is well known for its use in myasthenia gravis.

For the most part, I rarely have to add more than a beta blocker and a volume expander for patients like you. But follow-up is important because dosing frequently requires periodic titration.

I hope this helps you understand your condition better.

Suggested Reading

Benditt DG, Ferguson DW, Grubb BP, et al. Tilt table testing for assessing syncope. American College of Cardiology. J Am Coll Cardiol 1996; 28:263-275

Bickerstaff ER. Impairment of consciousness in migraine. Lancet 1961; 278:1057-1059.

Cheshire WP, Goldstein DP. Autonomic uprising: the tilt table test in autonomic medicine. Clin Auton Res 2019; 29:215-230.

Cutsforth-Gregory JK. Postural tachycardia syndrome and neurally mediated syncope. Continuum (Minneap, Minn) 2020;6:93-115.

Freeman R, Wieling W, Axelrod FB, et al. Consensus statement on the definition of orthostatic hypotension, neurally mediated syncope and the postural tachycardia syndrome. Clin Auton Res 2011; 21:69-72.

Low PA, Sandroni P, Joyner M, Shen W-K. Postural tachycardia syndrome (POTS). J Cardiovasc Electrophysiol 2009; 20:352-358.

Mayuga K, Butters K, Fouad-Tarazi F. Early versus late postural tachycardia: a re-evaluation of a syndrome. Clin Auton Res 2008; 18:155-157.

SHOULD I CONSIDER GOING TO AN INPATIENT HEADACHE CENTER?

ALEXANDER FEOKTISTOV, MD, PHD

I have been experiencing severe headache over the past 5 days and none of my medications seem to be helping. Is there anything that could be done?

There are several effective preventive and acute medications used in migraine management, but occasionally patients may find themselves in a situation when none of the usual treatments provide relief. A good example would be status migrainosus – a migraine complication that is defined as an intractable and prolonged migraine attack lasting over 72 hours despite adequate treatment, associated with severe headache, light and sound sensitivity, nausea, and occasionally vomiting. In cases like that, the patient might need to be admitted to a hospital, preferably to a specialized inpatient headache unit for parenteral treatment to abort an ongoing refractory headache cycle.

How long should I wait before being admitted?

The duration of the hospital stay depends on the severity of the symptoms and the treatment attempted. When we discuss adequate acute treatment, it is important to recognize that it should involve migraine-specific therapy including (if appropriate) triptans, ergotamine-containing medications, NSAIDs, gepants, or ditans. If there is no response to the above therapies, the person might first attempt to use a "cycle breaker" medication, such as a short course of a corticosteroid like prednisone, methylprednisolone, or dexamethasone. If the pain and other migraine-associated symptoms persist, then the next step might be hospitalization. Overall that decision process should not take more than 5-7 days.

Do I have to stay in the hospital? Could that treatment be tried at home?

Inpatient treatment provides a unique opportunity to utilize highly specific and effective parenteral migraine therapies that may require close monitoring of vital signs, blood tests, ECG, and other measures. Some of the medications, such as intravenous infusions of dihydroergotamine, are administered every 8 hours for a few days with close monitoring of blood pressure, which makes it difficult to administer at home. Another important aspect of the specialized inpatient headache treatment is the ability to apply several treatment modalities and combine various treatments during the same hospital stay which frequently would require significantly longer times to arrange and coordinate. These might include evaluation and management by pain management specialists and psychology teams, and the use of non-drug treatments such as biofeedback and acupuncture.

Should I consider going to an Emergency Room or Urgent Care first?

At times going to ER or urgent care can be helpful especially for patients with episodic migraine who have developed status migrainosus. Many patients, to achieve sustainable results, may require repeated administration of medications and a prolonged stay from 2-3 days and up to over a week in some cases. Emergency rooms are not set up to provide extended care, in which case patients would be better cared for at the specialized inpatient headache unit.

What are the other common reasons for hospitalization?

Up to 60% of all headache-related hospitalizations are for detoxification therapy from pain relievers containing opioids and barbiturates. Unfortunately, in clinical practice, we are still seeing a great number of patients with acute medication overuse or medication overuse headaches. In all these situations one of the most critical steps is the discontinuation of the drugs that patients have been overusing. Of course, some of the medications such as over-the-counter pain relievers, non-steroidal anti-inflammatory drugs, triptans, and ergotamine-containing medications can be discontinued on an outpatient basis. But for those patients who have been overusing opioids or barbiturates as well as those patients who have failed outpatient detoxification protocols, an inpatient treatment program might provide significantly better results. Frequently, patients may need to be closely monitored in the milieu of the headache inpatient unit for signs of medication withdrawal which should be managed promptly.

Other common reasons for inpatient treatment could be a prolonged, disabling and an intractable course of headaches that requires more aggressive treatment, the presence of severe and poorly controlled nausea and vomiting, or the presence of unusual neurological symptoms. These may require detailed examination and diagnostic investigation. Occasionally initiation of certain preventive medications that require specific patient education and monitoring, such as initiation of treatment with monoaminoxidase inhibitors, may require hospitalization. Patients with intractable migraine and significant comorbidities, including psychiatric ones, may require close monitoring and therefore hospitalization.

What type of treatments could be considered during the hospitalization?

In most dedicated inpatient headache units, a multidisciplinary approach is emphasized. This may consist of detoxification from overused acute headache treatments, acute and around-the-clock parenteral therapy to treat the headache, initiation or adjustment of prophylactic therapy, as well as potential interventional treatment modalities like nerve blocks. Non-pharmacological options such as biofeedback, physical, acupuncture, psychological evaluation, and counseling may also be introduced.

How do you perform the detoxification therapy from opioids and barbiturates?

While most triptans, ergots, non-steroidal agents (NSAIDs) and over-the-counter medications could be simply discontinued, detoxification of opioids and butalbital requires gradual medication cessation and close monitoring for potential withdrawal symptoms.

There are different ways where opioid detoxification can be accomplished which may include a gradual dose decrease every few days or weeks depending on the initial dose. Higher doses and prolonged opioid overuse will require a more gradual dose decrease. Some patients may benefit from switching from a short-acting opioid to a long-acting one, followed by a gradual dose reduction and eventual cessation. The most common opioid withdrawal symptoms include restlessness, anxiety, insomnia, nightmares, muscle aches, rhinorrhea, mydriasis, nausea, and occasionally vomiting. These symptoms can last over 5-10 days and sometimes longer. The withdrawal symptoms could be managed with the addition of clonidine, muscle relaxants, and NSAIDs.

For those patients overusing barbiturates like butalbital, the withdrawal symptoms could be more severe and dangerous and may include severe anxiety and restlessness, agitation, nausea, vomiting, tachycardia (rapid heart rate), and even seizures. Patients who are overusing high doses of barbiturates should be monitored closely and the withdrawal symptoms managed promptly. One of the ways to discontinue butalbital-containing products is to switch the medication to phenobarbital, substituting 30 mg of phenobarbital for every 100 mg of butalbital used. The phenobarbital dose then should be reduced by 30 mg/day every three days as tolerated. Once again, the use of adjunctive therapy is important to manage possible withdrawal symptoms as well as underlying headaches.

It is also important to recognize that medication cessation may at first cause temporary worsening of the headache. Therefore, having available diverse pain management options is critical and should include medication therapies, interventional treatment modalities, and non-pharmacological treatment options.

Is there anything else that could be done to manage the headache while being admitted?

The advantage of inpatient treatment is that multiple symptoms could be managed and addressed at the same time. The primary headache disorder with which the patient was admitted is treated during the inpatient stay. When appropriate some patients may benefit from the intravenous administration of dihydroergotamine through a program known as the DHE-45 protocol. This protocol was first described in 1986 and consists of slow intravenous infusions over 60-120 minutes of 0.5-1 mg of dihydroergotamine (DHE) every 8 hours for a total of 9 doses. One of the common side effects of the treatment is nausea, therefore pre-medication of each dose with an antiemetic drug like ondansetron, prochlorperazine, or metoclopramide is recommended. Considering that dihydroergotamine is a potent vasoconstrictor, vital signs are monitored closely for any evidence of hypertension before and during DHE infusion. If hypertension does occur, the dihydroergotamine infusion is discontinued until the blood pressure is controlled.

Some may also benefit from intravenous administration of ketorolac 30 mg every 6-12 hours. We found that certain muscle relaxants such as orphenadrine 30-60 mg IV every 12 hours can be very beneficial adjunctive therapy especially for patients with a co-existing myofascial pain syndrome seen in up to 70% of patients with chronic migraine. Another effective and well-tolerated treatment option is the intravenous infusion of magnesium sulfate 1 g every 8-12 hours. We have had success using infusions of valproate sodium 500-750 mg IV every 12 hours and intravenous slow injections of diphenhydramine 25-50 mg every 6-12 hours. Some of these medications may produce sedation and close monitoring is important.

Some patients may benefit from a trial of droperidol 0.625-2.5 mg IV every 12 hours. We do recommend evaluating QTc interval on the EKG before starting the infusion and monitoring the EKG closely while using droperidol. Considering that droperidol may contribute to QT prolongation it should be avoided in those patients whose QTc interval has been prolonged.

Most of these medications can be combined and used on the same day. We frequently alternate these medications every 4-6 hours as appropriate. Finally, some patients may benefit from short-term use of corticosteroids like methylprednisolone 80-100 mg IM or IV for 1-2 doses.

Is there anything else that could be done in the hospital besides intravenous medications?

Some patients with specific headache presentations such as the severe or predominantly occipital location of pain, or comorbid severe neck and shoulders pain may benefit from a variety of interventional procedures such as greater and lesser occipital nerve blocks or trigger point injections. These can be performed at the bedside. For those with a suspected cervicogenic etiology, a diagnostic cervical facet medial branch nerve block could be performed. If positive results are achieved, this could be followed by a therapeutic procedure such as medial branch radiofrequency ablation. Other nerve blocks that may be utilized include supraorbital and supratrochlear nerve blocks, sphenopalatine ganglion blocks, and auriculotemporal nerve blocks. Some of these interventions can be done by a trained headache specialist or a neurologist, while others may require evaluation by a pain management specialist.

Is there a role for non-pharmacological interventions?

In addition to pharmacotherapy and interventional treatment modalities, patients could also be evaluated by a psychologist with assessment of pain coping skills and development of new pain coping strategies. We found this to be especially valuable in patients with medication overuse headache. Other non-pharmacological methods might be beneficial such as biofeedback, acupuncture, and physical therapy.

The significance of the educational component of the inpatient headache program that allows a patient to gain a better understanding of their condition and methods of management must not be underestimated. It is also often beneficial to demonstrate that there are other patients with similar or even worse headache problems out there. That realization that they are not alone in their journey can be very powerful.

That sounds like a lot of options that could be tried during the hospital stay! For how long I should expect to be hospitalized?

Depending on a specific clinical situation, the need for detoxification therapy, and overall response to treatment, one might expect to be in the hospital between 3 and 10 days.

Suggested Reading

Diamond S, Freitag FG, Maliszewski M. Inpatient treatment of headache: Long-term results. Headache 1986; 26:189-197.

Feoktistov A. Inpatient Treatment of Headaches. Headache and Migraine Biology and Management, Academic Press, 2015, 285-291

Freitag FG, Lake A 3rd, Lipton R, Cady R, Diamond S, Silberstein S; US Headache Guidelines Consortium, Section on Inpatient Treatment Chairpersons. Inpatient treatment of headache: an evidence-based assessment. Headache 2004;44:342-60.

Lake AE, Saper JR, Madden SF. Comprehensive inpatient treatment for intractable migraine: A prospective long-term outcome study. Headache 1993; 33:55-62

Marmura MJ, Hou A. Inpatient Management of Migraine. Neurol Clin 2019;37:771-788.

Rapoport A, Stang P, Gutterman DL. Cady R, Markley H, Weeks R, Saiers J, Fox AW. Analgesic rebound headache in clinical practice: data from a physician survey. Headache 1996; 36:14-19

Silberstein SD, Silberstein JR. Chronic daily headache: Long-term prognosis following inpatient treatment with repetitive IV DHE. Headache 1992; 32:439-445.

How can a Pain Physician Help Me with My Headaches?

Yury Khelemsky, M.D.

What role does a pain physician play in the treatment of my headaches?

The interventional pain physician can be an indispensable part of a comprehensive headache management team. Although such teams are still a rarity, their emergence makes it apparent to the involved patients and practitioners alike that a collaborative multispecialty approach is indispensable in the management of complex medical phenomena, such as headache.

There are areas of care that are usually attended to by headache neurologists and some that are uniquely the realm of pain physicians. Sometimes the roles may overlap. For example, both headache neurologists and pain physicians can perform certain procedures such as supraorbital and occipital nerve blocks. Both can discuss and prescribe medications or administer infusions. If the pain physician and neurologist work closely together, this overlap can bolster the availability of these services to the patient. The result is timely treatment, which is of critical importance. Coordinating types and goals of care among multiple providers allows the patient to avoid any gaps in understanding and education. Furthermore, receiving care from practitioners with varied training backgrounds provides the patient with a more rounded and perhaps insightful assessment and treatment plan for their condition.

Pain physicians are qualified to perform procedures that may be helpful with a wide variety of headaches such as migraine, tension-type, cluster, post-traumatic, and cervicogenic headaches. Some may also provide relief of certain facial pain disorders. These procedures include blocks of the trigeminal nerve and its branches, occipital nerve blocks, cervical medial branch blocks, sphenopalatine ganglion blocks, trigger point injections, and temporomandibular joint (TMJ) injections. Epidural blood patches may provide relief of headaches due to spinal fluid leaks. Various ablative techniques including radiofrequency ablation and cryoablation, and implantation of devices for peripheral nerve stimulation and spinal cord stimulation may be utilized to provide relief in patients with headaches that are refractory to other therapies.

Is there a relationship between my headaches and neck pain?

Neck pain is very common in the general population, and it is almost universal in people who suffer from chronic headaches. Up to 90% of those with migraine and tension headaches have concomitant neck pain. There is likely bidirectionality in the relationship between headache and neck pain, meaning that sometimes headache can cause neck pain and sometimes neck pain can provoke headache. Such relationships can be explained through an understanding of the neuroanatomical connections of the head and neck. Often it is difficult to clinically identify which is the primary source of the initial trouble, and multiple different treatment strategies may be required to address pain in both locations.

The term "referred" pain is used when pain is felt in a place that is different from its anatomic source. For example, pain that is felt in the head (including the face) that comes from the neck is known as cervicogenic headache (headache generated by the cervical spine). The mechanism of such headaches involves the trigeminocervical complex, a relay station on the neurologic highway where travelers from the cervical system (neck) and trigeminal system (head) intermix and affect each other. Pain from the neck may not only be the primary source of head discomfort, as we discussed representing a case of referred pain, but alternatively may activate or "trigger" an underlying headache condition such as migraine.

One would think that the longer someone has pain and headaches, the less they feel it. However, unfortunately, the exact opposite is true. These systems aren't just on and off switches, they become sensitized, which means that an environment more conducive to pain is created over time.

Typically, neck pain that is relevant to the headache patient is the result of chronic tension in the muscles of the neck, as well as inflammation of the small joints of the cervical spine, known as the facet joints. The joints, ligaments, tendons, and local muscles may become inflamed due to stress or poor posture, often related to suboptimal work ergonomics, or due to injury to the neck. A cervical sprain or "whiplash" injury is a good example of the latter. Cervical spine inflammation and resulting pain is transmitted via the medial branch nerves into the trigeminocervical complex.

Consequently, the medial branches are frequent targets of procedures aimed at treating neck pain and headache. Some branches of nerves from the upper cervical spine contribute to the occipital nerves which may also provide a site for procedural treatment.

Which procedures are available to help with my headaches?

Nerve blocks provide the starting point of interventional pain management. These involve injections of numbing medications (e.g., local anesthetics) alone or mixed with steroids around nerves responsible for pain. Immediate pain relief is due to the direct action of the local anesthetic, but sometimes pain relief is delayed as the pain circuit may involve structures other than just the nerves being treated. As these structures become more sensitive (prone to pain) over time, the pain relief can be delayed. Just like when one turns off the fire under a cast iron skillet, it can take time for the skillet to cool down. It may take a series of injections to gradually desensitize the pain circuit and reduce chronic inflammation. If nerve blocks provide only short- lived relief, the nerves can be treated with radiofrequency ablation (heat), pulsed radiofrequency (electrical modulation), or cryoablation (cold) to provide longer lasting relief.

Blocks of the trigeminal nerve and its branches (i.e., supraorbital, auriculotemporal, infraorbital, zygomaticotemporal, mental, etc.) have been used to help pain related to migraine, hemicrania continua, trigeminal neuralgia, and peripheral neuralgias.

Blocks of the occipital nerves have been used in patients with migraine and cluster headache, occipital neuralgia, and cervicogenic headache.

Sphenopalatine ganglion blocks target a small bundle of nerves located in the sinuses. These nerves are likely involved with a variety of headaches and facial pain, such as migraine and cluster headache. Blocks can either be done directly with a needle or by a simply putting some numbing medicine into the nostril (via a variety of methods including using long q-tips or specialized injection devices).

The temporomandibular joint (TMJ) can cause both cause jaw and facial pain, as well as trigger underlying headaches. Temporomandibular joint dysfunction is a term that encompasses issues arising from the joint and surrounding structures. The TMJ joint may be injected with steroids, lubricants (hyaluronic acid) or regenerative compounds, such as platelet rich plasma (PRP), while the surrounding muscles can be treated with botulinum toxin.

Cervical medial branch blocks (cMBBs) are useful in the treatment of chronic neck pain, cervicogenic headache, tension headache and migraine headache. These are performed in the back of the neck under x-ray guidance. Unlike epidural injections, the needle does *not* go into the spine as the targets are on the outer surface of the bones. If the blocks result in pain relief that is helpful, but transient, a radiofrequency ablation procedure can then be performed. This is also done with a special needle, may result in 6-12 months of pain relief, and can be repeated if necessary.

For patients suffering from low pressure headaches due to a leak of cerebrospinal fluid (CSF), epidural blood patching can be performed. This involves taking the patient's own blood and injecting it into the epidural space in order to seal the leak. Patients who have spontaneous leaks, that is, not caused by a previous procedure like an epidural or a lumbar puncture (e.g., spinal tap) often require several of these blood patches, especially if the exact source of the leak cannot be identified.

Trigger point injections and fascial injections target the muscles and the fascia, which can become painful because of headaches or act as triggers for them. These can be done with ultrasound guidance to ensure precision, as well as avoidance of unrelated surrounding structures.

Stimulation of peripheral nerves (i.e., supraorbital, occipital, vagal, etc.) with implantable devices is also an option for some patients. These procedures are done by either pain physicians or functional neurosurgeons. Spinal cord stimulation, a technique that has been well established in the treatment of many types of pain, has also been used in some patients with severe persistent migraine headaches, but remains experimental at this time.

Why are several different treatments being done at the same time to help with my headaches?

It is rare that a person with difficult to treat pain previously unresponsive to various treatment will find a silver bullet – that is, a single therapy that will result in a perfect outcome. The concept of multimodal analgesia comes from the observation that combinations of treatments for complex pain tend to work better than single therapies. Optimally, each treatment should target a different point in the pain pathway. For example, many patients with refractory migraine can achieve treatment success with a combination of medications, botulinum toxin injections, nerve blocks, lifestyle modification and physical therapy. Indeed, each patient is unique and requires a thoughtful multidisciplinary approach aimed at both treatment of active issues, as well as development of strategies to prevent these issues from recurring in the future.

Suggested Reading

Abdel-Kader A, Khelemsky Y. Interventional Treatment of Head and Neck Pain. In Natbony L, Green M, editors. *Integrative Pain Medicine: An Evidence Based Guide for Clinicians*. Switzerland: Springer International Publishing 2021: pp 215-258.

Renton T, Beke A. A Narrative Review of Therapeutic Peripheral Nerve Blocks for Chronic Orofacial Pain Conditions. *J Oral Facial Pain Headache* 2022;36(1):49-58

Robbins MS. Clinic-based Procedures for Headache. *Continuum (Minneap Minn)* 2021;27:732-745.

Velásquez-Rimachi V, Chachaima-Mar J, Cárdenas-Baltazar EC, et al. Greater occipital nerve block for chronic migraine patients: A meta-analysis. *Acta Neurol Scand* 2022;146:101-114.

How Do I Get into a Research Study?

Peter McAllister, MD

Medical Director, New England Institute
for Neurology and Headache
Chief Medical Officer, New England Institute for
Clinical Research and Ki Clinical Research
Stamford, Connecticut

In the last five years, there has been a veritable explosion of exciting new treatments for migraine and cluster headache. From the anti-CGRP monoclonal antibodies to the gepants, ditans to neurostimulators, the lives of countless persons with migraine disease have been dramatically improved by the availability of these groundbreaking products. But how did they get here, these new medicines? Did they just show up on the market, declaring themselves safe, effective and ready for consumption? The answer, of course, is no: all new medications require an arduous, multi-phase process of clinical research, focusing on both clinical efficacy and safety and tolerability. And to state the obvious: clinical trials are only successful when they recruit volunteers – patients willing and able to comply with the study rules, knowing (in most cases) they may receive the medication or a placebo. This is where you, the patient, come in. Without research study participants, there would be no new medications.

The Basics of Clinical Research

When a novel compound is discovered, research begins in the laboratory. This basic "bench" work identifies the unique characteristics of a medicine, such as which receptor(s) it binds to, and how it may be metabolized. Animal studies generally follow, often beginning with rodents such as mice and working up the phylogenetic chain (rabbits, dogs, and then monkeys, for example). Here, scientists learn about pharmacokinetics (what the body does to the drug), pharmacodynamics (what the drug does to the body and how it interacts with other drugs) along with its safety profile. At this point the research transitions to humans, with a phase 1 study. In this phase, a small number of healthy volunteers (that is, those who do not have the disease for which the pharmaceutical is being evaluated) take the study medication over a wide range of doses, and have their blood sampled frequently for a period of time (for example, every hour for 12 or 24 hours). In a phase 1 study scientists learn more about what the drug does to the body, and what the body does to the drug. Efficacy (how well a drug works) is not generally a consideration in this phase, but rather basic biochemistry, physiology and safety issues are of paramount concern.

If a drug passes through phase 1 without any red flags – primarily safety issues – a phase 2 study is undertaken, in which a moderate sized group of persons (say 200-500) with the disease being studied is administered one or two doses (or more, or less- it varies) of either the study medication or a placebo (commonly referred to as a sugar pill; if the compound is an injectable then an inert fluid is administered). This is performed in a blinded fashion, meaning the participants do not know whether they received the study drug or the placebo. If fact, the investigator is also kept in the dark, and the allocation of drug or placebo is random, which is why these studies are referred to as randomized, double-blind, placebo-controlled trials. While safety and tolerability are still a main concern, in phase 2, clinicians also get a signal of whether the compound in question actually works (demonstrates efficacy) when compared to the placebo at the study termination when the blind is broken and statisticians analyze the data. If (and only if) there is demonstrated efficacy coupled with good safety and tolerability, then the pharmaceutical enters the final stage for approval, a large (500+ to many thousand participant) randomized, double-blind, placebo-controlled, multi-center phase 3 trial. In fact, the United States Food and Drug Administration (FDA) generally requires *two* phase 3 studies, with both showing statistical superiority of the study drug versus placebo (again, with a favorable safety and tolerability profile), before it gives the green light for approval. The process is similar in the European Union (their FDA equivalent is called the EMA) and other developed countries (Health Canada and Japan's PMDA are two examples), with rigorous clinical studies required for drug or medical device approval. Thus, the progression from drug discovery to regulatory agency approval is long, involved and expensive, but is designed to ensure, to the extent possible, that a new medication works and won't likely hurt the consumer.

Where Do I Fit In?

As mentioned, many thousands of clinical trial participants are required to pass all the hurdles outlined above. There is simply no path for a novel compound to get out on the market unless patients are willing to step up and take part in the process. You – the potential study subject - are key to the success of the whole process. Fortunately, being a study partner has many positive aspects, along with a few potential downsides. The key is knowing what you are getting into so you can make an informed decision about whether to participate or not.

Clinical Research Participation – the Pluses and Minuses

The advantages of study participation are numerous: access to medicines or medical devices often several years before the general public; free trial-related medical care, which, depending on the study, may include a physical exam, blood tests, electrocardiogram, and possibly MRI or other imaging; the knowledge that you are doing something positive for science, and helping those suffering from the same condition as you; lastly, in most clinical trials, participants are financially compensated for their time and travel expenses.

The downsides to participating in a clinical research study include the possibility of having an adverse reaction to the medicine. In over twenty years of conducting clinical trials in migraine and other headache disorders, I have encountered numerous adverse events (abbreviated "AEs"), nearly all of which were judged to be mild or moderate, and often not related to the medicine under study. I have not encountered any serious adverse events (SAEs) related to a study compound in a headache trial, but of course that is not to say that such an event in impossible. It is important to note that AEs and SAEs are not uncommon in clinical research, and not all (in fact, generally very few) are actually related to the study drug. For example, if a study participant slices her finger while cutting vegetables and needs stitches, that is considered an adverse event (AE), but not one related to the medication under study. Likewise, if a subject is involved in a motor vehicle accident, and needs emergency surgery, that would be an SAE, but again, not related to the trial compound (unless of course sedation was a side-effect and the subject fell asleep at the wheel). Normal life events happen for the months (or in some cases years) during which a trial is conducted, and when an AE or SAE occurs investigators must decide whether the medication under study was a causal factor or not. In a recent clinical trial I was involved in, there were two deaths – a homicide and an accidental drowning – and while tragic, neither had anything to do with the compound we were studying.

Another issue with being in a trial is adhering to the protocol. In many migraine studies, participants are asked to keep track of their headaches, usually by logging into a smartphone-like device. If you don't record enough entries (say 80% compliance), you may be asked to withdraw. Some patients find this an arduous chore, and elect not to go into a trial. Finally, while in a clinical trial you may be prohibited from taking certain medicines, or using recreational or medical marijuana, even if approved for use in your state.

So How Do I Get into a Clinical Trial?

Study entry begins with a thorough review of the consent form. This document is read to prospective participants by the investigator or his/her designated study coordinator. Above all, the patient's safety and well-being are of paramount concern, and the informed consent document reflects this. The document describes in detail all the potential concerns, risks, benefits and side-effects of participation. For example, if blood is drawn during the study, the consent form states that pain, bruising or other adverse events may result from the venipuncture. The patients is given ample opportunity to ask questions, and when all are satisfactorily answered, they sign the consent form. The signing obligates them to nothing – it simply acknowledges that they have read and understand the consent form. Consent to participate in a clinical trial may be withdrawn at any time, for any reason.

You may be surprised to learn that the hardest part of clinical study participation is actually getting in. The rules regarding who can get into a particular study are worked out between the sponsor (pharmaceutical company, device manufacturer, university) and the FDA, who jointly develop inclusion and exclusion criteria. A potential subject has to meet all the inclusion criteria, and not have any of the exclusion criteria for study admission. Inclusion criteria include demographics. For example, a particular trial seeks adults ages 18-50 with chronic migraine (15 or more headaches days per month, with eight of those meeting criteria for migraine), who have not responded to two or more preventive medicines. So, if you are 51 years old, have episodic migraine, and have not failed two or more preventives, you are not eligible for the trial.

Exclusion criteria define those who are not eligible for participation. Common criteria here include unstable medical or psychiatric conditions, substance abuse, a history of cancer in the last five years, and having headache types other than the one under study. You may also be denied study entry if your blood tests, electrocardiogram or other tests come back significantly abnormal. Most trials exclude subjects with positive urine drug screens. Patients who are pregnant, planning to conceive, or who are not willing to use a reliable form of birth control for the duration of the trial are excluded.

How do I Find a Clinical Study for My Condition?

Over the years, our center has conducted online surveys about the decision process that a patient uses when choosing to participate in one our studies or not. We have found that the biggest concern is that the patient will be a "guinea pig", or a "lab rat". That is, patients are concerned primarily about safety – of the drug under study, the tests, and the process itself. When skeptical would-be participants are educated about research (that the FDA is strongly biased toward ensuring safety over efficacy considerations, that the entire process is explained and transparent, that they can withdraw at any time), many – but certainly not all – are converted and agree to enroll. We have found over the years that once a patient completes their first clinical research study, they "get it". At the final study visit their first question often is, "when is the next study starting?"

The best online site for locating research studies near you is www.clinicaltrials.gov. All sponsors of "legit" research trials in the United States (and many international ones as well) have to register on this site. It is user-friendly, with a Google-like search engine which allows one to enter multiple search terms including the disease (say, cluster headache), your location (by zip code) and other criteria (for example "pediatric", "actively recruiting", "preventive" and more).

Randomized, double-blind, placebo-controlled clinical research trials are how ground-breaking new treatments gain approval and ultimately make it to your local pharmacy. These endeavors require, first and foremost, participants. Being part of a clinical trial can be a positive and rewarding experience, a chance to give back and helps others with your condition. If one is fully informed and the process is transparent, fear and anxiety are greatly reduced. We need more patients to enroll in our trials. In fact, we need more participation from those not typically enrolled, including (specifically for migraine trials) more men, people of color, and other demographics, those economically disadvantaged and members of the LGBTQ community. Pediatric studies are notoriously difficult to enroll, given the added layer of parental involvement. Outreach efforts to find and educate these groups would be welcome. There has never been a healthier time to be alive, and clinical research – the process of testing exciting new medicines – is one major reason.

Suggested reading

https://www.cancer.org/treatment/treatments-and-side-effects/clinical-trials/what-you-need-to-know/what-does-a-clinical-trial-involve.html , accessed 8/22/2021

https://clinicaltrials.gov/ , accessed 8/22/2021

Friedman L, Furburg C, DeMets D. Fundamentals of Clinical Trials, 4th Edition. Springer, 12/2020.

https://www.health.harvard.edu/blog/thinking-joining-clinical-trial-heres-need-know-2016090110187 , accessed 8/22/2021

https://www.nih.gov/health-information/nih-clinical-research-trials-you/finding-clinical-trial, accessed 8/22/2021

Turner JR. A Concise Guide to Clinical Trials. Turner Medical Communications, LLC, 9/1/2011

CONTRIBUTORS

Ashley Alex, MD
Assistant Professor of Neurology
University at Buffalo Jacobs School of Medicine
Buffalo, New York

Jacob M. Appel MD JD
Associate Professor of Psychiatry
and Medical Education Icahn School of
Medicine at Mount Sinai
New York, New York

Cynthia E. Armand, MD
Assistant Professor of Neurology
Albert Einstein College of Medicine/Montefiore Medical Center
Bronx, New York

Sait Ashina, MD
Assistant Professor of Neurology and Anesthesia
Harvard Medical School
Beth Israel Deaconess Medical Center
Boston, Massachusetts

Sheena K Aurora
Adjunct Clinical Associate Professor,
Division of Pain, Stanford University
Full time employee Impel Neuropharma

Shannon Babineau MD
Clinical Assistant Professor of Neurology and Pediatrics Sidney Kimmel
Medical College of Thomas Jefferson University
Staff Child Neurologist, Atlantic Medical Group
Morristown, New Jersey

Mark Barber, MD, MPH
Assistant Professor of Neurology
Division of Headache Medicine
Icahn School of Medicine at Mount Sinai
New York, New York

Jennifer P. Bassiur DDS
Associate Professor of Dental Medicine (Oral Surgery)
Columbia University Medical Center
New York, New York

Olivia Begasse de Dhaem, MD, FAHS
Director of Neurology Mentorship and Community Engagement
Assistant Neurology Program Director
Westchester Medical Center
Hawthorne, New York

Jan Lewis Brandes, MD, MS, FAAN, FAHS
Director and Founder, Nashville Neuroscience Group
Assistant Clinical Professor, Department of Neurology, Vanderbilt University School of Medicine
Nashville, Tennessee

Susan W. Broner, MD
Assistant Professor Clinical Neurology
Weill Cornell Medical College
Medical Director
Weill Cornell Medicine Headache Program
New York, New York

Cristina Cabret-Aymat, MD
Neurology/ Headache and Facial Pain
Ochsner, North Shore Region
Covington, Louisiana

Roger K. Cady, MD
Co-Founder of Headache Care Center
and Primary Care Network
Springfield, Missouri

Monica Chan, MD
Fellow in Headache Medicine
Icahn School of Medicine at Mt. Sinai
New York, New York

Murray Choueka, MD
Fellow in Headache Medicine
Department of Neurology
Icahn School of Medicine at Mt. Sinai
New York, New York

Rachel Colman MD
Assistant Professor Neurology
University of Connecticut School of Medicine
Hartford Healthcare Headache Center
Ayer Neuroscience Institute
Norwich, Connecticut

Wade M. Cooper, DO
Associate Professor of Neurology
and Anesthesiology
University of Michigan
Ann Arbor, Michigan

Merle Diamond, MD
President, Medical Director Diamond Headache Clinic & Diamond Headache
Inpatient Unit at AMITA Health
Saint Joseph Hospital
Chicago, Illinois

Mohamed Elshorafa, MD
Assistant Professor of Headache Medicine and Child Neurology
Department of Neurology
The Icahn School of Medicine at Mt. Sinai
New York, New York

Kathleen Farmer-Cady, PsyD
Co-Founder of Headache Care Center
and Primary Care Network
Springfield, Missouri

Alexander Feoktistov MD, PhD
Director, Synergy Integrative Headache Center
Associate Professor
Chicago Medical School
Rosalind Franklin University of Medicine and Science
Chicago, Illinois

Olga Fermo, MD
Senior Associate Consultant
Department of Neurology
Mayo Clinic Florida
Jacksonville, Florida

Grace Forde, M.D.
Director of Neurological Services
North American Partners in Pain Management
Lake Success, New York

Robert H. Fryer MD, PhD
Associate Professor of Neurology
Columbia University Medical Center
New York, New York

Jack Gladstein, MD
Professor of Pediatrics and Neurology
University of Maryland School of Medicine
Baltimore, Maryland

Jasmin Marie Harpe, MD, MPH
Headache Fellow
John R. Graham Headache Center
BWH/MGH/Harvard Headache Fellowship
Boston, Massachusetts

Wilson Heredia MD
Assistant Professor of Neurology
Center for Headache and Pain Medicine
Department of Neurology
Icahn School of Medicine at Mount Sinai
New York, New York

W. Howell Jarrard MD
Assistant Professor of Neurology
Medical University of South Carolina
Charleston, South Carolina

Georgia Kane, MD
Director of Headache Center of Excellence at the Tampa VA
Assistant Professor
University of South Florida, College of Medicine
Tampa, Florida

Robert Kaniecki, MD
Director UPMC Headache Center
Associate Professor of Neurology
University of Pittsburgh School of Medicine
Pittsburgh, Pennsylvania

Yury Khelemsky, M.D.
Program Director, Pain Medicine Fellowship
Associate Professor
Department of Anesthesiology, Perioperative
and Pain Medicine
Department of Neurology
Icahn School of Medicine at Mount Sinai
New York, New York

Britany Klenofsky, MD
Assistant Professor of Neurology
Division of Headache Medicine
Icahn School of Medicine at Mount Sinai
New York, New York

Stephen Krieger, MD, FAAN
Professor of Neurology
Icahn School of Medicine at Mount Sinai
New York, New York

Dr. Anand Kumar
Assistant Professor of Neurology
Banaras Hindu University
Varanasi, India

Vincent T. Martin, MD
Director, Headache & Facial Pain Center
Professor of Medicine
University of Cincinnati College of Medicine
Cincinnati, Ohio

Paul G. Mathew, MD, DNBPAS, FAAN, FAHS
Assistant Professor of Neurology
Harvard Medical School
Massachusetts General Brigham Health Care/Harvard Vanguard Medical Associates
Boston, Massachusetts

Alexander Mauskop, MD, FAAN
Professor of Clinical Neurology
SUNY Downstate Medical Center
Director, New York Headache Center
New York, New York

Allison Navis, MD
Assistant Professor
Division Neuro-Infectious Diseases
Icahn School of Medicine at Mount Sinai
New York, New York

Peter McAllister, MD
Medical Director, New England Institute for Neurology and Headache
Chief Medical Officer, New England Institute for Clinical Research and Ki Clinical Research
Stamford, Connecticut

Kate Mullin, MD
Associate Medical Director
New England Institute for Neurology and Headache
Stamford, Connecticut

Robert Myers DO
Headache Specialist and Neurologist
Hoboken, New Jersey

Stephanie J. Nahas, MD, MSEd
Associate Professor, Department of Neurology
Thomas Jefferson University
Philadelphia, Pennsylvania

Lauren R. Natbony, MD
Assistant Clinical Professor of Neurology
Division of Headache Medicine
Icahn School of Medicine at Mount Sinai
New York, New York

Allison Navis, MD
Assistant Professor
Division Neuro-Infectious Diseases
Icahn School of Medicine at Mount Sinai
New York City

Anna Pace, MD
Assistant Professor
Department of Neurology
Center for Headache and Facial Pain
Icahn School of Medicine at Mount Sinai
New York, New York

Alan M. Rapoport, M.D.
Professor of Neurology
The David Geffen School of Medicine at UCLA
Los Angeles, California
Past President, The International Headache Society

John F. Rothrock MD
Professor and Vice Chair
Department of Neurology
George Washington University School of Medicine
Washington, DC

Neha Vijayvargiya Safi, MD
Multiple Sclerosis Fellow
Icahn School of Medicine at Mount Sinai
New York, New York

Huma U Sheikh, MD
CEO, NY Neurology Medicine, PC
Assistant Professor of Neurology
Icahn School of Medicine at Mount Sinai

Risako Shirane, MD MSc
Fellow in Headache Medicine
Department of Neurology
Yale School of Medicine
New Haven, Connecticut

Suhail Sidhu, MD
Creighton University School of Medicine,
Omaha, Nebraska

Nomita Sonty, M.Phil, Ph.D
Associate Professor of Medical Psychology
Departments of Anesthesiology & Psychiatry
College of Physicians and Surgeons
Columbia University
New York, New York
Mark Stillman, MD
Cleveland, OH

Stewart J. Tepper, MD, FAHS
Professor of Neurology
Geisel School of Medicine at Dartmouth
Director, Dartmouth Headache Center
Dartmouth-Hitchcock Medical Center
Lebanon, New Hampshire

Dr. Pravin Thomas
Consultant Neurologist
Clinical Lead and Program Director, Comprehensive Headache and Facial Pain Center,
Narayana Health
Bangalore, India

Terrence Tian, DO, MPH
Lufkin Fellow of Headache Medicine
Department of Neurology
Division of Headache Medicine
Icahn School of Medicine at Mt. Sinai
New York, New York

María-Carmen Wilson, MD
Associate Professor of Neurology
University of Queensland/Ochsner Medical School
Covington, Louisiana